Dietary Plant Origin Bio-Active Compounds, Intestinal Functionality and Microbiome

Dietary Plant Origin Bio-Active Compounds, Intestinal Functionality and Microbiome

Editor

Elad Tako

MDPI • Basel • Beijing • Wuhan • Barcelona • Belgrade • Manchester • Tokyo • Cluj • Tianjin

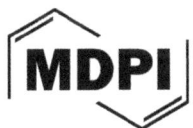

Editor
Elad Tako
Cornell University
USA

Editorial Office
MDPI
St. Alban-Anlage 66
4052 Basel, Switzerland

This is a reprint of articles from the Special Issue published online in the open access journal *Nutrients* (ISSN 2072-6643) (available at: https://www.mdpi.com/journal/nutrients/special_issues/bioactive_compounds_intestinal_functionality_microbiome).

For citation purposes, cite each article independently as indicated on the article page online and as indicated below:

LastName, A.A.; LastName, B.B.; LastName, C.C. Article Title. *Journal Name* **Year**, *Volume Number*, Page Range.

ISBN 978-3-03943-865-5 (Hbk)
ISBN 978-3-03943-866-2 (PDF)

Cover image courtesy of Elad Tako.

© 2020 by the authors. Articles in this book are Open Access and distributed under the Creative Commons Attribution (CC BY) license, which allows users to download, copy and build upon published articles, as long as the author and publisher are properly credited, which ensures maximum dissemination and a wider impact of our publications.
The book as a whole is distributed by MDPI under the terms and conditions of the Creative Commons license CC BY-NC-ND.

Contents

About the Editor vii

Elad Tako
Dietary Plant-Origin Bio-Active Compounds, Intestinal Functionality, and Microbiome
Reprinted from: *Nutrients* **2020**, *12*, 3223, doi:10.3390/nu12113223 1

**Gizela A. Pereira, Frhancielly S. Sodré, Gilson M. Murata, Andressa G. Amaral,
Tanyara B. Payolla, Carolina V. Campos, Fabio T. Sato, Gabriel F. Anhê and Silvana Bordin**
Fructose Consumption by Adult Rats Exposed to Dexamethasone In Utero Changes the
Phenotype of Intestinal Epithelial Cells and Exacerbates Intestinal Gluconeogenesis
Reprinted from: *Nutrients* **2020**, *12*, 3062, doi:10.3390/nu12103062 5

Johnathon Carboni, Spenser Reed, Nikolai Kolba, Adi Eshel, Omry Koren and Elad Tako
Alterations in the Intestinal Morphology, Gut Microbiota, and Trace Mineral Status Following
Intra-Amniotic Administration (*Gallus gallus*) of Teff (*Eragrostis tef*) Seed Extracts
Reprinted from: *Nutrients* **2020**, *12*, 3020, doi:10.3390/nu12103020 23

**Lotta Nylund, Salla Hakkola, Leo Lahti, Seppo Salminen, Marko Kalliomäki, Baoru Yang
and Kaisa M. Linderborg**
Diet, Perceived Intestinal Well-Being and Compositions of Fecal Microbiota and Short Chain
Fatty Acids in Oat-Using Subjects with Celiac Disease or Gluten Sensitivity
Reprinted from: *Nutrients* **2020**, *12*, 2570, doi:10.3390/nu12092570 41

Tom Warkentin, Nikolai Kolba and Elad Tako
Low Phytate Peas (*Pisum sativum* L.) Improve Iron Status, Gut Microbiome, and Brush Border
Membrane Functionality In Vivo (*Gallus gallus*)
Reprinted from: *Nutrients* **2020**, *12*, 2563, doi:10.3390/nu12092563 55

**Pieter Van den Abbeele, Lynn Verstrepen, Jonas Ghyselinck, Ruud Albers,
Massimo Marzorati and Annick Mercenier**
A Novel Non-Digestible, Carrot-Derived Polysaccharide (cRG-I) Selectively Modulates the
Human Gut Microbiota while Promoting Gut Barrier Integrity: An Integrated In Vitro Approach
Reprinted from: *Nutrients* **2020**, *12*, 1917, doi:10.3390/nu12071917 73

**Pieter Van den Abbeele, Jonas Ghyselinck, Massimo Marzorati, Agusti Villar,
Andrea Zangara, Carsten R. Smidt and Ester Risco**
In Vitro Evaluation of Prebiotic Properties of a Commercial Artichoke Inflorescence Extract
Revealed Bifidogenic Effects
Reprinted from: *Nutrients* **2020**, *12*, 1552, doi:10.3390/nu12061552 95

**Agata Jabłońska-Trypuć, Urszula Wydro, Elżbieta Wołejko, Joanna Rodziewicz and
Andrzej Butarewicz**
Possible Protective Effects of TA on the Cancerous Effect of Mesotrione
Reprinted from: *Nutrients* **2020**, *12*, 1343, doi:10.3390/nu12051343 107

Katarzyna Petka, Tomasz Tarko and Aleksandra Duda-Chodak
Is Acrylamide as Harmful as We Think? A New Look at the Impact of Acrylamide on the
Viability of Beneficial Intestinal Bacteria of the Genus *Lactobacillus*
Reprinted from: *Nutrients* **2020**, *12*, 1157, doi:10.3390/nu12041157 125

Agata Jabłońska-Trypuć, Urszula Wydro, Elżbieta Wołejko, Grzegorz Świderski and Włodzimierz Lewandowski
Biological Activity of New Cichoric Acid–Metal Complexes in Bacterial Strains, Yeast-Like Fungi, and Human Cell Cultures In Vitro
Reprinted from: *Nutrients* **2020**, *12*, 154, doi:10.3390/nu12010154 . . . . **147**

Bárbara Pereira da Silva, Nikolai Kolba, Hércia Stampini Duarte Martino, Jonathan Hart and Elad Tako
Soluble Extracts from Chia Seed (*Salvia hispanica* L.) Affect Brush Border Membrane Functionality, Morphology and Intestinal Bacterial Populations In Vivo (*Gallus gallus*)
Reprinted from: *Nutrients* **2019**, *11*, 2457, doi:10.3390/nu11102457 . . . . **169**

Estefanía Valero-Cases, Débora Cerdá-Bernad, Joaquín-Julián Pastor and María-José Frutos
Non-Dairy Fermented Beverages as Potential Carriers to Ensure Probiotics, Prebiotics, and Bioactive Compounds Arrival to the Gut and Their Health Benefits
Reprinted from: *Nutrients* **2020**, *12*, 1666, doi:10.3390/nu12061666 . . . . **187**

About the Editor

Elad Tako holds degrees in animal science (B.S.), endocrinology (M.S.), and physiology/nutrigenomics (Ph.D.), with previous appointments at the Hebrew University of Jerusalem, North Carolina State University, and Cornell University. As an Associate Professor with the Department of Food Science at Cornell University, Dr. Tako's research focuses on various aspects of trace mineral deficiencies, emphasizing molecular, physiological and nutritional factors and practices that influence the intestinal micronutrient absorption. With over 100 peer-reviewed publications and presentations, he leads a research team focused on understanding the interactions between dietary factors, physiological and molecular biomarkers, the microbiome, and intestinal functionality. His research accomplishments include the development of the Gallus gallus intra-amniotic administration procedure, and establishing recognized approaches for using animal models within mineral bioavailability and intestinal absorption screening processes. He has also developed a zinc status physiological blood biomarker (red blood cell Linoleic Acid: Dihomo–Linolenic Acid Ratio), and molecular tissue biomarkers to assess the effect of dietary mineral deficiencies on intestinal functionality, and how micronutrients dietary deficiencies alter gut microbiota composition and function.

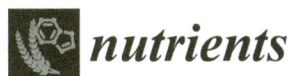

Editorial

Dietary Plant-Origin Bio-Active Compounds, Intestinal Functionality, and Microbiome

Elad Tako

Department of Food Science, Cornell University, Stocking Hall, Ithaca, NY 14853-7201, USA; et79@cornell.edu

Received: 5 October 2020; Accepted: 17 October 2020; Published: 22 October 2020

Abstract: In recent years, plant-origin bio-active compounds in foods (staple crops, fruit, vegetables, and others) have been gaining interest, and processes to consider them for public health recommendations are being presented and discussed in the literature. However, at times, it may be challenging to demonstrate causality, and there often is not a single compound–single effect relationship. Furthermore, it was suggested that health benefits may be due to metabolites produced by the host or gut microbiome rather than the food constituent per se. Over the years, compounds that were investigated were shown to increase gut microbial diversity, improve endothelial function, improve cognitive function, reduce bone loss, and many others. More recently, an additional and significant body of evidence further demonstrated the nutritional role and potential effects that plant-origin bio-active compounds might have on intestinal functionality (specifically the duodenal brush border membrane, morphology, and the abundance of health-promoting bacterial populations). Hence, the special issue "Dietary Plant-Origin Bio-Active Compounds, Intestinal Functionality, and Microbiome" comprises 11 peer-reviewed papers on the most recent evidence regarding the potential dietary intake and effects of plant-origin bio-active compounds on intestinal functionality, primarily in the context of brush border functional proteins (enzymes and transporters), mineral (and other nutrients) dietary bioavailability, and the intestinal microbiome. Original contributions and literature reviews further demonstrated the potential dietary relevance that plant bio-active compounds hold in human health and development. This editorial provides a brief and concise overview that addresses and summarizes the content of the *Dietary Plant-Origin Bio-Active Compounds, Intestinal Functionality, and Microbiome* special issue.

Keywords: plant origin; bio-active compounds; intestine; microbiome

---

The purpose of the current special issue is to further expand and add research knowledge of the vital role dietary plant-origin bio-active compounds hold in various nutrition-related physiological and metabolic pathways. In addition, the purpose is to further contribute to the knowledge regarding the relationship between plant-origin bio-active compounds, the intestinal morphology and functionality, and potential effects on the intestinal microbiome.

Plant-based diets contain a plethora of metabolites that may impact on health and disease prevention. Most are focused on the potential bioactivity and nutritional relevance of several classes of phytochemicals, such as polyphenols, flavonoids, carotenoids, phyto-estrogens, and frucrooligo-saccharides [1]. These compounds are found in fruit, vegetables, and herbs [2]. Daily intakes of some of these compounds may exceed 100 mg. Moreover, intestinal bacterial activity may transform complex compounds such as anthocyanins, procyanidins, and isoflavones into simple phenolic metabolites [3]. The colon is thus a rich source of potentially active phenolic acids that may impact both locally and systemically on gut health. Furthermore, non-digestible fiber (prebiotics) are dietary substrates that selectively promote proliferation and/or activity of health-promoting bacterial populations in the colon [4]. Prebiotics, such as inulin, raffinose, and stachyose, have a proven ability to promote the abundance of intestinal bacterial populations, which may provide additional health benefits to the host [5–10]. Furthermore, various pulse seed soluble (fiber) extracts are responsible for improving gastrointestinal motility, intestinal functionality and morphology, and mineral absorption [9,11]. Studies have indicated that the consumption of seed-origin soluble extracts can up-regulate the expression of brush border membrane (BBM) proteins that contribute for digestion and absorption of nutrients. The soluble extracts can positively affect intestinal health by increasing the mucus production, goblet cells number/diameter, villus surface area, and crypt depth [9,10]. These functional and morphological effects appear to occur due to the increased motility of the digestive tract, leading to hyperplasia and/or hypertrophy of muscle cells. Plant-origin soluble extracts may act, directly or indirectly, as a factor that increases mineral solubility and, therefore, dietary bioavailability. This occurs due to fiber fermentation and bacterial production of short chain fatty acids (SCFA) that reduces intestinal pH, inhibits the growth of potentially pathogenic bacterial population and increases the solubility and, therefore, absorption of minerals. The SCFA can increase the proliferation of epithelial cells, which, in return, increase the absorptive surface area, which contributes to the absorption of nutrients [12,13]. Several phenolic acids and other phytochemicals affect the expression and activity of enzymes involved in the production of inflammatory mediators of pathways thought to be important in the development of gut disorders including colon cancer. However, it is still unclear as to which of these compounds are beneficial to gut health. Hence, the aim of the current special issue is to further explore the interactions between dietary plant-origin bio-active compounds, their potential effects on the intestinal bacterial populations, and overall intestinal functionality and gut health.

This monograph, based on a special issue of Nutrients, contains 11 manuscripts—1 review and 10 original publications—that reflect the wide spectrum of currently conducted research in the field of dietary plant-origin bio-active compounds, intestinal functionality, and microbiome. The manuscripts in this special issue collection include contributors and researchers from multiple countries, including USA, Canada, Australia, Brazil, Poland, Finland, Belgium, Netherlands, and Spain. The presented manuscripts cover a wide variety and range of topics in the field of dietary plant-origin bio-active compounds, intestinal functionality, and microbiome, with emphasis on diet and intestinal well-being and compositions of fecal microbiota and short chain fatty acids in oat and by using subjects with celiac disease or gluten sensitivity [14]. The demonstration of low phytate peas (Pisum sativum L.)-based diets improve iron status, gut microbiome, and brush border membrane functionality in vivo (Gallus gallus) [15]. The presentation of novel non-digestible, carrot-derived polysaccharide (cRG-I) and how it selectively modulates the human gut microbiota while promoting gut barrier integrity (an integrated in vitro approach) [16]. The in vitro evaluation of prebiotic properties of a commercial artichoke inflorescence extract revealed bifidogenic effects [17]. The discussion of possible protective effects of traumatic acid (TA) on the cancerous effect of mesotrione [18]. Is Acrylamide as a harmful as we think? A new look at the impact of Acrylamide on the viability of beneficial intestinal bacteria of the genus *Lactobacillus* [19] The biological activity of new cichoric acid–metal complexes in bacterial strains, yeast-like fungi, and human cell cultures in vitro [20]. The presentation of how soluble extracts from chia seed (*Salvia hispanica* L.) affect brush border membrane functionality, morphology and intestinal bacterial populations in vivo (*Gallus gallus*) [21]. The fructose consumption by adult rats exposed to dexamethasone in utero changes the phenotype of intestinal epithelial cells and exacerbates intestinal gluconeogenesis [22]. Alterations in the intestinal morphology, gut microbiota, and trace mineral status following intra-amniotic administration (Gallus gallus) of teff (Eragrostis tef) seed extracts [23]. Non-dairy fermented beverages as potential carriers to ensure probiotics, prebiotics, and bio-active compounds arrival to the gut and their health benefits [24]. These wide spectra of topics further demonstrate the importance and relevance of dietary plant-origin bio-active compounds, and their effects on intestinal functionality and microbiome.

This special issue and collection of manuscripts is a useful summary of progress in various areas related to dietary plant-origin bio-active compounds, intestinal functionality, and microbiome. It also points to additional research needs, including recommendations for future research in the field, and to better understand the dietary role that dietary plant-origin bio-active compounds hold and regarding human nutrition and overall health.

Funding: This research received no external funding

Conflicts of Interest: The author declares no conflict of interest.

References

1. Upadhyay, S.; Dixit, M. Role of Polyphenols and Other Phytochemicals on Molecular Signaling. *Oxid. Med. Cell. Longev.* **2015**, 504253. [CrossRef] [PubMed]
2. Shinwari, K.J.; Rao, P.S. Trends in Food Science & Technology. Stability of bioactive compounds in fruit jam and jelly during processing and storage: A review. *Trends Food Sci. Technol.* **2018**, *75*, 181–193.
3. Hartono, K.; Reed, S.; Ayikarkor Ankrah, N.; Tako, T. Alterations in gut microflora populations and brush border functionality following intra-amniotic daidzein administration. *RSC Adv.* **2015**, *5*, 6407–6412. [CrossRef]
4. Slavin, J. Fiber and Prebiotics: Mechanisms and Health Benefits. *Nutrients* **2013**, *5*, 1417–1435. [CrossRef] [PubMed]
5. Tako, E.; Rutzke, M.A.; Glahn, R.P. Using the domestic chicken (Gallus gallus) as an in vivo model for Fe bioavailability. *J. Poult. Sci.* **2010**, *89*, 514–521. [CrossRef] [PubMed]
6. Pacifici, S.; Song, J.; Zhang, C.; Wang, Q.; Kolba, N.; Tako, E. Intra Amniotic Administration of Raffinose and Stachyose Affects the Intestinal Brush Border Functionality and Alters Gut Microflora Populations. *Nutrients* **2017**, *9*, 304. [CrossRef] [PubMed]
7. Hou, T.; Kolba, N.; Tako, E. Intra-Amniotic Administration (Gallus gallus) of Cicer arietinum and Lens culinaris Prebiotics Extracts and Duck Egg White Peptides Affects Calcium Status and Intestinal Functionality. *Nutrients* **2017**, *9*, 785. [CrossRef]
8. Hou, T.; Tako, E. The In Ovo Feeding Administration (Gallus Gallus)—An Emerging In Vivo Approach to Assess Bioactive Compounds with Potential Nutritional Benefits. *Nutrients* **2018**, *10*, 418. [CrossRef]
9. Morais Dias, D.; Kolba, N.; Hart, J.; Ma, M.; Sha, S.; Lakshmanan, N.; Nutti Regini, M.; Duarte Martino, H.; Tako, E. Soluble extracts from carioca beans (Phaseolus vulgaris L.) affect the gut microbiota and iron related brush border membrane protein expression in vivo (Gallus gallus). *Food Res. Int.* **2019**, *120*, 172–180. [CrossRef]
10. Beasley, J.T.; Johnson, A.A.T.; Kolba, N.; Bonneau, J.P.; Ohayon, M.N.; Koren, O.; Tako, E. Nicotianamine-chelated iron improves micronutrients physiological status and gastrointestinal health in vivo (*Gallus gallus*). *Sci. Rep.* **2020**, *10*, 2297. [CrossRef]
11. Wang, X.; Kolba, N.; Tako, E. Alterations in gut microflora populations and brush border functionality following intra-amniotic administration (*Gallus gallus*) of wheat bran prebiotics extracts. *Food Funct.* **2019**, 19. [CrossRef] [PubMed]
12. Reed, S.; Neuman, H.; Moscovich, S.R.; Koren, O.; Tako, E. Chronic Zinc Deficiency AltersChick Gut Microbiota Composition and Function. *Nutrients* **2015**, *7*, 9768–9784. [CrossRef] [PubMed]
13. Reed, S.; Knez, M.; Uzan, A.; Stangoulis, J.; Koren, O.; Tako, E. Alterations in the gut (*Gallus gallus*) microbiota following the consumption of zinc biofortified wheat (*Triticum aestivum*)-based diet. *J. Agric. Food Chem.* 2018. [CrossRef] [PubMed]
14. Nylund, L.; Hakkola, S.; Lahti, L.; Salminen, S.; Kalliomäki, M.; Yang, B.; Linderborg, K.M. Diet, Perceived Intestinal Well-Being and Compositions of Fecal Microbiota and Short Chain Fatty Acids in Oat-Using Subjects with Celiac Disease or Gluten Sensitivity. *Nutrients* **2020**, *12*, 2570. [CrossRef] [PubMed]
15. Warkentin, T.; Kolba, N.; Tako, E. Low Phytate Peas (Pisum sativum L.) Improve Iron Status, Gut Microbiome, and Brush Border Membrane Functionality In Vivo (*Gallus gallus*). *Nutrients* **2020**, *12*, 2563. [CrossRef]
16. Van den Abbeele, P.; Verstrepen, L.; Ghyselinck, J.; Albers, R.; Marzorati, M.; Mercenier, A. A Novel Non-Digestible, Carrot-Derived Polysaccharide (cRG-I) Selectively Modulates the Human Gut Microbiota while Promoting Gut Barrier Integrity: An Integrated In Vitro Approach. *Nutrients* **2020**, *12*, 1917. [CrossRef]
17. Van den Abbeele, P.; Ghyselinck, J.; Marzorati, M.; Villar, A.; Zangara, A.; Smidt, C.R.; Risco, E. In Vitro Evaluation of Prebiotic Properties of a Commercial Artichoke Inflorescence Extract Revealed Bifidogenic Effects. *Nutrients* **2020**, *12*, 1552. [CrossRef]

18. Jabłońska-Trypuć, A.; Wydro, U.; Wołejko, E.; Rodziewicz, J.; Butarewicz, A. Possible Protective Effects of TA on the Cancerous Effect of Mesotrione. *Nutrients* **2020**, *12*, 1343. [CrossRef]
19. Petka, K.; Tarko, T.; Duda-Chodak, A. Is Acrylamide as Harmful as We Think? A New Look at the Impact of Acrylamide on the Viability of Beneficial Intestinal Bacteria of the Genus Lactobacillus. *Nutrients* **2020**, *12*, 1157. [CrossRef]
20. Jabłońska-Trypuć, A.; Wydro, U.; Wołejko, E.; Świderski, G.; Lewandowski, W. Biological Activity of New Cichoric Acid–Metal Complexes in Bacterial Strains, Yeast-Like Fungi, and Human Cell Cultures In Vitro. *Nutrients* **2020**, *12*, 154. [CrossRef]
21. Pereira da Silva, B.; Kolba, N.; Stampini Duarte Martino, H.; Hart, J.; Tako, E. Soluble Extracts from Chia Seed (Salvia hispanica L.) Affect Brush Border Membrane Functionality, Morphology and Intestinal Bacterial Populations In Vivo (*Gallus gallus*). *Nutrients* **2019**, *11*, 2457. [CrossRef] [PubMed]
22. Pereira, G.; Sodré, F.; Murata, G.; Amaral, A.; Payolla, T.; Campos, C.; Sato, F.; Anhê, G.; Bordin, S. Fructose consumption by adult rats exposed to dexamethasone in utero changes the phenotype of intestinal epithelial cells and exacerbates intestinal gluconeogenesis. *Nutrients* **2020**, 3062, in press. [CrossRef] [PubMed]
23. Carboni, J.; Reed, S.; Kolba, N.; Eshel, A.; Koren, O.; Tako, E. Alterations in the Intestinal Morphology, Gut Microbiota, and Trace Mineral Status Following Intra-Amniotic Administration (*Gallus gallus*) of Teff (*Eragrostis tef*) Seed Extracts. *Nutrients* **2020**, *12*, 3020. [CrossRef] [PubMed]
24. Valero-Cases, E.; Cerdá-Bernad, D.; Pastor, J.J.; Frutos, M.J. Non-Dairy Fermented Beverages as Potential Carriers to Ensure Probiotics, Prebiotics, and Bioactive Compounds Arrival to the Gut and Their Health Benefits. *Nutrients* **2020**, *12*, 1666. [CrossRef] [PubMed]

Publisher's Note: MDPI stays neutral with regard to jurisdictional claims in published maps and institutional affiliations.

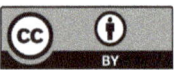

© 2020 by the author. Licensee MDPI, Basel, Switzerland. This article is an open access article distributed under the terms and conditions of the Creative Commons Attribution (CC BY) license (http://creativecommons.org/licenses/by/4.0/).

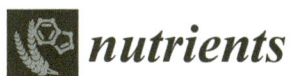

Article

Fructose Consumption by Adult Rats Exposed to Dexamethasone In Utero Changes the Phenotype of Intestinal Epithelial Cells and Exacerbates Intestinal Gluconeogenesis

Gizela A. Pereira [1], Frhancielly S. Sodré [1], Gilson M. Murata [1], Andressa G. Amaral [1], Tanyara B. Payolla [1], Carolina V. Campos [2], Fabio T. Sato [1], Gabriel F. Anhê [2] and Silvana Bordin [1,*]

1. Department of Physiology and Biophysics, Institute of Biomedical Sciences, University of Sao Paulo, Sao Paulo, 05508-000 SP, Brazil; gizela.usp@gmail.com (G.A.P.); frhanshirley@gmail.com (F.S.S.); gilmasa@gmail.com (G.M.M.); andressa_amaral@usp.br (A.G.A.); tany_line@yahoo.com.br (T.B.P.); fabiotakeosato@gmail.com (F.T.S.)
2. Department of Pharmacology, Faculty of Medical Sciences, State University of Campinas, Campinas, 13083-887 SP, Brazil; ca.v.campos20@gmail.com (C.V.C.); anhegf@unicamp.br (G.F.A.)
* Correspondence: sbordin@icb.usp.br; Tel.: +55-11-3091-7245

Received: 3 September 2020; Accepted: 2 October 2020; Published: 7 October 2020

Abstract: Fructose consumption by rodents modulates both hepatic and intestinal lipid metabolism and gluconeogenesis. We have previously demonstrated that in utero exposure to dexamethasone (DEX) interacts with fructose consumption during adult life to exacerbate hepatic steatosis in rats. The aim of this study was to clarify if adult rats born to DEX-treated mothers would display differences in intestinal gluconeogenesis after excessive fructose intake. To address this issue, female Wistar rats were treated with DEX during pregnancy and control (CTL) mothers were kept untreated. Adult offspring born to CTL and DEX-treated mothers were assigned to receive either tap water (Control-Standard Chow (CTL-SC) and Dexamethasone-Standard Chow (DEX-SC)) or 10% fructose in the drinking water (CTL-fructose and DEX-fructose). Fructose consumption lasted for 80 days. All rats were subjected to a 40 h fasting before sample collection. We found that DEX-fructose rats have increased glucose and reduced lactate in the portal blood. Jejunum samples of DEX-fructose rats have enhanced phosphoenolpyruvate carboxykinase (PEPCK) expression and activity, higher facilitated glucose transporter member 2 (GLUT2) and facilitated glucose transporter member 5 (GLUT5) content, and increased villous height, crypt depth, and proliferating cell nuclear antigen (PCNA) staining. The current data reveal that rats born to DEX-treated mothers that consume fructose during adult life have increased intestinal gluconeogenesis while recapitulating metabolic and morphological features of the neonatal jejunum phenotype.

Keywords: intrauterine growth restriction (IUGR); fructose; dexamethasone; intestinal gluconeogenesis

1. Introduction

The consumption of fructose-sweetened beverages has significantly increased during the last decades and a great number of observational studies have associated this nutritional habit with increased cardiometabolic risk [1]. In accordance with this hypothesis, experimental studies have described that rats consuming high amounts of fructose or sucrose develop glucose intolerance and increased hepatic gluconeogenesis [2–4].

The mechanisms underlying the metabolic effects of excessive fructose intake rely on its hepatic as well as its intestinal metabolism [5]. The small intestine absorbs fructose through a facilitated glucose transporter member 5 (GLUT5)-dependent mechanism and partially metabolizes it into lactate, glucose, and fatty acids that are sequentially secreted to the portal circulation [6,7]. However, intestinal fructose metabolism capacity is limited and when high amounts of fructose are consumed, a considerable fraction reaches the liver [7]. Hepatic metabolism of fructose, in turn, produces glyceraldehyde-3-phosphate that is driven to either gluconeogenesis or de novo lipogenesis (DNLG) [8].

Besides its metabolism to intermediates that feed gluconeogenesis and DNLG, fructose was described to modulate the expression of key metabolic genes [5]. Fructose consumption increased the expression of GLUT5 and gluconeogenic enzymes glucose-6-phosphatae (G6Pase) and fructose-1,6-bisphosphatase (FBP1) in the small intestine [9,10]. Excessive fructose intake was also reported to increase the hepatic expression of the gluconeogenesis enzymes G6Pase, FBP1, and phosphoenolpyruvate carboxykinase (PEPCK) [11–14], and the DNLG enzymes acetyl-CoA carboxylase (ACC), fatty acid synthase (FAS), and stearoyl-CoA desaturase-1 (SCD1) [15].

We have recently demonstrated that the modulation of key metabolic genes induced by fructose in the liver can interact with other factors, such as birth weight. Fructose supplementation of rats born small due to maternal treatment with dexamethasone (DEX) induced an expected increase in the expression of PEPCK, FAS, and ACC, but failed to increase the expression of genes involved in very low density lipoproteins (VLDL) assembly and secretion, leading to an exacerbation in hepatic steatosis [16].

In addition to low birth weight, in utero exposure to DEX is recognized to program the energy metabolism during adult life. Offspring born to DEX-treated mothers develop glucose intolerance and increased hepatic PEPCK expression as soon as the 21st day of life [17]. Additionally, pancreatic postnatal development of rats born to DEX-treated mothers is hallmarked by lower pancreatic b-cell mass and higher pancreatic a-cell mass and glucagon levels [18]. Treatment of pregnant mice with DEX was also described to epigenetically impair brown adipose tissue (BAT) thermogenesis and energy expenditure in the offspring, leading to increased adiposity and insulin resistance [19].

Aside from the liver, several studies have reported the expression of G6Pase and PEPCK in the small intestine of humans and rats, deeming this organ relevant in endogenous glucose production (EGP) [20–22]. Significant contribution of the small intestine to EGP is particularly relevant after a fasting period of at least 40 h, the period of time necessary for an increase in both G6Pase and PEPCK in the jejunum [23–25].

The present study has been undertaken to evaluate if prenatal exposure to DEX and excessive consumption of fructose during adult life could interact to modulate small intestine gluconeogenesis. To achieve this aim, we have evaluated key enzymatic and biochemical end-points indicative of intestinal gluconeogenesis as well as morphological aspects of the jejunum in 40 h fasted rats born to DEX-treated mothers and/or exposed to liquid fructose during adulthood.

2. Materials and Methods

2.1. Experimental Design and Diet

Eight-week-old nulliparous Wistar rats were acquired from the Animal Breeding Center at the Institute of Biomedical Sciences, University of Sao Paulo (Protocol # 5367250619). The animals were housed and mated with male rats as previously described [16].

After mating, pregnant rats were randomly assigned to receive 0.1 mg/kg/day dexamethasone (DEX) diluted in the drinking water from the 14th to the 19th day of pregnancy or remain untreated (CTL). On the 80th day of life, male offspring of DEX-treated and CTL dams were divided into two additional groups that were either kept with tap water or 10% fructose (w/v) solution ad libitum for the next 80 days. All offspring received standard chow ad libitum from the weaning to the 160th day of life.

The different groups were thereafter designed as follows: offspring born to CTL mothers that received only standard chow (SC) and tap water during adult life (CTL-SC); offspring born to DEX-treated mothers that received only SC and tap water during adult life (DEX-SC); offspring born to CTL mothers that received SC plus 10% fructose during adult life (CTL-fructose); and offspring born to DEX-treated mothers that received SC plus 10% fructose during adult life (DEX-fructose). On the 160th day of life, the animals were subjected to a 40 h fasting before euthanasia. During fasting, standard chow was removed and 10% fructose was replaced by tap water.

2.2. Pyruvate Tolerance Test (PTT)

Rats were fasted for 40 h and a 20% sodium pyruvate solution was injected intraperitoneal (i.p.) at a dosage of 2 g/kg of body mass. Glucose concentration was determined in blood extracted from the tail before (0 min) and 15, 30, 60, and 90 min after pyruvate injection (tail blood samples were chosen as representative of systemic blood). The area under the curve (AUC) of tail blood glucose levels vs. time was calculated using each individual baseline (basal glycemia) to estimate whole-body gluconeogenesis. We also collected portal blood samples at the end of the PTT (90 min after pyruvate challenge) to estimate the ability of the small intestine to convert pyruvate into glucose.

2.3. Tissue Sampling and Preparation

The rats were anesthetized with isoflurane. Proper level of anesthesia was assured by loss of pedal reflex. The abdominal cavity then was opened and portal blood was punctured. Euthanasia was performed by rupture of the diaphragm (with surgical scissors) followed by immediate cardiac puncture of the systemic blood. Systemic and portal blood samples were collected in EDTA-coated tubes and centrifuged at 2000 rpm for 20 min at 4 °C. Plasma samples were removed and used for biochemical analysis.

Intestinal segments were harvested from the proximal jejunum (5 cm beyond the ligament of Treitz), opened at the mesenteric border, pinned flat on a cork mat, and gently washed in ice-cold 0.1 M phosphate-buffered saline solution (PBS). The time elapsed between euthanasia and jejunum samples harvesting was approximately 2 min. The segments were transversally cut into two samples. In one sample, the mucosa was scraped and frozen under −80 °C for subsequent molecular and biochemical analyses (described below).

The second jejunum sample was immediately fixed with 10% buffered formaldehyde for 24 h, dehydrated in alcohol, diaphanized in xylol, and embedded in paraffin. Nonserial longitudinal sections (5–7 μm thick) were subjected to hematoxylin–eosin (HE) staining for morphometric analysis. In some rats, the entire small intestine was dissected and its length (cm) was measured and expressed as the relative length to tibia length [26].

2.4. Analysis of Blood Parameters

Plasma glucose, triglycerides, lactate, and cholesterol determinations were performed using commercially available kits (Labtest Diagnóstica SA, Lagoa Santa, MG, Brazil).

2.5. Enzymatic Activity

The activities of phosphoenolpyruvate carboxykinase (PEPCK; EC 4.1.1.32), glucose-6-phosphatase (G6Pase; EC 3.1.3.9), and hexokinase (HK; EC 2.7.1.1) were measured using spectrophotometric assays at 340 nm, following standard methods described elsewhere [27–29]. Protein concentration of each sample was determined by the Bradford method, and enzymatic activities were normalized by protein content.

2.6. Molecular Analyses

Scraped mucosal cells were processed for both qPCR and Western blotting (WB), as previously described [16]. The nitrocellulose membranes for WB were stained with Ponceau S before incubation with the primary antibodies. The stained membranes were allowed to dry at room temperature, scanned, and subjected to optical density (OD) quantification. All the lanes (from the top to the bottom) of labeled proteins were scanned to better represent the total amount of protein actually loaded in the gel. Subsequently, these values were applied to normalize the OD data of the target proteins detected in the respective membranes. This method was validated as an appropriate loading control [30]. The primary antibodies used were as follows: anti-GLUT2 (cat. # sc-9117) from Santa Cruz Biotechnology (Santa Cruz, CA, USA) and anti-GLUT5 (cat. # IM-0292) from Rhea Biotech (Campinas, SP, Brazil).

Total RNA was extracted using QIAzol reagent and used for reverse transcription with random primers for the analysis of mRNA expression. The primer sequences and accession numbers were as follows: *G6pc* (NM_013098) 5′-ACCTTCTTCCTGTTTGGTTTCGC-3′ and 5′-CGGTACATGCTGGAGTTGAGGG-3′; *Pck1* (NM_198780) 5′-TGGTCTGGACTTCTCTGCCAAG-3′ and 5′-AATGATGACCGTCTTGCTTTCG-3′; *Ggt1* (NM_053840) 5′-ACCCGACTTCATCGCTGTG-3′ and 5′-GCATGTTCTCCAGAGTCCCAC-3′; *Rpl37a* (X14069) 5′-CAAGAAGGTCGGGATCGTCG-3′; and 5′-ACCAGGCAAGTCTCAGGAGGTG-3′. Values of mRNA expression were normalized using the internal control gene *Rpl37a*. Fold changes were calculated by the $2^{-\Delta\Delta CT}$ method.

2.7. Morphometric Analysis of the Jejunum Wall

The morphometric analyses were performed blindly using AxioVision Release 4.8-SP2 software (Carl Zeiss Microscopy, Jena, Germany) and consisted of the evaluation of the villus height and crypt depth. The height of each villus was measured from the top of the villus to the crypt transition, and the crypt depth was defined as the invagination between two villi. These analyses were performed in five fields at 100× magnification from different jejunum regions, including 2–3 villus/crypt per field, totaling 10–15 villus/crypt per animal [31].

2.8. Immunohistochemical Evaluation of Cell Proliferation

Antigen retrieval was performed in citric acid (10 mM, pH 6.0) at 95 °C for 40 min, followed by cooling for 30 min. After antigen retrieval, sections were incubated with 3% hydrogen peroxide diluted in methanol for 30 min to quench endogenous peroxidase, then rinsed with deionized water followed by PBS, pH 7.4. Sections then were incubated with 6% defatted milk for 30 min, at 37 °C, to block nonspecific staining. The anti-PCNA monoclonal antibody, from Dako-Agilent (Santa Clara, CA, USA; Cat. No. M0879), was diluted 1:1000 in PBS plus 1% bovine serum albumin (BSA) and incubated on sections overnight at 4 °C. All sections were washed three times in PBS for 5 min each time, then incubated with secondary antibody conjugated with horseradish peroxidase labeled polymer (EnVision + Dual link System-HRP) for 30 min at room temperature. 3,3′-diaminobenzidine (DAB) was used to visualize the antigen/antibody complex and the specimens were then lightly counterstained with hematoxylin. Negative control samples were performed by substituting the primary antibody with antibody diluent. We analyzed 10 crypts from each section under a 400× magnification [32]. Cell proliferation rate was expressed as percentage of PCNA-positive cells.

2.9. Statistical Analyses

Comparisons were performed using two-way ANOVA, followed by a Tukey's multiple comparison test. The two factors considered for the two-way ANOVA were in utero exposure to DEX (either exposed or not) and treatment of 10% fructose during adulthood (either treated or not). When making comparisons between two groups, the unpaired Student's *t*-test was used. Statistical analyses were conducted using GraphPad Prism software version 8.4.3 (GraphPad Software, Inc., San Diego, CA, USA). All results are presented as the means ± standard error of the mean (SEM). Results with p values lower than 0.05 were considered significant.

3. Results

3.1. Consumption of Fructose by Rats Born to DEX-Treated Mothers Modifies Body Composition but Does Not Modulate Small Intestine Length

As reported by us in previous studies [16,33], rats born to DEX-treated mothers displayed reduced birth weight (18% lower than CTL; $p = 0.033$) (Figure 1A). The body weights of the 40 h fasted offspring with 160 days of age were influenced by both in utero exposure to DEX and treatment with 10%

fructose ($p < 0.0001$ and $p = 0.0002$, respectively). The post hoc analysis revealed that DEX-SC were lighter (9%; $p < 0.01$) while CTL-fructose were heavier (10%; $p < 0.001$) when compared to age-matched CTL-SC. In addition, DEX-fructose rats were lighter than the SC-fructose group (13%; $p < 0.0001$) (Figure 1B).

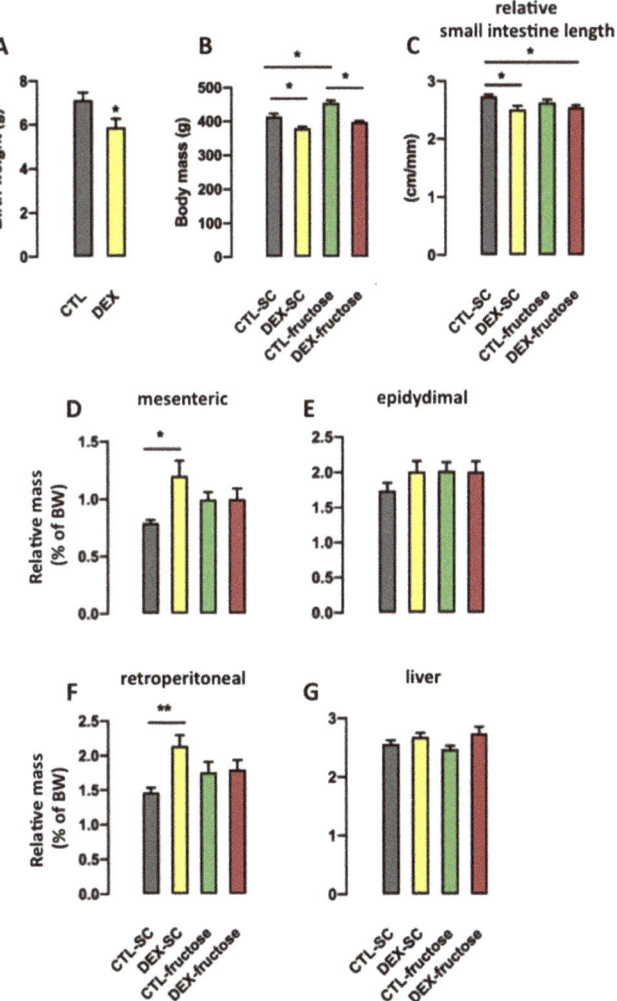

Figure 1. Morphometrical parameters of rats exposed to dexamethasone (DEX) in utero. Body weight was measured at birth (**A**) and at the end of treatment (**B**) in nonfasted rats. Fasted rats were euthanized at the end of the 80th day of fructose consumption, and the small intestine length relative to tibia length (**C**), and fat pads (mesenteric, (**D**); epidydimal, (**E**); retroperitoneal, (**F**)) and liver (**G**) masses relative to body weight were also measured. Results are presented as mean ± standard error of the mean (S.E.M.). * $p < 0.05$, ** $p < 0.01$ ($n = 10$–20). Offspring born to control (CTL) mothers that received only standard chow (SC) and tap water during adult life (CTL-SC); offspring born to DEX-treated mothers that received only SC and tap water during adult life (DEX-SC); offspring born to CTL mothers that received SC plus 10% fructose during adult life (CTL-fructose); and offspring born to DEX-treated mothers that received SC plus 10% fructose during adult life (DEX-fructose).

Small intestine length, relative to tibia length, was influenced by in utero exposure to DEX ($p = 0.0035$). The post hoc analysis revealed that both DEX-SC and DEX-fructose had shorter small intestine when compared to CTL-SC (respectively 8% and 7% shorter; $p < 0.05$) (Figure 1C).

Mesenteric adiposity was influenced by the factor in utero exposure to DEX in the 40 h fasted offspring ($p = 0.0264$). However, the post hoc analysis revealed a specific increase of mesenteric adiposity in 40 h fasted DEX-SC (42% higher than CTL-SC; $p < 0.05$) (Figure 1D). The treatments had no effect on epididymal adiposity (Figure 1E). Retroperitoneal adiposity of the 40 h fasted adult offspring presented changes that were similar to those seen for mesenteric adiposity. The post hoc analysis revealed a specific increase of retroperitoneal adiposity of the 40 h fasted DEX-SC (50% higher than CTL-SC; $p < 0.01$) (Figure 1F). The relative weight of the liver was not affected by the treatments (Figure 1G).

3.2. Biochemical Changes Detected in Rats Born to DEX-Treated Mothers That Consume Fructose during Adulthood Indicates Increased Intestinal Gluconeogenesis

Both in utero exposure to DEX and treatment with 10% fructose during adulthood affected systemic glucose levels after a 40 h fasting ($p = 0.046$ and $p = 0.039$, respectively). However, the post hoc analysis revealed that systemic glucose levels were increased exclusively in 40 h fasted DEX-fructose (28% higher than CTL-SC; $p < 0.05$) (Figure 2A). Similarly, in utero exposure to DEX and treatment with 10% fructose during adulthood influenced systemic triglyceride levels after a 40 h fast ($p = 0.0025$ and $p < 0.0001$, respectively). In regard to this, the post hoc analysis indicated that systemic triglyceride levels were increased in 40 h fasted DEX-fructose when compared to CTL-SC, DEX-SC, and CTL-fructose (respectively 108%, 62%, and 36%; $p < 0.0001$, $p < 0.001$, and $p < 0.05$). Systemic triglycerides were also increased in 40 h fasted CTL-fructose (52% higher than CTL-SC; $p < 0.05$) (Figure 2B). Total systemic cholesterol levels after 40 h fasting were not altered in any of the four groups studied (Figure 2C).

Both in utero exposure to DEX and treatment with 10% fructose during adulthood also modified portal glucose levels after a 40 h fasting ($p < 0.0001$ and $p = 0.045$, respectively). Our post hoc analysis revealed that portal glucose levels were increased in 40 h fasted DEX-fructose (144% higher than CTL-SC and 83% higher than CTL-fructose; $p < 0.0001$ and $p < 0.01$). The portal glucose levels were also increased in 40 h fasted DEX-SC (102% higher than CTL-SC; $p < 0.05$) (Figure 2D). Portal lactate levels detected after a 40 h fasting were only influenced by in utero exposure to DEX ($p < 0.05$). The post hoc analysis revealed a specific reduction of portal lactate levels in 40 h fasted DEX-fructose rats (26% lower than CTL-SC; $p < 0.05$) (Figure 2E).

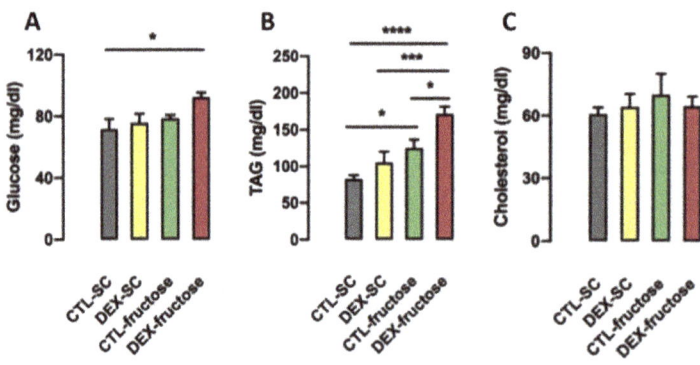

Figure 2. *Cont.*

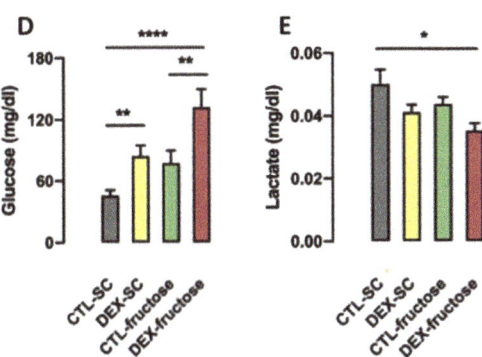

Figure 2. Effects of fructose on biochemical parameters of systemic and portal blood in rats exposed to dexamethasone (DEX) in utero. Systemic blood samples were collected to measure glucose (**A**), triacylglycerol (**B**), and total cholesterol (**C**). Portal hepatic vein samples were collected to measure glucose (**D**) and lactate (**E**). Results are presented as mean ± standard error of the mean (S.E.M.). * $p < 0.05$, ** $p < 0.01$, *** $p < 0.001$, **** $p < 0.0001$ ($n = 8$–12). Offspring born to control (CTL) mothers that received only standard chow (SC) and tap water during adult life (CTL-SC); offspring born to DEX-treated mothers that received only SC and tap water during adult life (DEX-SC); offspring born to CTL mothers that received SC plus 10% fructose during adult life (CTL-fructose); and offspring born to DEX-treated mothers that received SC plus 10% fructose during adult life (DEX-fructose).

3.3. Rats Born to DEX-Treated Mothers That Consume Fructose during Adulthood Display Increased Portal Glucose Levels after Challenge with Exogenous Pyruvate

We next performed the pyruvate tolerance test with the attempt to clarify if the higher portal glucose levels seen in 40 h fasted DEX-fructose rats were due to increased gluconeogenesis. The glucose levels in tail blood samples were assessed at different time points after pyruvate injection (Figure 3A). Treatment with 10% fructose during adulthood influenced the area under the curve (AUC) values in 40 h fasted rats ($p < 0.0001$). Our post hoc analysis indicated that whole-body gluconeogenesis is increased in fructose-treated rats irrespective of maternal treatment with DEX. This can be concluded because the AUC values of both CTL-fructose and DEX-fructose rats were similar to each other and higher than those of CTL-SC (respectively 174% and 227% higher; $p = 0.0227$ and $p = 0.0016$) (Figure 3B).

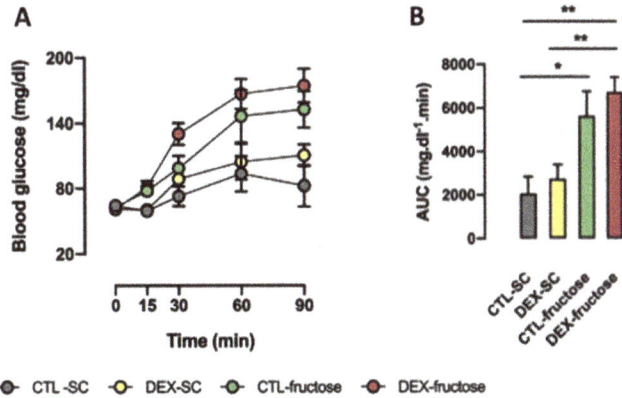

Figure 3. *Cont.*

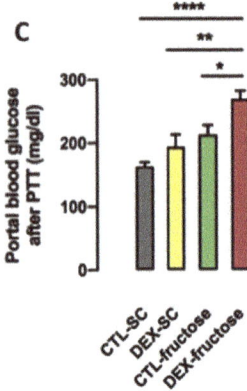

Figure 3. Whole-body and intestinal use of pyruvate as a gluconeogenesis substrate by rats exposed to dexamethasone (DEX) in utero and treated with fructose during adult life. The 40 h fasted rats received an i.p. injection containing sodium pyruvate. The blood from the tail was collected before and 15, 30, 60, and 90 min after intraperitoneal (i.p.) injection for glucose measurements (**A**) and the area under the curve (AUC) was calculated above each individual baseline (**B**). Glucose levels were also measured in portal blood at the end of the pyruvate tolerance test (PTT) (**C**). Results are presented as mean ± standard error of the mean (S.E.M.) * $p < 0.05$, ** $p < 0.01$, **** $p < 0.0001$ ($n = 8$). Offspring born to control (CTL) mothers that received only standard chow (SC) and tap water during adult life (CTL-SC); offspring born to DEX-treated mothers that received only SC and tap water during adult life (DEX-SC); offspring born to CTL mothers that received SC plus 10% fructose during adult life (CTL-fructose); and offspring born to DEX-treated mothers that received SC plus 10% fructose during adult life (DEX-fructose).

Glucose levels in portal blood 90 min after challenge with pyruvate were influenced by both in utero exposure to DEX and treatment with 10% fructose during adulthood ($p = 0.0043$ and $p = 0.0001$, respectively). In contrast to the changes in whole-body gluconeogenesis, our post hoc analysis revealed increased portal glucose levels after challenge with pyruvate exclusively in DEX-fructose rats (65% higher than CTL-SC, 26% higher than CTL-fructose, and 39% higher than DEX-SC; $p < 0.001$, $p = 0.0301$, and $p = 0.0055$) (Figure 3C).

3.4. Rats Born to DEX-Treated Mothers That Consume Fructose during Adulthood Display Increased PEPCK Expression and Activity in the Jejunum

The expression of *G6pc* (the gene that encodes G6Pase) in the jejunum was not affected in any of the four groups after a 40 h fasting (Figure 4A). The activity of G6Pase in the jejunum of the 40 h fasted rats was influenced by in utero exposure to DEX ($p = 0.035$) but no specific differences were found in the post hoc analysis (Figure 4B).

The expression of *Pck1* (the gene that encodes PEPCK) in the jejunum of the 40 h fasted rats was modulated by in utero exposure to DEX ($p = 0.005$). In this case, our post hoc analysis indicated a marked increase of *Pck1* expression in the jejunum of the 40 h DEX-fructose (88% higher than CTL-SC; $p < 0.05$) (Figure 4C). As with changes in expression, PEPCK activity in the jejunum of the 40 h fasted rats was regulated by in utero exposure to DEX ($p = 0.043$). Our post hoc analysis indicated a specific increase of PEPCK activity in the jejunum of the 40 h fasted DEX-fructose group (14% higher than CTL-SC; $p < 0.05$) (Figure 4D). The expression of fructose 1,6-bisphosphatase (*Fbp1*) was also evaluated but no differences were found among the groups (data not shown).

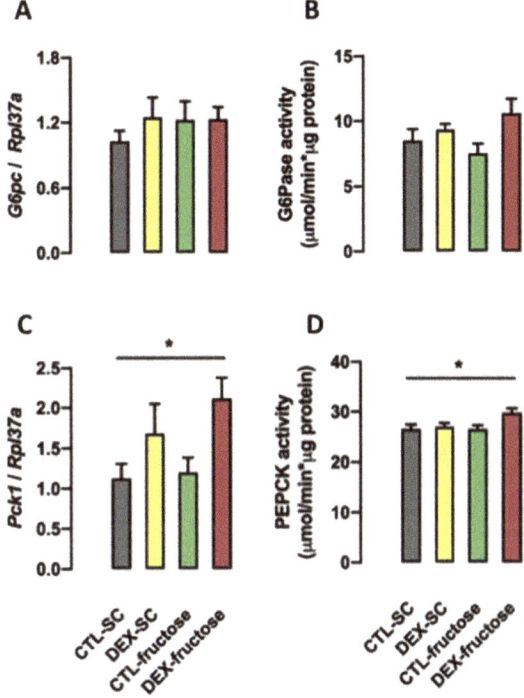

Figure 4. Expression and activity of enzymes involved in intestinal gluconeogenesis. Scraped epithelium of jejunum fragments was isolated and processed for qPCR detection of G6pc (**A**) and Pck1 (**C**) gene expression, as well as for maximum activities of the corresponding enzymes G6Pase (**B**) and PEPCK (**D**). Results are presented as mean ± standard error of the mean (S.E.M.). * $p < 0.05$ ($n = 6$–12). Offspring born to control (CTL) mothers that received only standard chow (SC) and tap water during adult life (CTL-SC); offspring born to dexamethasone (DEX)-treated mothers that received only SC and tap water during adult life (DEX-SC); offspring born to CTL mothers that received SC plus 10% fructose during adult life (CTL-fructose); and offspring born to DEX-treated mothers that received SC plus 10% fructose during adult life (DEX-fructose).

3.5. Rats Born to DEX-Treated Mothers That Consume Fructose during Adulthood Display Reduced HK Activity and Increased GLUT5 and GLUT2 Expression in the Jejunum

Both in utero exposure to DEX and treatment with 10% fructose during adulthood influenced hexokinase (HK) activity in the jejunum of the 40 h fasted rats ($p = 0.0362$ and $p = 0.0004$, respectively). The post hoc analysis revealed that reductions in HK activity in the jejunum of the 40 h fasted rats were specific for the DEX-fructose group (46% lower than CTL-SC, 51% lower than DEX-SC, and 44% lower than CTL-fructose; $p < 0.001$, $p < 0.0001$, and $p < 0.01$) (Figure 5A).

The expression of glutathione S-transferase 1 (*Gtt1*) in the jejunum of the 40 h fasted rats was influenced by in utero exposure to DEX ($p < 0.0001$). The post hoc analysis revealed that 40 h fasted DEX-SC rats had increased expression of *Gtt1* in the jejunum (90% higher than CTL-SC; $p < 0.05$). Increased expression of *Gtt1* in the jejunum was also found in 40 h fasted DEX-fructose (170% higher than CTL-fructose and 156% higher than CTL-SC; $p < 0.001$) (Figure 5B).

The content of facilitated glucose transporter member 2 (GLUT2) in the jejunum of the 40 h fasted rats was altered by treatment with 10% fructose during adulthood ($p = 0.0017$). The post hoc analysis revealed that the increase of GLUT2 content in the jejunum of the 40 h fasted rats was specific for DEX-fructose (60% higher than CTL-SC and 73% higher than DEXA-SC; $p < 0.01$) (Figure 5C).

The content of GLUT5 in the jejunum of the 40 h fasted rats was also influenced by in utero exposure to DEX ($p = 0.0299$). The post hoc analysis revealed a specific increase of GLUT5 content in the jejunum of the 40 h fasted DEX-fructose (75% higher than CTL-fructose; $p < 0.05$) (Figure 5D).

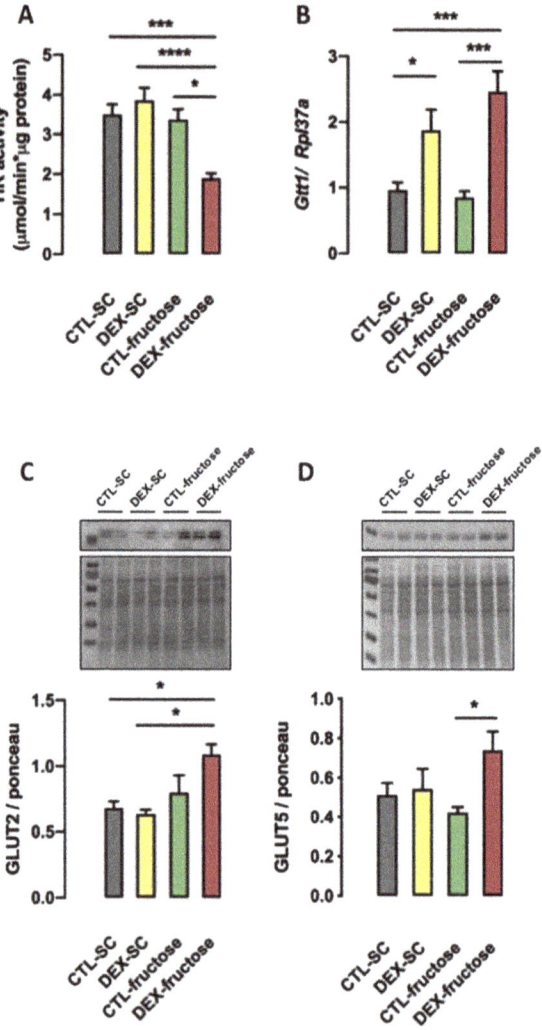

Figure 5. In utero dexamethasone (DEX) exposure alters glucose metabolism and phenotypic features of the jejunum epithelia. Scraped epithelium of jejunum fragments was isolated and processed for measurement of maximum hexokinase activity (**A**), expression of glutathione S-transferase 1 (Ggt1) by quantitative polymerase chain reaction (qPCR) (**B**), and Western blot of facilitated glucose transporter member 2 (GLUT2) (**C**) and facilitated glucose transporter member 5 (GLUT5) (**D**). Results are presented as mean ± standard error of the mean (S.E.M.). * $p < 0.05$, *** $p < 0.001$, **** $p < 0.0001$ ($n = 6$–12). Offspring born to control (CTL) mothers that received only standard chow (SC) and tap water during adult life (CTL-SC); offspring born to DEX-treated mothers that received only SC and tap water during adult life (DEX-SC); offspring born to CTL mothers that received SC plus 10% fructose during adult life (CTL-fructose); and offspring born to DEX-treated mothers that received SC plus 10% fructose during adult life (DEX-fructose).

3.6. Rats Born to DEX-Treated Mothers That Consume Fructose during Adulthood Display Morphological Changes in the Jejunum Epithelium

We have also assessed the mean crypt depth and the mean villous height, two aspects of the jejunum epithelium that are vital for its absorptive capacity. Images of the HE-stained jejunum sections are shown from each of the four different groups of 40 h fasted adult offspring (Figure 6A–D).

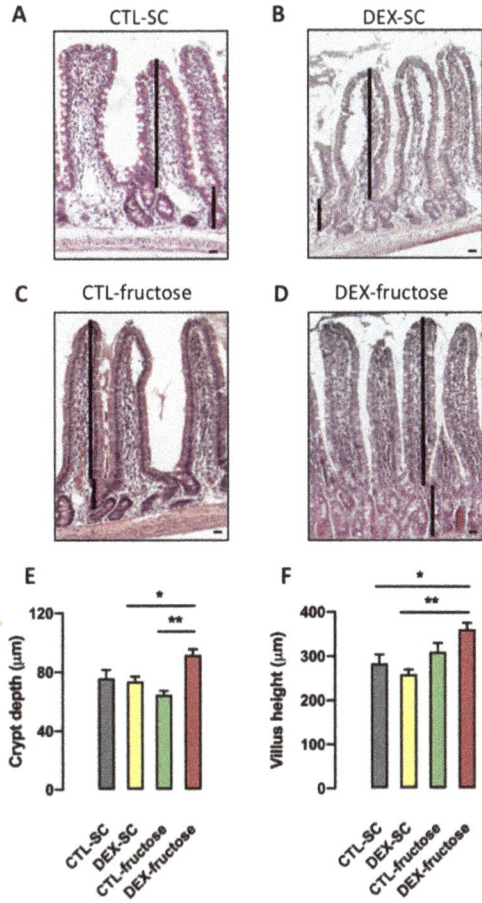

Figure 6. Morphometric analysis of the jejunum wall. The figure shows representative sections of villus and crypts of the four experimental groups (**A–D**). The height of each villus was measured from the top of the villus to the crypt transition (**E**), and the crypt depth was defined as the invagination between two villi (**F**). Results are presented as mean ± standard error of the mean (S.E.M.). * $p < 0.05$, ** $p < 0.01$ ($n = 5$). Offspring born to control (CTL) mothers that received only standard chow (SC) and tap water during adult life (CTL-SC); offspring born to dexamethasone (DEX)-treated mothers that received only SC and tap water during adult life (DEX-SC); offspring born to CTL mothers that received SC plus 10% fructose during adult life (CTL-fructose); and offspring born to DEX-treated mothers that received SC plus 10% fructose during adult life (DEX-fructose).

The mean crypt depth in the jejunum epithelium of 40 h fasted rats was modulated by in utero exposure to DEX ($p = 0.0119$). On the other hand, the post hoc analysis revealed that crypt depth was only increased in the jejunum epithelium of 40 h fasted DEX-fructose rats (25% higher than DEX-SC and 43% higher than CTL-fructose; $p < 0.05$ and $p < 0.01$) (Figure 6E).

Villous height was influenced by treatment with 10% fructose during adulthood ($p = 0.0017$). Similar to crypt depth, the post hoc analysis revealed that villous height was only increased in the jejunum epithelium of 40 h fasted DEX-fructose (27% higher than CTL-SC and 39% higher than DEX-SC; $p < 0.05$ and $p < 0.01$) (Figure 6F).

The proliferative potential in the jejunum epithelium was evaluated by assessing the relative number of PCNA-positive cells. Representative images of the jejunum sections stained with anti-PCNA antibody are shown from each of the four different groups of 40 h fasted adult offspring (Figure 7A–D). The hematoxylin-counterstained section that served as a negative control (by omission of the primary antibody) is shown in Figure 7E.

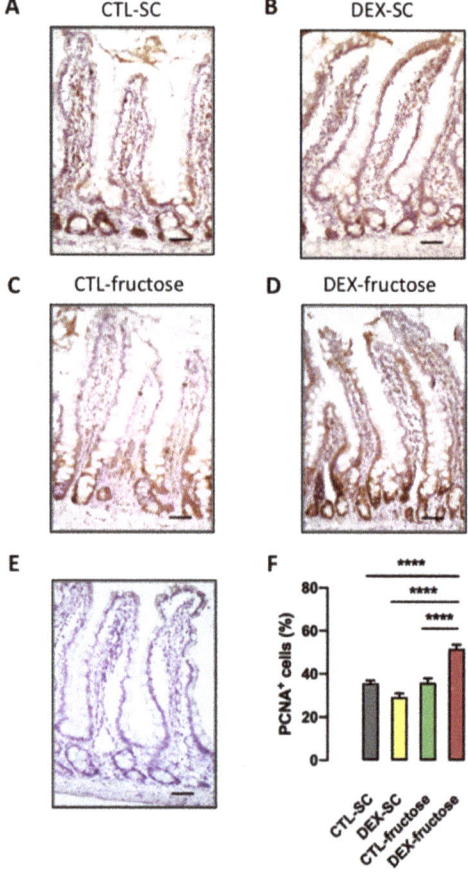

Figure 7. Jejunum was removed for immunohistochemical detection of proliferating cell nuclear antigen (PCNA). The figure shows representative sections of PCNA staining (**A–D**) and negative control sample (**E**). Sections were used to calculate the percentage of PCNA-positive cells in crypt cells (**F**). Results are presented as mean ± standard error of the mean (S.E.M.). **** $p < 0.0001$ ($n = 5$). Offspring born to control (CTL) mothers that received only standard chow (SC) and tap water during adult life (CTL-SC); offspring born to dexamethasone (DEX)-treated mothers that received only SC and tap water during adult life (DEX-SC); offspring born to CTL mothers that received SC plus 10% fructose during adult life (CTL-fructose); and offspring born to DEX-treated mothers that received SC plus 10% fructose during adult life (DEX-fructose).

Both factors, in utero exposure to DEX and treatment with 10% fructose during adulthood, influenced cell proliferation rate in the jejunum epithelium of the 40 h fasted rats ($p = 0.0158$ and $p < 0.0001$, respectively). The post hoc analysis revealed a particular increase in the cell proliferation rate of the jejunum epithelium of 40 h fasted DEX-fructose (48% higher than CTL-SC, 78% higher than DEX-SC, and 43% higher than CTL-fructose; $p < 0.0001$) (Figure 7F).

4. Discussion

In utero exposure to DEX is well known for programming metabolic changes in the adult offspring of rats. The metabolic imprinting caused by excessive exposure to DEX during fetal life is hallmarked by glucose intolerance, increased whole-body gluconeogenesis, and upregulation of PEPCK expression in the liver [17,33,34]. Recently, we have also described that in utero exposure to DEX exacerbates hepatic steatosis caused by fructose consumption during adult life [16]. The present study further contributes to this topic by revealing that rats born to DEX-treated mothers present exacerbated intestinal gluconeogenesis after consuming excessive fructose during adult life.

Changes in key endpoints support the above claim; increased PEPCK expression and activity in the jejunum and increased portal glucose levels were detected after a 40 h fasting in rats born to DEX-treated mothers that consumed fructose during adult life. An additional finding that supports the proposition that in utero exposure to DEX increases gluconeogenesis capacity is the higher portal glucose levels detected in DEX-fructose rats 90 min after the challenge with pyruvate, a known gluconeogenesis substrate. The 40 h fasting that preceded our sample collection and the PTT was performed because it has been previously described that intestinal gluconeogenesis does not significantly occur during shorter periods of food deprivation [25].

Another finding that supports the notion that intestinal gluconeogenesis is increased in rats born to DEX-treated mothers that consume fructose during adulthood is the increase in GLUT2 content in the jejunum of DEX-fructose rats, with parallel reduction in HK activity. GLUT2 is classically recognized for mediating the basolateral transport of glucose to the capillary vessels that feed the portal vein [35]. Our interpretation is that enterocytes of DEX-fructose rats have increased ability to synthesize glucose de novo (due to increased PEPCK) and release the newly synthesized glucose to the portal bloodstream (due to increased GLUT2 expression). Lower HK activity in the enterocytes of the DEX-fructose rats may contribute to the increased intestinal glucose release by reducing their rate of conversion of newly synthesized glucose back to glucose-6-phosphate.

In parallel with the above-mentioned biochemical changes that evidence increased intestinal gluconeogenesis, DEX-fructose rats exhibited lower portal lactate levels. This is particularly relevant because 10% fructose solution was replaced by water during the 40 h fasting. Thus, the current experiments do not support the notion that in utero exposure to DEX increases intestinal conversion of fructose into glucose but instead indicate that the jejunum of 40 h fasted adult DEX-fructose rats may increase the use of lactate as substrate for gluconeogenesis.

Interestingly, previous studies have reported that the small intestine of the fasted adult rat preferentially uses glutamine and glycerol, instead of lactate, as substrates for gluconeogenesis [23]. On the other hand, the small intestine of suckling rats is able to convert lactate into glucose [36]. Considering this, our data suggest that the small intestine of the offspring born to DEX-treated mothers that chronically consume fructose during adult life preserves a metabolic feature of the newborn small intestine.

Although it is challenging to presume the functional relevance of the increased GLUT5 in the jejunum of DEX-fructose rats after a 40 h fasting, this particular result reinforces the proposition that the small intestine of the adult offspring born to DEX-treated mothers preserves phenotypic features of the newborn after chronic exposure to fructose. Supporting this suggestion, it was previously demonstrated that DEX exacerbates GLUT5 expression induced by fructose in samples of small intestine of neonatal rats [37]. It is important to note that in utero exposure to DEX alone is not sufficient to stimulate GLUT5 content in the jejunum of the offspring. Such findings have also been previously reported in other studies [38] and support the notion that the two factors together (both in utero exposure to DEX and fructose consumption) seem to be necessary for enhancing jejunal GLUT5 content.

With regard to the morphological impact of DEX on the small intestine early in life, it has been previously reported that the lactating pups treated with DEX during lactation exhibit transitory changes in the small intestine epithelial architecture. Pups treated with DEX between the 11th and the 21st days of life display increased villous height and crypt depth in the jejunum soon after weaning. These changes are no longer detected by the age of 50 days [39]. Hence, we conclude that aside from the metabolic/biochemical features, morphological changes transiently described in the lactating pups exposed to DEX during early life are sustained in the adult offspring born to DEX-treated mothers only after consumption of excessive fructose.

We have also found that the frequency of PCNA-positive cells in the jejunum epithelial surface, a parameter that spontaneously reduces in the jejunum of the adult rat as the age advances beyond 90 days of life [40], is exacerbated in the 160-day-old DEX-fructose rats. Instead, *Ggt1* expression, an enzyme that plays a crucial role in de novo synthesis of intracellular GSH and ROS removal [41], is increased in the jejunum of adult rats born to DEX-treated mothers, irrespective of fructose consumption. Notably, GGT1 inhibition was associated with increased apoptosis in smooth muscle cells [42]. Thus, intestinal epithelial cells of the adult DEX-fructose offspring are unique in such a way that they combine long-term pro-proliferative and antiapoptotic adaptations.

Another interesting metabolic feature exhibited in the 40 h fasted DEX-fructose rats is the increased circulating triglyceride levels. Although we are not able to discern the hepatic or the intestinal origin of the lipoproteins that contribute to this phenomenon, it is important to take into account that intestinal production of triglyceride-enriched lipoprotein accounts for up to 40% of the triglycerides in fasting rats [43]. Moreover, chronic consumption of a fructose-enriched diet was described to increase the intestinal production of chylomicrons during fasting periods [44].

In summary, the present study supports the proposition that consumption of fructose by adult rats exposed to DEX during fetal life leads to an exacerbation in intestinal gluconeogenesis and retention of morphological features in the jejunum that are commonly found during neonatal life. These data provide a new mechanism to explain the increased prevalence of metabolic disturbances in humans that are born with low birth weight.

Author Contributions: Conceptualization, S.B. and G.A.P.; methodology, G.A.P., F.S.S., G.M.M., A.G.A., T.B.P., C.V.C., and F.T.S.; validation, G.A.P., F.S.S., G.M.M., and A.G.A; formal analysis, G.A.P., G.M.M., and A.G.A.; investigation, G.A.P. and F.S.S.; resources, S.B. and G.F.A.; data curation, S.B., G.M.M., and A.G.A.; writing—original draft preparation, G.A.P., A.G.A., and G.F.A.; writing—review and editing, S.B. and G.F.A.; supervision, S.B.; funding acquisition, S.B. and G.F.A. All authors have read and agreed to the published version of the manuscript.

Funding: This study was supported by the Research Foundation of the State of Sao Paulo (FAPESP Grants 2013/07607-8 and 2019/03196-0) and the National Council of Research (CNPq).

Acknowledgments: We acknowledge the technical support of Mariana M. Onari, Tiffany. B. Watanabe, Lais O.C. Lima, and Amanda M.S. Silva. We also thank Charles Serpellone Nash for carefully reviewing the manuscript.

Conflicts of Interest: The authors declare no conflicts of interest, financial or otherwise, associated with this article. The authors are responsible for the writing and content of the article.

References

1. Tappy, L.; Lê, K.A. Metabolic effects of fructose and the worldwide increase in obesity. *Physiol. Rev.* **2010**, *90*, 23–46. [CrossRef]
2. Faria, J.A.; de Araújo, T.M.; Razolli, D.S.; Ignácio-Souza, L.M.; Souza, D.N.; Bordin, S.; Anhê, G.F. Metabolic impact of light phase-restricted fructose consumption is linked to changes in hypothalamic AMPK phosphorylation and melatonin production in rats. *Nutrients* **2017**, *9*, 332. [CrossRef]
3. Oron-Herman, M.; Kamari, Y.; Grossman, E.; Yeger, G.; Peleg, E.; Shabtay, Z.; Shamiss, A.; Sharabi, Y. Metabolic syndrome: Comparison of the two commonly used animal models. *Am. J. Hypertens.* **2008**, *21*, 1018–1022. [CrossRef]

4. Bizeau, M.E.; Thresher, J.S.; Pagliassotti, M.J. A high-sucrose diet increases gluconeogenic capacity in isolated periportal and perivenous rat hepatocytes. *Am. J. Physiol. Endocrinol. Metab.* **2001**, *280*, E695–E702. [CrossRef]
5. Merino, B.; Fernández-Díaz, C.M.; Cózar-Castellano, I.; Perdomo, G. Intestinal fructose and glucose metabolism in health and disease. *Nutrients* **2019**, *12*, 94. [CrossRef]
6. Douard, V.; Ferraris, R.P. Regulation of the fructose transporter GLUT5 in health and disease. *Am. J. Physiol. Endocrinol. Metab.* **2008**, *295*, E227–E237. [CrossRef]
7. Jang, C.; Hui, S.; Lu, W.; Cowan, A.J.; Morscher, R.J.; Lee, G.; Liu, W.; Tesz, G.J.; Birnbaum, M.J.; Rabinowitz, J.D. The small intestine converts dietary fructose into glucose and organic acids. *Cell Metab.* **2018**, *27*, 351–361.e3. [CrossRef]
8. Theytaz, F.; de Giorgi, S.; Hodson, L.; Stefanoni, N.; Rey, V.; Schneiter, P.; Giusti, V.; Tappy, L. Metabolic fate of fructose ingested with and without glucose in a mixed meal. *Nutrients* **2014**, *6*, 2632–2649. [CrossRef]
9. Oh, A.R.; Sohn, S.; Lee, J.; Park, J.M.; Nam, K.T.; Hahm, K.B.; Kim, Y.B.; Lee, H.J.; Cha, J.Y. ChREBP deficiency leads to diarrhea-predominant irritable bowel syndrome. *Metabolism* **2018**, *85*, 286–297. [CrossRef]
10. Iizuka, K. The Role of carbohydrate response element binding protein in intestinal and hepatic fructose metabolism. *Nutrients* **2017**, *9*, 181. [CrossRef]
11. Kim, M.S.; Krawczyk, S.A.; Doridot, L.; Fowler, A.J.; Wang, J.X.; Trauger, S.A.; Noh, H.L.; Kang, H.J.; Meissen, J.K.; Blatnik, M.; et al. ChREBP regulates fructose-induced glucose production independently of insulin signaling. *J. Clin. Investig.* **2016**, *126*, 4372–4386. [CrossRef]
12. Koo, H.Y.; Wallig, M.A.; Chung, B.H.; Nara, T.Y.; Cho, B.H.; Nakamura, M.T. Dietary fructose induces a wide range of genes with distinct shift in carbohydrate and lipid metabolism in fed and fasted rat liver. *Biochim. Biophys. Acta* **2008**, *1782*, 341–348. [CrossRef]
13. Geidl-Flueck, B.; Gerber, P.A. Insights into the hexose liver metabolism-glucose versus fructose. *Nutrients* **2017**, *9*, 1026. [CrossRef]
14. Balakumar, M.; Raji, L.; Prabhu, D.; Sathishkumar, C.; Prabu, P.; Mohan, V.; Balasubramanyam, M. High-fructose diet is as detrimental as high-fat diet in the induction of insulin resistance and diabetes mediated by hepatic/pancreatic endoplasmic reticulum (ER) stress. *Mol. Cell. Biochem.* **2016**, *423*, 93–104. [CrossRef]
15. Chan, S.M.; Sun, R.Q.; Zeng, X.Y.; Choong, Z.H.; Wang, H.; Watt, M.J.; Ye, J.M. Activation of PPARα ameliorates hepatic insulin resistance and steatosis in high fructose-fed mice despite increased endoplasmic reticulum stress. *Diabetes* **2013**, *62*, 2095–2105. [CrossRef]
16. Payolla, T.B.; Teixeira, C.J.; Sato, F.T.; Murata, G.M.; Zonta, G.A.; Sodré, F.S.; Campos, C.V.; Mesquita, F.N.; Anhê, G.F.; Bordin, S. In Utero dexamethasone exposure exacerbates hepatic steatosis in rats that consume fructose during adulthood. *Nutrients* **2019**, *11*, 2114. [CrossRef]
17. Nyirenda, M.J.; Lindsay, R.S.; Kenyon, C.J.; Burchell, A.; Seckl, J.R. Glucocorticoid exposure in late gestation permanently programs rat hepatic phosphoenolpyruvate carboxykinase and glucocorticoid receptor expression and causes glucose intolerance in adult offspring. *J. Clin. Investig.* **1998**, *101*, 2174–2181. [CrossRef]
18. Santos-Silva, J.C.; da Silva, P.M.R.; de Souza, D.N.; Teixeira, C.J.; Bordin, S.; Anhê, G.F. In utero exposure to dexamethasone programs the development of the pancreatic β- and α-cells during early postnatal life. *Life Sci.* **2020**, *255*, 117810. [CrossRef]
19. Chen, Y.T.; Hu, Y.; Yang, Q.Y.; Son, J.S.; Liu, X.D.; de Avila, J.M.; Zhu, M.J.; Du, M. Excessive Glucocorticoids During Pregnancy Impair Fetal Brown Fat Development and Predispose Offspring to Metabolic Dysfunctions. *Diabetes* **2020**, *9*, 1662–1674. [CrossRef]
20. Mithieux, G.; Vidal, H.; Zitoun, C.; Bruni, N.; Daniele, N.; Minassian, C. Glucose-6-phosphatase mRNA and activity are increased to the same extent in kidney and liver of diabetic rats. *Diabetes* **1996**, *45*, 891–896. [CrossRef]
21. Rajas, F.; Bruni, N.; Montano, S.; Zitoun, C.; Mithieux, G. The glucose-6 phosphatase gene is expressed in human and rat small intestine: Regulation of expression in fasted and diabetic rats. *Gastroenterology* **1999**, *117*, 132–139. [CrossRef]
22. Rajas, F.; Croset, M.; Zitoun, C.; Montano, S.; Mithieux, G. Induction of PEPCK gene expression in insulinopenia in rat small intestine. *Diabetes* **2000**, *49*, 1165–1168. [CrossRef] [PubMed]
23. Croset, M.; Rajas, F.; Zitoun, C.; Hurot, J.M.; Montano, S.; Mithieux, G. Rat small intestine is an insulin-sensitive gluconeogenic organ. *Diabetes* **2001**, *50*, 740–746. [CrossRef]

24. Mithieux, G.; Bady, I.; Gautier, A.; Croset, M.; Rajas, F.; Zitoun, C. Induction of control genes in intestinal gluconeogenesis is sequential during fasting and maximal in diabetes. *Am. J. Physiol. Endocrinol. Metab.* **2004**, *286*, E370–E375. [CrossRef] [PubMed]
25. Penhoat, A.; Fayard, L.; Stefanutti, A.; Mithieux, G.; Rajas, F. Intestinal gluconeogenesis is crucial to maintain a physiological fasting glycemia in the absence of hepatic glucose production in mice. *Metabolism* **2014**, *63*, 104–111. [CrossRef]
26. Berg, B.; Harmison, C.R. Growth, disease, and aging in the rat. *J. Geront.* **1957**, *13*, 370–377. [CrossRef]
27. Opie, L.H.; Newsholme, E.A. The activities of fructose 1,6-diphosphatase, phosphofructokinase and phosphoenolpyruvate carboxykinase in white muscle and red muscle. *Biochem. J.* **1967**, *103*, 391–399. [CrossRef]
28. Trinder, P. Determination of blood glucose using an oxidase-peroxidase system with a non-carcinogenic chromogen. *J. Clin. Pathol.* **1969**, *22*, 158–161. [CrossRef]
29. Zammit, V.A.; Newsholme, E.A. The maximum activities of hexokinase, phosphorylase, phosphofructokinase, glycerol phosphate dehydrogenases, lactate dehydrogenase, octopine dehydrogenase, phosphoenolpyruvate carboxykinase, nucleoside diphosphatekinase, glutamate-oxaloacetate transaminase and arginine kinase in relation to carbohydrate utilization in muscles from marine invertebrates. *Biochem. J.* **1976**, *160*, 447–462.
30. Romero-Calvo, I.; Ocón, B.; Martínez-Moya, P.; Suárez, M.D.; Zarzuelo, A.; Martínez-Augustin, O.; de Medina, F.S. Reversible Ponceau staining as a loading control alternative to actin in Western blots. *Anal. Biochem.* **2010**, *401*, 318–320. [CrossRef]
31. Prakatur, I.; Miskulin, M.; Pavic, M.; Marjanovic, K.; Blazicevic, V.; Miskulin, I.; Domacinovic, M. Intestinal morphology in broiler chickens supplemented with propolis and bee pollen. *Animals* **2019**, *9*, 301. [CrossRef] [PubMed]
32. Uni, Z.; Geyra, A.; Ben-Hur, H.; Sklan, D. Small intestinal development in the young chick: Crypt formation and enterocyte proliferation and migration. *Br. Poult. Sci.* **2000**, *41*, 544–551. [CrossRef] [PubMed]
33. Pantaleão, L.C.; Murata, G.; Teixeira, C.J.; Payolla, T.B.; Santos-Silva, J.C.; Duque-Guimaraes, D.E.; Sodré, F.S.; Lellis-Santos, C.; Vieira, J.C.; de Souza, D.N.; et al. Prolonged fasting elicits increased hepatic triglyceride accumulation in rats born to dexamethasone-treated mothers. *Sci. Rep.* **2017**, *7*, 10367. [CrossRef] [PubMed]
34. Nyirenda, M.J.; Welberg, L.A.; Seckl, J.R. Programming hyperglycaemia in the rat through prenatal exposure to glucocorticoids-fetal effect or maternal influence? *J. Endocrinol.* **2001**, *170*, 653–660. [CrossRef]
35. Miyamoto, K.; Takagi, T.; Fujii, T.; Matsubara, T.; Hase, K.; Taketani, Y.; Oka, T.; Minami, H.; Nakabou, Y. Role of liver-type glucose transporter (GLUT2) in transport across the basolateral membrane in rat jejunum. *FEBS Lett.* **1992**, *314*, 466–470. [CrossRef]
36. Hahn, P.; Wei-Ning, H. Gluconeogenesis from lactate in the small intestinal mucosa of suckling rats. *Pediatr. Res.* **1986**, *20*, 1321–1323. [CrossRef]
37. Douard, V.; Cui, X.L.; Soteropoulos, P.; Ferraris, R.P. Dexamethasone sensitizes the neonatal intestine to fructose induction of intestinal fructose transporter (Slc2A5) function. *Endocrinology* **2008**, *149*, 409–423. [CrossRef]
38. Drozdowski, L.A.; Iordache, C.; Clandinin, M.T.; Todd, Z.S.C.; Gonnet, M.; Wild, G.; Uwiera, R.R.E.; Thomson, A.B.R. Dexamethasone and GLP-2 administered to rat dams during pregnancy and lactation have late effects on intestinal sugar transport in their postweaning offspring. *J. Nutr. Biochem.* **2008**, *19*, 49–60. [CrossRef]
39. Drozdowski, L.A.; Iordache, C.; Clandinin, M.T.; Wild, G.; Todd, Z.; Thomson, A.B.R. A combination of dexamethasone and glucagon-like peptide-2 increase intestinal morphology and glucose uptake in suckling rats. *J. Pediatr. Gastroenterol. Nutr.* **2006**, *42*, 32–39. [CrossRef]
40. Wang, L.; Li, J.; Li, Q.; Zhang, J.; Duan, X.-L. Morphological changes of cell proliferation and apoptosis in rat jejunal mucosa at different ages. *World J. Gastroenterol.* **2003**, *9*, 2060–2064. [CrossRef]
41. Uchida, H.; Nakajima, Y.; Ohtake, K.; Ito, J.; Morita, M.; Kamimura, A.; Kobayashi, J. Protective effects of oral glutathione on fasting-induced intestinal atrophy through oxidative stress. *World J. Gastroenterol.* **2017**, *23*, 6650–6664. [CrossRef] [PubMed]
42. Ghavami, S.; Mutawe, M.M.; Schaafsma, D.; Yeganeh, B.; Unruh, H.; Klonisch, T.; Halayko, A.J. Geranylgeranyl transferase 1 modulates autophagy and apoptosis in human airway smooth muscle. *Am. J. Physiol. Lung Cell Mol. Physiol.* **2012**, *302*, L420–L428. [CrossRef] [PubMed]

43. Ockner, R.K.; Hughes, F.B.; Isselbacher, K.J. Very low density lipoproteins in intestinal lymph: Origin, composition, and role in lipid transport in the fasting state. *J. Clin. Investig.* **1969**, *48*, 2079–2088. [CrossRef] [PubMed]
44. Haidari, M.; Leung, N.; Mahbub, F.; Uffelman, K.D.; Kohen-Avramoglu, R.; Lewis, G.F.; Adeli, K. Fasting and postprandial overproduction of intestinally derived lipoproteins in an animal model of insulin resistance. Evidence that chronic fructose feeding in the hamster is accompanied by enhanced intestinal de novo lipogenesis and ApoB48-containing lipoprotein overproduction. *J. Biol. Chem.* **2002**, *277*, 31646–31655. [PubMed]

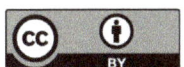 © 2020 by the authors. Licensee MDPI, Basel, Switzerland. This article is an open access article distributed under the terms and conditions of the Creative Commons Attribution (CC BY) license (http://creativecommons.org/licenses/by/4.0/).

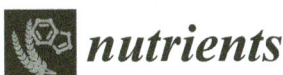

Article

Alterations in the Intestinal Morphology, Gut Microbiota, and Trace Mineral Status Following Intra-Amniotic Administration (*Gallus gallus*) of Teff (*Eragrostis tef*) Seed Extracts

Johnathon Carboni [1], Spenser Reed [2,3], Nikolai Kolba [2], Adi Eshel [4], Omry Koren [4] and Elad Tako [2,*]

1. Department of Biological Sciences, Cornell University, Ithaca, NY 14853, USA; jrc438@cornell.edu
2. Department of Food Science, Cornell University, Stocking Hall, Ithaca, NY 14853-7201, USA; smr292@email.arizona.edu (S.R.); nk598@cornell.edu (N.K.)
3. Department of Family Medicine, Kaiser Permanente Fontana Medical Centers, Fontana, CA 92335, USA
4. Azrieli Faculty of Medicine, Bar-Ilan University, 1311502 Safed, Israel; adizimer@gmail.com (A.E.); omry.koren@biu.ac.il (O.K.)
* Correspondence: et79@cornell.edu; Tel.: +1-607-255-0884

Received: 20 August 2020; Accepted: 30 September 2020; Published: 2 October 2020

Abstract: The consumption of teff (*Eragrostis tef*), a gluten-free cereal grain, has increased due to its dense nutrient composition including complex carbohydrates, unsaturated fatty acids, trace minerals (especially Fe), and phytochemicals. This study utilized the clinically-validated *Gallus gallus* intra amniotic feeding model to assess the effects of intra-amniotic administration of teff extracts versus controls using seven groups: (1) non-injected; (2) 18Ω H_2O injected; (3) 5% inulin; (4) teff extract 1%; (5) teff extract 2.5%; (6) teff extract 5%; and (7) teff extract 7.5%. The treatment groups were compared to each other and to controls. Our data demonstrated a significant improvement in hepatic iron (Fe) and zinc (Zn) concentration and LA:DGLA ratio without concomitant serum concentration changes, up-regulation of various Fe and Zn brush border membrane proteins, and beneficial morphological changes to duodenal villi and goblet cells. No significant taxonomic alterations were observed using 16S rRNA sequencing of the cecal microbiota. Several important bacterial metabolic pathways were differentially enriched in the teff group, likely due to teff's high relative fiber concentration, demonstrating an important bacterial-host interaction that contributed to improvements in the physiological status of Fe and Zn. Therefore, teff appeared to represent a promising staple food crop and should be further evaluated.

Keywords: teff; staple food crops; prebiotics; probiotics; iron deficiency; zinc deficiency; gut microbiota

1. Introduction

Iron (Fe) and zinc (Zn) deficiencies are prevalent public health crises worldwide but especially so in Africa, Latin America, and other parts of the developing world [1,2]. The etiology of these deficiencies includes a lack of substantial meat consumption in combination with a reliance on relatively poor sources of dietary Fe and Zn including grains and cereals. As it pertains to the latter, intrinsic dietary factors that limit Fe and Zn bioavailability such as phytic acid and polyphenolic compounds are often present in increased quantities in staple food crops [3–5]. Despite this, other intrinsic dietary factors such as prebiotic-like compounds have the potential to offset the inhibitor-like effects of phytate and polyphenols, thus improving mineral bioavailability [6].

Teff (*Eragrostis tef*), a staple cereal grain mainly consumed by peoples of Eritrea and Ethiopia, is gaining notoriety due to its dense nutrient composition including complex carbohydrates, unsaturated fatty acids, trace minerals (especially Fe), and phytochemicals [7,8]. Teff contains high amounts of phytates and polyphenols, although this amount varies by species and is comparable to values reported for other wholegrain cereals. Despite this, a recent study demonstrated that the prevalence of Fe and Zn deficiencies was much lower in Ethiopia relative to other African nations such as Kenya, Nigeria, and South Africa, likely due to the disproportionate dietary intake of teff relative to other cereal grains [9]. Furthermore, as teff is a gluten free cereal grain with high levels of trace minerals, it is well tolerated by individuals with food allergies and other gastrointestinal disorders, such as inflammatory bowel diseases, which negatively impact gut mineral absorption [7].

In addition to its favorable micronutrient profile, the fiber content of teff is uniquely high, especially when compared to other staple food crops such as sorghum, rice, maize, and wheat [7]. Constituents of fiber, such as the prebiotics inulin and raffinose, survive initial digestion in the upper gastrointestinal tract and become subsequently fermented by specific resident commensal bacteria in the colon [10]. This fermentation leads to the production of short-chain fatty acids (SCFA) [11]. SCFAs inhibit the growth of harmful pathogens, decrease intestinal pH, upregulate epithelial cell differentiation, thus increasing villus surface area, and upregulate brush-border membrane (BBM) gene expression [12]. In sum, these effects enhance gut mineral bioavailability and absorption [6,13–16]. Additionally, it has been suggested that specific polyphenolic compounds found in teff—such as ferulic acid, vanillic acid, cinnamic acid, and coumaric acid—exert a prebiotic effect and may improve trace mineral gut absorption [17].

The consumption of teff continues to rise as demand for well-tolerated, highly nutritious staple food crops continues to increase worldwide, especially as it pertains to biofortification efforts and other population-wide strategies for combating Fe and Zn deficiency [18]. Given the nutritional advantages of teff, especially its high concentration of trace minerals, it is important to evaluate other intrinsic factors that influence absorption and bioavailability. Therefore, using the validated, well-established *Gallus gallus* in vivo model [6,12–15,19,20], we sought to assess the effects of the intra-amniotic administration of teff seed extracts on serum and tissue Fe and Zn status, as well as on multiple parameters that influence trace mineral absorption and bioavailability, i.e., intrinsic phytate and polyphenolic concentration, enterocyte gene expression of various trace mineral dependent proteins, and brush border membrane morphology. Additionally, 16S rRNA gene sequencing of cecal contents was utilized to analyze potential alterations in intestinal microbiota structure and function from teff extracts. We hypothesize that intra-amniotic administration of teff extracts will indeed exert a prebiotic effect leading to increased serum and tissue Fe and Zn concentrations, favorable alterations in brush border membrane function and morphology, and positively restructure the gut microbiota.

2. Materials and Methods

2.1. Sample Preparation

Teff seeds (*Eragrostis tef*), purchased at a local grocer in Ithaca, NY were used in the study (Bob's Red Mill, Milwaukie, OR, USA). To obtain flour, seeds were ground up in three replicates, using a Kinematica Polymix PX-MFC 90 D analytical mill (Kinematica, Luzern, Switzerland) to a particle size of 50 µm.

2.2. Extraction of Prebiotics From Teff

The extraction of prebiotics was performed [6,20,21]. Briefly, the teff flour samples were dissolved in distilled water (50 g/L) (60 °C, 60 min) and then centrifuged at 3000× g (4 °C) for 25 min to remove particulate matter. The supernatant was collected and dialyzed (MWCO 12–14 kDa) exhaustively against distilled water for 48 h. The dialysate was collected and then lyophilized to yield a fine off-white powder.

2.3. Iron, Zinc, Calcium and Magnesium Analysis

Either a 500 mg sample of teff flour, a 100 mg sample of liver tissue (wet weight), or 50 µL of serum were pre-digested in boro-silicate glass tubes with 3 mL of a concentrated ultra-pure nitric acid and perchloric acid mixture (60:40 v/v) for 16 h at room temperature. Samples were then placed in a digestion block (Martin Machine, Ivesdale, IL, USA) and heated incrementally over 4 h to a temperature of 120 °C with refluxing. After incubating at 120 °C for 2 h, 2 mL of concentrated ultra-pure nitric acid was subsequently added to each sample before raising the digestion block temperature to 145 °C for an additional 2 h. The temperature of the digestion block was then raised to 190 °C and maintained for at least 10 minutes before samples were allowed to cool at room temperature. Digested samples were re-suspended in 20 mL of ultrapure water prior to analysis using ICP-AES (inductively coupled plasma-atomic emission spectroscopy; Thermo iCAP 6500 Series, Thermo Scientific, Cambridge, United Kingdom) with quality control standards (High Purity Standards, Charleston, SC, USA) following every 10 samples. Yttrium purchased from High Purity Standards (10M67-1) was used as an internal standard. All samples were digested and measured with 0.5 µg/mL of Yttrium (final concentration) to ensure batch-to-batch accuracy and to correct for matrix inference during digestion. Serum LA:DGLA ratio, a novel measure of Zn status, was determined as previously published [21].

2.4. Phytate Analysis

A 500 mg sample from teff flour and teff extract were first extracted in 10 mL of 0.66 M hydrochloric acid under constant motion for 16 h at room temperature. A 1 mL aliquot of total extract was collected using a wide bore pipet tip and then centrifuged (16,000× g) for 10 min to pellet debris. A 0.5 mL sample of supernatant was then neutralized with 0.5 mL 0.75 M sodium hydroxide and stored at −20 °C until the day of analysis. A phytate/total phosphorous kit (K-PHYT; Megazyme International, Ireland) was used to measure liberated phosphorous by phytase and alkaline phosphatase. Phosphorous was quantified by colorimetric analysis as molybdenum blue with phosphorous standards read at a wavelength of 655 nm against the absorbance of a reagent blank. Total phytate concentrations were calculated with Mega-Calc™ by subtracting free phosphate concentrations in the extracts from the total amount of phosphorous that is exclusively released after enzymatic digestion.

2.5. Protein and Fiber Analysis

Protein and fiber analyses were performed as previously published by Wiesinger et al. [22]. Briefly, the total nitrogen concentrations were measured in a 500 mg sample of teff flour or teff extract by the Dumas combustion method at A&L Great Lakes Laboratories (Fort Wayne, IN, USA) in accordance with AOAC method 968.06. Complete methodology is indicated in the supplementary materials.

2.6. Polyphenol Extraction

Next, 5 mL of methanol:water (50:50 v/v) was added to either 500 mg of teff flour or teff extract, and vortexed for one minute before incubating in a sonication water bath for 20 min at room temperature. Samples were again vortexed and placed on a compact digital Rocker (Labnet International, Inc., Edison, NJ, USA) at room temperature for 60 min before centrifuging at 4000× g for 15 min. Supernatants were filtered with a 0.2 µm Teflon™ syringe filter and stored at −20 °C until chemical analysis.

Liquid Chromatography-Mass Spectroscopy (LC-MS) Analysis of Polyphenols

Extracts and standards were analyzed as previously published [23]. Briefly, samples were analyzed with an Agilent 1220 Infinity Liquid Chromatograph (LC; Agilent Technologies, Inc., Santa Clara, CA, USA) coupled to an Advion expressionL® compact mass spectrometer (CMS; Advion Inc., Ithaca, NY, USA). Advion Mass Express™ software was used to control the LC and CMS instrumentation and data acquisition. Individual polyphenols were identified and confirmed by comparison of m/z and LC retention times with authentic standards. Polyphenol standard curves for flavonoids were derived from integrated areas under UV absorption peaks from 5 replications. Standard curves for caffeic acid, ferulic, and protocatechuic acids were constructed from MS ion intensities using 5 replications. The complete methodology is indicated in the supplementary materials.

2.7. Animals and Study Design

Cornish-cross fertile broiler eggs ($n = 79$) were obtained from a commercial hatchery (Moyer's chicks, Quakertown, PA, USA). The eggs were incubated under optimal conditions at the Cornell University Animal Science poultry farm incubator. All animal protocols were approved by Cornell University Institutional Animal Care and Use committee (ethic approval code: 2007-0129). Prebiotics in powder form were separately diluted in 18 MΩ H_2O to determine the concentrations necessary to maintain an osmolarity value (OSM) of less than 320 OSM to ensure that the *Gallus gallus* embryos would not be dehydrated upon injection of the solution. At day 17 of embryonic incubation, eggs containing viable embryos were weighed and divided into 7 groups ($n = 11$–15). All treatment groups were assigned eggs of similar weight frequency distribution. Each group was then injected with the specified solution (1 mL per egg) with a 21-gauge needle into the amniotic fluid, which was identified by candling. The 7 groups were assigned as follows: (1) non-injected; (2) 18Ω H_2O; (3) 5% inulin; (4) teff extract 1%; (5) teff extract 2.5%; (6) teff extract 5%; and (7) teff extract 7.5%. After all eggs were injected, the injection holes were sealed with cellophane tape and the eggs were placed in hatching baskets such that each treatment was equally represented at each incubator location. Immediately after hatch (21 days) and from each treatment group, chicks were euthanized by CO_2 exposure and their small intestine, blood, pectoral muscle, cecum, and liver were collected.

2.8. Blood Analysis and Hb Measurements

Blood was collected using micro-hematocrit heparinized capillary tubes (Fisher Scientific, Waltham, MA, USA). Blood Hb concentrations were determined spectrophotometrically using the QuantiChrom™ Hemoglobin Assay (DIHB-250, BioAssay Systems, Hayward, CA, USA) following the kit manufacturer's instructions.

2.9. Isolation of Total RNA From Duodenum and Liver Tissue Samples

Total RNA was isolated as previously published [23]. Briefly, total RNA was extracted from 30 mg of the proximal duodenal tissue or liver tissue ($n = 8$) using Qiagen RNeasy Mini Kit (RNeasy Mini Kit, Qiagen Inc., Valencia, CA, USA) according to the manufacturer's protocol. All steps were carried out under RNase free conditions. RNA was quantified by absorbance at A 260/280. Integrity of the 18S ribosomal RNAs was verified by 1.5% agarose gel electrophoresis followed by ethidium bromide staining. DNA contamination was removed using TURBO DNase treatment and removal kit from AMBION (Austin, TX, USA). The complete methodology is indicated in the supplementary materials.

2.10. Real-Time Polymerase Chain Reaction (RT-PCR)

RT-PCR was performed as previously published [23]. Briefly, in order to create the cDNA, a 20 µL reverse transcriptase (RT) reaction was completed in a BioRad C1000 touch thermocycler using the Improm-II Reverse Transcriptase Kit (Catalog #A1250; Promega, Madison, WI, USA). The concentration of cDNA obtained was determined by measuring the absorbance at 260 nm and 280 nm using an extinction coefficient of 33 (for single stranded DNA). Genomic DNA contamination was assessed using a real-time RT-PCR assay for the reference of genes samples. The complete methodology is indicated in the supplementary materials.

2.10.1. Primer Design

Primer design was conducted as previously published [13] and as indicated in the supplementary materials. The sequences and the description of primers used in this study are summarized in Table 1.

Table 1. DNA Sequences of the primers used in this study.

Analyte	Forward Primer (5'→3')	Reverse Primer (5'→3')	Base Pair	GI Identifier
\multicolumn{5}{c}{Calcium Metabolism}				
TRPV6	GCTCCCAGAACCTTCTCTATTT	CCAGGTAATCCTGAGCTCTAATG	123	418307
PMCA1b	TGCAGATGCTGTGGGTAAAT	CCATAAGGCTTCCGCAATAGA	100	374244
NXC1	CCTGACGGAGAAATAAGGAAGA	CCCAGGAGAAGACACAGATAAA	114	395760
\multicolumn{5}{c}{Iron Metabolism}				
DMT1	TTGATTCAGAGCCTCCCATTAG	GCGAGGAGTAGGCTTGTATTT	101	206597489
Ferroportin	CTCAGCAATCACTGGCATCA	ACTGGGCAACTCCAGAAATAAG	98	61098365
DcytB	CATGTGCATTCTCTTCCAAAGTC	CTCCTTGGTGACCGCATTAT	103	20380692
\multicolumn{5}{c}{Inflammatory Response}				
IL-1β	CTCACAGTCCTTCGACATCTTC	TGTTGAGCCTCACTTTCTGG	119	88702685
IL-6	ACCTCATCCTCCGAGACTTTA	GCACTGAAACTCCTGGTCTT	105	302315692
TNF-α	GACAGCCTATGCCAACAAGTA	TTACAGGAAGGGCAACTCATC	109	53854909
\multicolumn{5}{c}{Magnesium Metabolism}				
MRS2	GCTGGTAACCGGGATTATGT	GCAGGAACATGAGGAGGTAAT	105	420820
TRPM6	ACAGATGCTGCTGACTGATATG	AAGATAGTGGGTGGTAGGAGAA	99	100859603
TRPM7	GCGTGGGATAGAGTTGACATT	TCACAAGGGCATCCAACATAG	100	427502
\multicolumn{5}{c}{Zinc Metabolism}				
ZnT1	GGTAACAGAGCTGCCTTAACT	GGTAACAGAGCTGCCTTAACT	105	54109718
ZnT7	GGAAGATGTCAGGATGGTTCA	CGAAGGACAAATTGAGGCAAAG	87	56555152
ZIP9	CTAAGCAAGAGCAGCAAAGAAG	CATGAACTGTGGCAACGTAAAG	100	237874618
Δ6 desaturase	GGCGAAAGTCAGCCTATTGA	AGGTGGGAAGATGAGGAAGA	93	261865208
\multicolumn{5}{c}{Hypertension}				
ACE	CATGGCCTTGTCTGTCTCC	GAGGTATCCAAAGGGCAGG	142	424059
AT1R	TCATCTGGCTCCTTGCTGG	AACCTAGCCCAACCCTCAG	138	396065
\multicolumn{5}{c}{BBM Functionality}				
AP	CGTCAGCCAGTTTGACTATGTA	CTCTCAAAGAAGCTGAGGATGG	138	45382360
SI	CCAGCAATGCCAGCATATTG	CGGTTTCTCCTTACCACTTCTT	95	2246388
SGLT1	GCATCCTTACTCTGTGGTACTG	TATCCGCACATCACACATCC	106	8346783
18s rRNA	GCAAGACGAACTAAAGCGAAAG	TCGGAACTACGACGGTATCT	100	7262899

2.10.2. Real-Time qPCR Design

All procedures were conducted as previously described [23]. Briefly, cDNA was used for each 10 µL reaction together with 2×BioRad SSO Advanced Universal SYBR Green Supermix (Cat #1725274, Hercules, CA, USA), which included buffer, Taq DNA polymerase, dNTPs, and SYBR green dye. The data on the expression levels of the genes were obtained as Cp values based on the "second derivative maximum" (automated method) as computed by Bio-Rad CFX Maestro 1.1 (Version 4.1.2433.1219, Hercules, CA, USA). The specificity of the amplified real-time RT-PCR products were verified by a melting curve analysis (60–95 °C) after 40 cycles, which should result in a number of different specific products, each with a specific melting temperature. The complete methodology is indicated in the supplementary materials.

2.11. Collection of Microbial Samples and Intestinal Contents DNA Isolation

The ceca were sterilely removed and contents were treated as described previously [23]. A full description of the method is indicated in the supplementary materials.

16S rRNA Gene Amplification, Sequencing and Analysis

16S rRNA gene amplification, sequencing, and analysis was performed as previously described [11]. Briefly, microbial genomic DNA was extracted from cecal samples using the PowerSoil DNA isolation kit, as described by the manufacturer (MoBio Laboratories Ltd., Carlsbad, CA, USA). Bacterial 16S rRNA gene sequences were PCR-amplified from each sample using the 515F-806R primers for the V4 hypervariable region of the 16S rRNA gene, including 12-base barcodes. The complete methodology is indicated in the supplementary materials.

2.12. Glycogen Analysis

Glycogen analysis was obtained from pectoralis muscle as previously described [8,23]. Briefly, the pectoral muscle samples were then homogenized in 8% perchloric acid. Samples were then centrifuged at 12,000× g at 4 °C for 15 min. The supernatant was removed and 1.0 mL of petroleum ether was added to each tube. After mixing, the petroleum ether fraction was removed and samples from the bottom layer were transferred to a new tube containing 300 µL of color reagent. All samples were read at a wavelength of 450 nm in ELISA reader and the amount of glycogen was calculated according to a standard curve. The amount of glycogen present in pectoral sample was determined by multiplying the weight of the tissue by the amount of glycogen per 1 g of wet tissue. A full description of the method is described in the supplementary materials.

2.13. Liver Ferritin Analysis

Liver ferritin analysis was conducted as previously described [8,23]. Briefly, 1 g of sample was diluted into 1 mL of 50 mM Hepes buffer, pH 7.4, and homogenized on ice for 2 min (5000× g). One mL of each homogenate was subjected to heat treatment for 10 min at 75 °C to aid isolation of ferritin (other proteins are not stable at that temperature). Subsequently, samples were immediately cooled down on ice for 30 min. Thereafter, samples were centrifuged for 30 min (13,000× g) at 4 °C until a clear supernatant was obtained and the pellet containing most of the insoluble denatured proteins was discarded. Native polyacrylamide gel electrophoresis was conducted using a 6% separating gel and a 5% stacking gel. Samples were run at a constant voltage of 100 V. Thereafter, gels were treated with either of the two stains: Coomasie blue G-250 stain, specific for proteins, or potassium ferricyanide ($K_3Fe(CN)_6$) stain, specific for Fe. The corresponding band found in the protein and Fe stained gel was considered to be ferritin. Measurements of the bands were conducted using the Quantity-One-1-D analysis program (Bio-Rad, Hercules, CA, USA). A full description of the method is described in the supplementary materials.

2.14. Tissue Morphology Examination

Villus epithelium analysis was performed as was previously described [23]. Samples were fixed in fresh 4% (*v*/*v*) buffered formaldehyde, dehydrated, cleared, and embedded in paraffin. Serial sections were cut at 5 µm and placed on glass slides. Intestinal sections were deparaffinized in xylene, rehydrated in a graded alcohol series, stained with Alcian Blue/Periodic acid-Schiff, and examined by light microscopy. The following variables were measured in the intestine: villus height, villus width, depth of crypts, paneth cells, goblet cell number, goblet cell diameter, types of goblet cells in the villi epithelium, goblet cells within the crypts, and the mucus layer thickness in each segment were performed with a light microscope using EPIX XCAP software (Standard version, Olympus, Waltham, MA, USA). The complete methodology is indicated in the supplementary materials.

2.15. Statistical Analysis

All values are expressed as means and standard deviation. Experimental treatments for the intra amniotic administration assay were arranged in a completely randomized design. The results were analyzed by ANOVA. For significant *p*-values, a post-hoc Duncan test was used to compare test groups. Statistical analysis was carried out using SPSS version 20.0 software. The level of significance was established at $p < 0.05$. For the microbiome results, Faith's Phylogenetic Diversity [24] was used to calculate bacterial richness within each sample. Differences between groups were analyzed by ANOVA. Beta diversity (between samples) was calculated using Jaccard distances and analyzed using a pairwise PERMANOVA test. Predictive metagenomic analysis (PICRUST) [25] was used to identify significant differences in predicted metabolic pathways between the groups. Statistically significant p-values associated with microbial clades and functions identified by LEfSe [26] were corrected for multiple comparisons using the Benjamini–Hochberg false discovery rate (FDR) correction.

3. Results

3.1. Concentration of Calcium, Iron, Magnesium, and Zinc in Teff Flour and in Teff Flour Extract

Fe and Zn concentrations were higher in the teff extract compared to the teff seed ($p < 0.05$, Table 2), whereas Ca and Mg concentrations were higher in the teff seed compared to the teff extract ($p < 0.05$, Table 2). The soluble fiber and total fiber content were higher in the teff extract compared to the teff seed, however the insoluble fiber content was higher in the teff seed compared to the teff extract ($p < 0.05$, Table 3). There were no significant differences in protein or phytic acid between the two groups. However, the content of phytate:Fe ratio was significantly greater in the teff seed relative to teff extract ($p < 0.05$).

Table 2. Concentrations of calcium, iron, magnesium, and zinc in teff flour and teff extract [1].

Treatment Group	Calcium (µg/g)	Iron (µg/g)	Magnesium (µg/g)	Zinc (µg/g)
Teff seed	2259.32 ± 24.73 [a]	60.64 ± 0.92 [b]	2023.49 ± 18.93 [a]	42.87 ± 0.42 [b]
Teff seed extract	2052.07 ± 123.95 [b]	128.23 ± 11.60 [a]	1088.87 ± 42.24 [b]	53.84 ± 4.50 [a]

[1] Values are means ± SEM, $n = 5$. [a,b] Treatment groups not indicated by the same letter are significantly different ($p < 0.05$).

Table 3. Dietary fiber, protein, phytic acid, and phytate:Fe ratio in teff flour and teff extract [1].

Treatment Group	Insoluble Fiber (g/100 g)	Soluble Fiber (g/100 g)	Total Fiber (g/100 g)	Protein (g/100 g)	Phytic Acid (g/100 g)	Phytic Acid:Iron Ratio
Teff seed	8.32 ± 0.23 [a]	2.10 ± 0.12 [b]	10.43 ± 0.11 [b]	10.02 ± 0.39 [a]	0.14 ± 0.02 [a]	1.74 ± 0.03 [a]
Teff seed extract	6.15 ± 0.61 [b]	6.98 ± 0.91 [a]	13.13 ± 0.30 [a]	10.86 ± 0.88 [a]	0.17 ± 0.11 [a]	0.41 ± 0.05 [b]

[1] Values are means ± SEM, $n = 5$. [a,b] Treatment groups not indicated by the same letter are significantly different ($p < 0.05$).

3.2. Polyphenol Profile of the Teff Seed Flour and Extract

The concentration of the five most prevalent polyphenolic compounds found in the teff variety are presented in Table 4. Teff seeds contained high levels of ferulic acid.

Table 4. Concentration of the five most common polyphenolic compounds in teff samples [1].

Polyphenolic Compounds	Mass (Da)	(M + H) (Da)	(M − H) (Da)	Retention Time (min)	Found in (MS mode)	
					Teff Seed (extract)	Teff Seed (flour)
Protocatechuic Acid	154.12	155.128	153.112	1.621	NEG	NEG
Caffeic Acid	180.16	181.168	179.152	2.958	POS/NEG	ND
Vanillic Acid	168.15	169.158	167.142	3.094	POS	ND
p- Coumaric Acid	164.16	165.168	164.152	3.895	POS/NEG	ND
Ferulic Acid	194.18	195.188	193.172	4.428	POS/NEG	POS

[1] Values are means ± SEM, $n = 5$. MAU: milli absorbance unit; min: minutes. Da: Dalton; M + H: Mass + Hydrogen; M − H: Mass − Hydrogen; MS: Mass Spectrometry; ND: Not Determined; POS: Positive. NEG: Negative.

3.3. Hemoglobin, Body Weight, Cecum Weight, and Cecum:Body Weight Ratio

There were no significant differences in hemoglobin concentrations between any of the treatment groups. The body weight of the non-injected group was significantly lower than all other groups ($p < 0.05$, Table 5). Among cecum weights and cecum:body weight ratio, the non-injected and 2.5% teff groups demonstrated significantly lower values when compared to all other groups ($p < 0.05$).

Table 5. Hemoglobin, body weight, cecum weight, and cecum:body weight ratio in all groups [1].

Treatment Group	Hemoglobin (g/dL)	Body Weight Average (g)	Cecum Weight Average (g)	Cecum:Body Weight Ratio
NI	8.747 ± 0.797 [a]	45.4 ± 1.3 [b]	0.5 ± 0.1 [b]	0.010 ± 0.002 [b]
18Ω H$_2$O	10.603 ± 0.591 [a]	46.9 ± 1.2 [a]	0.5 ± 0.1 [a]	0.011 ± 0.001 [a]
5% Inulin	8.860 ± 0.690 [a]	49.7 ± 0.9 [a]	0.6 ± 0.1 [a]	0.012 ± 0.001 [a]
1% Teff	9.575 ± 1.138 [a]	47.0 ± 1.0 [a]	0.6 ± 0.1 [a]	0.012 ± 0.001 [a]
2.5% Teff	8.410 ± 0.920 [a]	47.1 ± 1.1 [a]	0.5 ± 0.0 [b]	0.010 ± 0.001 [b]
5% Teff	8.501 ± 0.874 [a]	46.5 ± 1.3 [a]	0.7 ± 0.1 [a]	0.015 ± 0.002 [a]
7.5% Teff	9.569 ± 0.633 [a]	47.4 ± 1.4 [a]	0.6 ± 0.0 [a]	0.012 ± 0.001 [a]

[1] Values are means ± SEM, $n = 8$. [a,b] Treatment groups not indicated by the same letter are significantly different ($p < 0.05$). NI = non-injected.

3.4. Hepatic, Serum Fe, and Zn Concentrations: LA:DGLA Ratio

Liver Fe concentration was significantly higher in the inulin and 7.5% teff group compared to the non-injected control group ($p < 0.05$, Table 6). The 18ΩH$_2$O, 1% teff, 2.5% teff, and 5% teff groups had higher liver Fe concentration than the control group, although they were not significantly different from each other. The concentration of Zn in the liver was the highest in the 7.5% teff group (similar to the 5% inulin group), and significantly different from all other groups ($p < 0.05$). Serum Fe and Zn concentrations did not different amongst groups ($p > 0.05$). Figure 1 depicts the LA:DGLA ratio for the NI, 18ΩH$_2$O, and 7.5% teff groups. The 7.5% teff group demonstrated a significantly lower LA:DGLA ratio, signifying a relative increase in Zn status, compared to both control groups ($p < 0.05$). We have previously demonstrated the LA:DGLA ratio as a novel physiological biomarker of zinc status [19,21].

Table 6. Fe and Zn concentrations in liver and serum [1].

Treatment Groups	Liver		Serum	
	Iron (µg/g)	Zinc (µg/g)	Iron (µg/g)	Zinc (µg/g)
NI	32.47 ± 2.83 [b]	15.79 ± 0.95 [c]	2.09 ± 0.24 [a]	0.86 ± 0.08 [a]
18Ω H$_2$O	37.93 ± 4.93 [ab]	16.12 ± 0.96 [c]	2.00 ± 0.27 [a]	0.84 ± 0.07 [a]
5% Inulin	48.96 ± 4.39 [a]	18.23 ± 0.88 [abc]	2.76 ± 0.33 [a]	0.97 ± 0.08 [a]
1% Teff	37.40 ± 3.67 [ab]	17.61 ± 0.91 [bc]	2.22 ± 0.40 [a]	0.91 ± 0.08 [a]
2.5% Teff	36.39 ± 3.54 [ab]	22.82 ± 2.42 [ab]	2.09 ± 0.22 [a]	0.89 ± 0.06 [a]
5% Teff	39.40 ± 3.89 [ab]	23.37 ± 3.10 [ab]	2.83 ± 0.28 [a]	0.81 ± 0.07 [a]
7.5% Teff	46.44 ± 5.83 [a]	24.14 ± 3.33 [a]	2.88 ± 0.38 [a]	1.02 ± 0.07 [a]

[1] Values are means ± SEM, $n = 8$. [a,b,c] Treatment groups not indicated by the same letter are significantly different ($p < 0.05$). NI = non-injected.

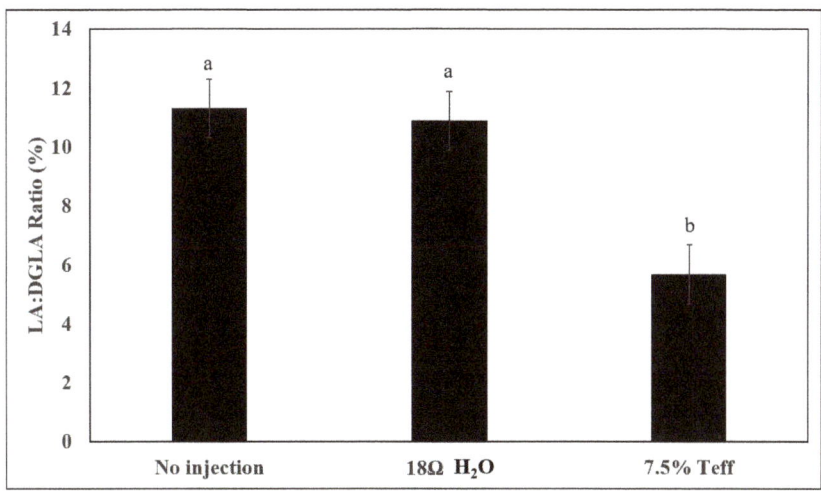

Figure 1. Effect of the intra-amniotic administration of experimental solutions and control on the Linoleic acid (LA): Dihomo-γ-linolenic acid (DGLA) ratio. Values are the means ± SEM, $n = 8$. [a,b] Treatment groups not indicated by the same letter are significantly different ($p < 0.05$).

3.5. Pectoral Muscle Glycogen Concentration

There were no significant differences in glycogen concentration observed between any of the treatment and control groups ($p > 0.05$, Table 7).

Table 7. Glycogen and liver ferritin concentrations [1].

Treatment Group	Glycogen (mg/g)	Liver Ferritin (AU)
NI	0.034 ± 0.011 [a]	1.974 ± 0.005 [a]
18Ω H$_2$O	0.022 ± 0.003 [a]	1.534 ± 0.519 [a]
5% Inulin	0.029 ± 0.005 [a]	0.148 ± 0.005 [b]
1% Teff	0.035 ± 0.006 [a]	1.491 ± 0.299 [a]
2.5% Teff	0.022 ± 0.007 [a]	0.275 ± 0.245 [b]
5% Teff	0.044 ± 0.017 [a]	0.031 ± 0.001 [b]
7.5% Teff	0.021 ± 0.007 [a]	0.034 ± 0.001 [b]

[1] Values are means ± SEM, $n = 8$. [a,b] Treatment groups not indicated by the same letter are significantly different ($p < 0.05$). NI = non-injected.

3.6. Liver Ferritin Concentration

The non-injected, water, and 1% teff groups had significantly greater levels of liver ferritin compared to all other treatment groups ($p < 0.05$, Table 7).

3.7. Duodenal Gene Expression of Relevant Proteins

Figure 2 depicts the gene expression of various proteins involved either directly involved in mineral metabolism or indirectly involved requiring these trace minerals as cofactors.

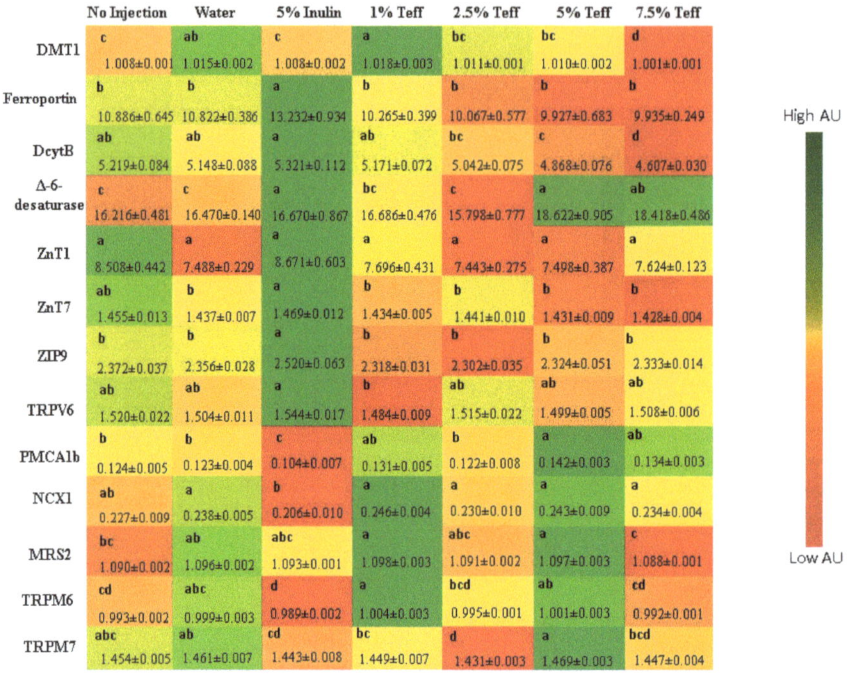

	No Injection	Water	5% Inulin	1% Teff	2.5% Teff	5% Teff	7.5% Teff
DMT1	c 1.008±0.001	ab 1.015±0.002	c 1.008±0.002	a 1.018±0.003	bc 1.011±0.001	bc 1.010±0.002	d 1.001±0.001
Ferroportin	b 10.886±0.645	b 10.822±0.386	a 13.232±0.934	b 10.265±0.399	b 10.067±0.577	b 9.927±0.683	b 9.935±0.249
DcytB	ab 5.219±0.084	ab 5.148±0.088	a 5.321±0.112	ab 5.171±0.072	bc 5.042±0.075	c 4.868±0.076	d 4.607±0.030
Δ-6-desaturase	c 16.216±0.481	c 16.470±0.140	a 16.670±0.867	bc 16.686±0.476	c 15.798±0.777	a 18.622±0.905	ab 18.418±0.486
ZnT1	a 8.508±0.442	a 7.488±0.229	a 8.671±0.603	a 7.696±0.431	a 7.443±0.275	a 7.498±0.387	a 7.624±0.123
ZnT7	ab 1.455±0.013	b 1.437±0.007	a 1.469±0.012	b 1.434±0.005	b 1.441±0.010	b 1.431±0.009	b 1.428±0.004
ZIP9	b 2.372±0.037	b 2.356±0.028	a 2.520±0.063	b 2.318±0.031	b 2.302±0.035	b 2.324±0.051	b 2.333±0.014
TRPV6	ab 1.520±0.022	ab 1.504±0.011	a 1.544±0.017	b 1.484±0.009	ab 1.515±0.022	ab 1.499±0.005	ab 1.508±0.006
PMCA1b	b 0.124±0.005	b 0.123±0.004	c 0.104±0.007	ab 0.131±0.005	b 0.122±0.008	a 0.142±0.003	ab 0.134±0.003
NCX1	ab 0.227±0.009	a 0.238±0.005	b 0.206±0.010	a 0.246±0.004	a 0.230±0.010	a 0.243±0.009	a 0.234±0.004
MRS2	bc 1.090±0.002	ab 1.096±0.002	abc 1.093±0.001	a 1.098±0.003	abc 1.091±0.002	a 1.097±0.003	c 1.088±0.001
TRPM6	cd 0.993±0.002	abc 0.999±0.003	d 0.989±0.002	a 1.004±0.003	bcd 0.995±0.001	ab 1.001±0.003	cd 0.992±0.001
TRPM7	abc 1.454±0.005	ab 1.461±0.007	cd 1.443±0.008	bc 1.449±0.007	d 1.431±0.003	a 1.469±0.003	bcd 1.447±0.004

High AU / Low AU

Figure 2. Effect of the intra-amniotic administration of experimental solutions on duodenal gene expression. Values are the means (AU: arbitrary units) ± SEM, n = 8. a–d Per gene, treatments groups not indicated by the same letter are significantly different ($p < 0.05$). DMT1, Divalent metal transporter 1; DcytB, Duodenal cytochrome b; ZnT1, Zinc transporter 1; ZnT7, Zinc transporter 7; ZIP9, Zinc transporter 9; TRPV6, Transient Receptor Potential Cation Channel Subfamily V Member 6; PMCA1b, Plasma Membrane Calcium ATP-pump; NCX1, Sodium Calcium Exchanger 1; MRS2, Magnesium transporter MRS2; TRPM6, Transient Receptor Potential Cation Channel Subfamily M member 6; TRPM7, Transient Receptor Potential Cation Channel Subfamily M member 7.

3.7.1. Fe-Related Proteins

For the proteins responsible directly for Fe uptake at the brush border membrane (BBM), ferroportin, and DMT1, the expression was higher in the 5% inulin group and 1% teff group, respectively. The expression of these proteins was lower in the animals receiving the higher teff concentrations. The expression of DctyB was also higher in the 5% inulin group, and decrease in a dose-dependent fashion in the groups receiving increasing teff concentration.

3.7.2. Zn-Related Proteins

The expression of proteins related to cellular Zn uptake, transport and storage—ZnT1, ZnT7, and ZIP9—was greatest in the non-injected and 5% inulin groups and was significantly lower in all concentrations of teff groups.

3.7.3. Ca-Related Proteins

The expression of proteins related to cellular Ca regulation—TRPV6, PMCA1b, and NXC1—were differentially expressed across groups. TRPV6, a BBM protein involved in the initial steps of Ca absorption in the gut, was highest in the 5% inulin group. The Ca efflux proteins, PMCA1b and NXC1, were expressed highest in the 5% teff group.

3.7.4. Mg-Related Proteins

The expression of the cellular membrane Mg influx proteins TRPM6 and TRPM7 was increased in the 1% teff and 5% teff groups, respectively. MRS2, a Mg-specific protein in the cellular mitochondria, was increased in both 1% and 5% teff groups.

3.7.5. Inflammatory Cytokines and BBM Proteins

Figure 3 depicts a panel of inflammatory cytokines and BBM proteins evaluated amongst the treatment groups. As a whole, the 5% inulin group had greater expression of all three cytokines relative to the control group, while a decreased expression was seen in the higher concentration teff groups ($p < 0.05$). Both aminopeptidase and sucrose isomaltase were expressed at a higher amount in the 5% inulin group. Likewise, the highest concentration teff group (7.5%) showed the lowest expression. For sodium-glucose transport protein 1, the 5% teff group had the highest expression, with the lowest expression observed in the 5% inulin group.

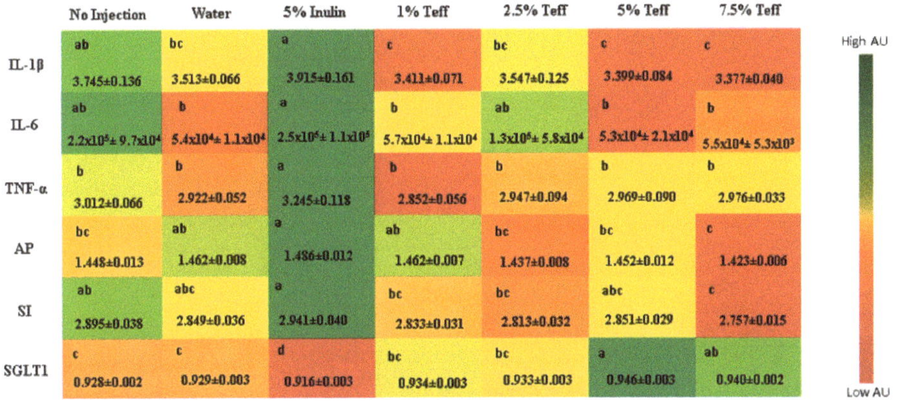

	No Injection	Water	5% Inulin	1% Teff	2.5% Teff	5% Teff	7.5% Teff
IL-1β	ab 3.745±0.136	bc 3.513±0.066	a 3.915±0.161	c 3.411±0.071	bc 3.547±0.125	c 3.399±0.084	c 3.377±0.040
IL-6	ab 2.2×10^5± 9.7×10^4	b 5.4×10^4± 1.1×10^4	a 2.5×10^5± 1.1×10^5	b 5.7×10^4± 1.1×10^4	ab 1.3×10^5± 5.8×10^4	b 5.3×10^4± 2.1×10^4	b 5.5×10^4± 5.3×10^3
TNF-α	b 3.012±0.066	b 2.922±0.052	a 3.245±0.118	b 2.852±0.056	b 2.947±0.094	b 2.969±0.090	b 2.976±0.033
AP	bc 1.448±0.013	ab 1.462±0.008	a 1.486±0.012	ab 1.462±0.007	bc 1.437±0.008	bc 1.452±0.012	c 1.423±0.006
SI	ab 2.895±0.038	abc 2.849±0.036	a 2.941±0.040	bc 2.833±0.031	bc 2.813±0.032	abc 2.851±0.029	c 2.757±0.015
SGLT1	c 0.928±0.002	c 0.929±0.003	d 0.916±0.003	bc 0.934±0.003	bc 0.933±0.003	a 0.946±0.003	ab 0.940±0.002

Figure 3. Effect of the intra-amniotic administration of experimental solutions on intestinal and heart gene expression. Values are the means (AU: arbitrary units) ± SEM, $n = 8$. a–c Per gene, treatments groups not indicated by the same letter are significantly different ($p < 0.05$). IL-1β, Interleukin 1 beta; IL-6, Interleukin 6; TNF-α, Tumor Necrosis Factor Alpha; AP, Amino peptidase; SGLT1, Sodium-Glucose transport protein 1; SI, Sucrose isomaltase.

3.8. Morphometric Analysis of Duodenal Villi, Depth of Crypts and Goblet Cells

Table 8 depicts the morphometric measurements for villi length and diameter, crypt depth, and mucus layer width. As a whole, the teff groups showed the most significant response with the 2.5% and 7.5% teff groups with the longest villus length, the 1% teff group with the greatest villus diameter, and the 1% teff group had the greatest intestinal crypt depth.

Table 8. Effect of the intra-amniotic administration of experimental teff solutions on duodenal villus and crypts measurements [1].

Treatment Group	Villus Length (μm)	Villus Diameter (μm)	Depth of Crypts (μm)
NI	223.29 ± 3.44 [ab]	53.15 ± 0.73 [b]	66.30 ± 1.33 [b]
18Ω H$_2$O	224.14 ± 4.10 [ab]	46.84 ± 0.69 [c]	53.42 ± 1.11 [c]
5% Inulin	274.11 ± 3.92 [b]	43.66 ± 0.64 [d]	51.30 ± 1.06 [c]
1% Teff	266.85 ± 4.39 [a]	56.22 ± 0.78 [a]	73.62 ± 1.40 [a]
2.5% Teff	263.66 ± 3.85 [a]	53.44 ± 0.75 [ab]	65.74 ± 1.26 [b]
5% Teff	302.83 ± 2.95 [ab]	54.80 ± 0.67 [ab]	67.75 ± 1.43 [b]
7.5% Teff	290.86 ± 3.12 [a]	50.00 ± 0.02 [ab]	66.38 ± 1.25 [b]

[1] Values are the means ± SEM, $n = 5$. a–d Treatment groups not indicated by the same letter are significantly different ($p < 0.05$). NI = non-injected.

Table 9 depicts the morphometric measurements of duodenal goblet cells. As above, the teff treatment groups demonstrated greatest benefit with the 2.5% teff group showing greatest goblet cell diameter, 1% and 2.5% teff groups showing greatest crypt goblet cell count per unit area, and 1% teff group with the greatest villus goblet cell count per unit area ($p < 0.05$). The NI and 5% inulin groups had significantly greater numbers of acidic villus goblet cells than did all other groups ($p < 0.05$). The quantity of neutral goblet cells was significantly greater in the NI group. However, the 2.5% teff group had the greatest amount of mixed villus goblet cell types ($p < 0.05$).

Table 9. Effect of the intra-amniotic administration of experimental teff solutions on duodenal goblet cells [1].

Treatment Group	Goblet Cell Diameter (μM)	Crypts Goblet Cell Number	Total Villus Goblet Cell Number	Villus Goblet Cell Number		
				Acidic	Neutral	Mixed
NI	6.50 ± 0.06 [cd]	9.53 ± 0.32 [b]	51.32 ± 1.34 [b]	10.22 ± 0.26 [a]	0.12 ± 0.03 [a]	0.13 ± 0.03 [c]
18Ω H$_2$O	6.37 ± 0.06 [de]	10.01 ± 0.22 [b]	44.83 ± 1.16 [c]	9.46 ± 0.23 [b]	0.00 ± 0.00 [b]	0.05 ± 0.03 [d]
5% Inulin	6.06 ± 0.04 [f]	12.27 ± 0.33 [a]	54.56 ± 1.40 [b]	10.65 ± 0.25 [a]	0.00 ± 0.00 [b]	0.02 ± 0.01 [d]
1% Teff	6.82 ± 0.05 [b]	12.15 ± 0.28 [a]	61.76 ± 1.56 [a]	9.37 ± 0.24 [b]	0.00 ± 0.00 [b]	0.22 ± 0.03 [b]
2.5% Teff	7.54 ± 0.05 [a]	11.81 ± 0.24 [a]	54.27 ± 1.20 [b]	6.21 ± 0.15 [d]	0.00 ± 0.00 [b]	0.32 ± 0.04 [a]
5% Teff	6.29 ± 0.06 [e]	10.11 ± 0.27 [b]	42.54 ± 0.93 [c]	8.33 ± 0.20 [c]	0.00 ± 0.00 [b]	0.18 ± 0.03 [bc]
7.5% Teff	6.64 ± 0.06 [bc]	9.51 ± 0.24 [b]	43.12 ± 0.98 [c]	7.81 ± 0.19 [c]	0.00 ± 0.00 [b]	0.16 ± 0.03 [bc]

[1] Values are the means ± SEM, $n = 5$. a–f Treatment groups not indicated by the same letter are significantly different ($p < 0.05$). NI = non-injected.

3.9. Analysis of the Gut Microbiota

Figure 4 represents the observed differences in gut microbial diversity among treatment groups. No significant differences were found in α-diversity using Faith's phylogenetic diversity (PD) among treatment groups (Figure 4A, $p > 0.05$). Variation between samples (β-diversity) was calculated by using Jaccard distances. The chick microbiotas in the Inulin treatment group were the least similar (biggest distances between samples) to one another compared to the other groups (Figure 4B,C, $p < 0.01$). The distances within the teff treatment groups, except 2.5%, were not significantly different from both the NI control and 18Ω H$_2$O groups, which indicates the constant influence of the treatment on the microbial population.

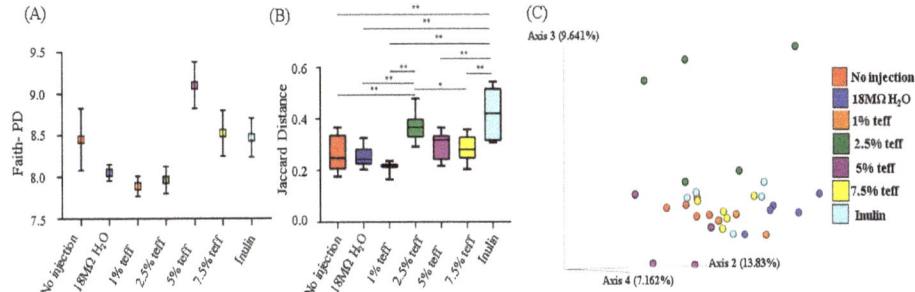

Figure 4. Microbial diversity of the cecal microbiome. (**A**) Measure of α- diversity using Faith's Phylogenetic Diversity; (**B**) Box-plots of Jaccard distances within the different groups; (**C**) Principal Coordinates Analysis (PCoA) based on Jaccard distances. Each dot represents one animal, and the colors represent the different treatment groups. $n = 5$, * = $p < 0.05$, ** = $p < 0.01$.

Although there were observed cecal microbiota shifts at the phylum and genera level, these differences were not significant (Figure 5, $p > 0.05$).

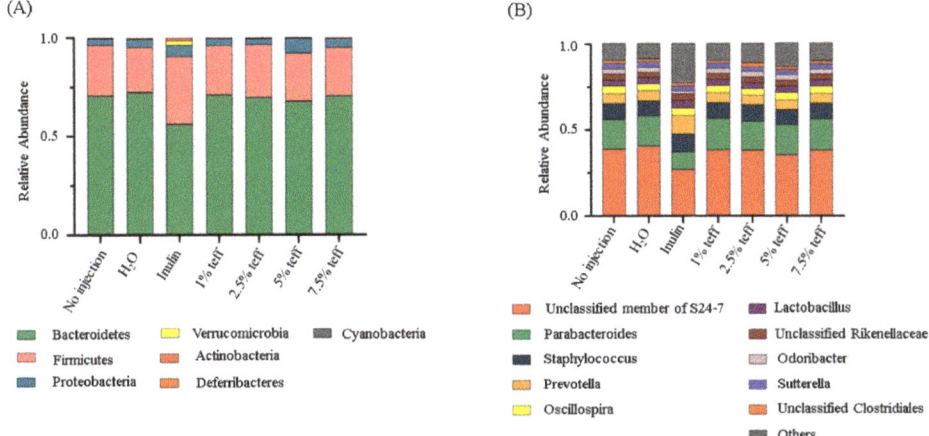

Figure 5. Compositional changes of the gut microbiota. (**A**) Phylum-level differences between the intra-amniotic administration measured at day of hatch (day 21); (**B**) Genus-level differences between the intra-amniotic administration groups as measure at day of hatch (day 21).

We also analyzed whether the genetic capacity of the microbiota could be affected by experimental teff solutions. Metagenome functional predictive analysis was carried out using PICRUSt software, feature abundance was normalized by 16S rRNA gene copy number, identified using the Greengenes database, and Kyoto Encyclopedia of Genes and Genomes (KEGG) orthologs prediction was calculated. Differentially-expressed pathways are displayed in Figure 6. In all but one bacterial metabolic pathway, mineral absorption and relative abundance were greater in teff treatment groups when compared to both NI control and 18Ω H_2O groups. Bacterial mineral absorption pathway was upregulated in the inulin group when compared to controls and teff treatment groups.

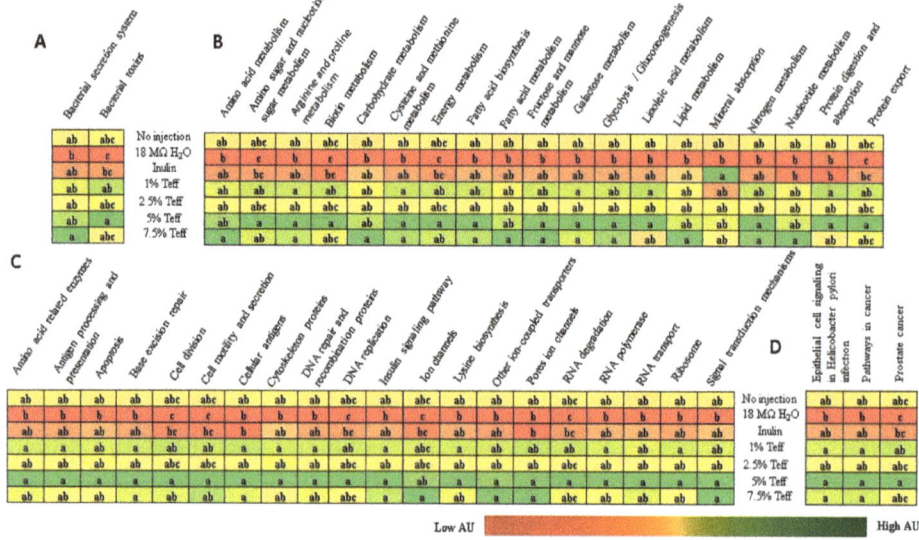

Figure 6. Predictive functional capacity of the cecal microbiota collected at hatch. (**A**) Bacterial processes; (**B**) metabolic processes; (**C**) cellular processes; and (**D**) human diseases. Treatment groups are indicated by their names and groups not indicated by the same letter are significantly different ($p < 0.05$).

4. Discussion

The implementation of teff as an advantageous staple food crop is rapidly growing due to its relative ease of cultivation, sensory quality of teff-based products, and favorable macro- and micronutrient composition [3,18,27]. Compared to other crops, teff does contain notable antinutrients, such as a higher concentration of phytic acid; however, processing methods such as fermentation can drastically lower phytic acid concentration and thus mineral inaccessibility. Despite this, the total polyphenolic content of many teff verities is lower than other food crops including sorghum and cowpea, while specific polyphenols have been shown to aid in mineral bioavailability, including ferulic, caffeic, and protocatechuic acids, which have been found in relatively higher quantities [4,7,8]. Polyphenolic analysis of the teff samples used in this study corroborated previous data demonstrating presence of ferulic, caffeic, and protocatechuic acids. The prevailing wisdom has been that phytate and polyphenolic compounds as a whole disproportionately limit trace mineral bioavailability despite the presence of other promoter-like compounds, such as prebiotics, which can counteract this effect [28–30]. We suggest a revised approach to this notion given the favorable physiologic and nutritional benefits afforded by intra-amniotic teff extract administration despite higher phytate concentration.

We have evaluated the effect of intra-amniotic teff extract administration on mineral status and other pertinent physiologic parameters. To our knowledge, ours is the first study to evaluate the effect of teff seed extract on mineral status, duodenal brush border membrane development, and functionality, as well as cecal microbiota. Intra-amniotic teff extract administration increased hepatic Fe and Zn concentrations, although serum Fe and Zn concentrations were not affected. Gene expression analysis demonstrated that teff extract up-regulated certain duodenal mineral transporters, such as DMT1 (BBM major Fe transporter) and ferroportin (BLM major Fe exporter), relative to control. Additionally, hepatic ferritin, the animal's primary form of cellular Fe storage, was decreased in all teff treatment groups except the 1% concentration, which could be explained by the prioritization of developing an embryo for hemoglobin synthesis versus storage. Indeed, previous intra-amniotic feeding trials have been unable to demonstrate a significant difference in Fe and Zn status, which are secondary to the relatively short treatment exposure time [6,13,23] that carries over to results for serum mineral status. However, the LA:DGLA ratio, a sensitive and specific biomarker of Zn status, was significantly lower in the higher concentration teff extract group demonstrating relative Zn repletion in this group [21,31]. Therefore, it appears that despite the short treatment exposure time, the significant increases in the hepatic Fe and Zn concentrations combined with lower LA:DGLA ratio in the 7.5% concentration group suggest that teff has potentially greater influence on mineral status than other intra amniotic nutritional solutions and purified extracts we have previously tested and thus may demonstrate superiority in delivering bioavailable Fe and Zn [13,32].

Further, the duodenal morphometric analysis demonstrated a significant ($p < 0.05$) effect on villus length, diameter, and crypt depth in all experimental teff groups. This effect was not concentration-dependent. Additionally, a significant ($p < 0.05$) increase in neutral and mixed duodenal goblet cells was observed in all teff groups when compared to both water-injected and non-injected controls. Increased number and size of duodenal goblet cells is a surrogate for increased luminal mucin production and secretion, which serves as a defensive barrier to pathogens and promotes epithelial cell function. Additionally, an improvement in villus architecture yields an increased surface area, thus improving the digestive enzyme and absorptive capacity [21,33,34]. The brush border gene expression analysis was mixed, with teff groups showing upregulated SGLT-1 expression while the inulin group showing a relative increase in SI and AP expression. Taken as a whole, this data demonstrates that the intra-amniotic administration of teff extract can modulate brush border membrane development and functionality. These results are in accordance with other intra amniotic administration trials that used isolated prebiotic polysaccharide compounds [12–15,32].

Together with beneficial changes in physiological parameters and brush border membrane functionality occurring as a result of intra-amniotic administration of teff extracts, we found low inter-individual variation among the different teff treatment groups (except of 2.5%) compared to the Inulin treatment. Significant differences in the composition of the cecal microbiotas were not observed. Using KEGG analysis, for the exception of bacterial mineral absorption, the functional capacity of the cecal microbiota demonstrated up-regulation in all bacterial metabolic pathways in the higher concentration teff groups. Given that brush border absorptive capacity was significantly increased in the teff groups, lower bacterial mineral metabolism in the teff group was likely due to less free Fe and Zn present in cecal contents for bacteria to utilize, and hence a compensatory upregulation in the bacterial mineral absorption pathway.

Several notable pathways upregulated in the teff groups included bacterial energy metabolism, sugar/carbohydrate metabolism, fatty acid biosynthesis, and protein synthesis. This was likely due, in part, to the large fiber content present in teff [7]. Indeed, relative to other staple food crops such as wheat, sorghum, and maize, teff contains several folds higher concentration of crude fiber, total, and soluble dietary fiber [7]. Fiber delivered to cecal bacteria exerts a prebiotic-like effect by allowing for the proliferation of butyrate- and other SCFA-producing bacteria. We demonstrated that bacterial fatty acid production was significantly increased in the teff extract groups. SCFAs have been shown to promote the proliferation and differentiation of intestinal mucosal epithelial cells [35,36]. Additionally, in the presence of increased dietary fiber, an overall increase in bacterial fermentation, reduction in intestinal luminal pH, and improvement in the solubilization of minerals such as Fe and Zn was observed in vivo [6,12,14]. Although we did not observe significant taxonomic shifts in the cecal microbiota of the animals receiving teff extract, the upregulation of many bacterial pathways relevant to Fe and Zn metabolism is a profound and novel finding. Additional studies are now warranted to assess cecal microbiota shifts post hatch and during a longer feeding trial.

5. Conclusions

The present study demonstrates that teff contains high amounts of fiber, phytic acid, and the polyphenols ferulic, caffeic, and protocatechuic acids, which have been shown to improve micronutrient absorption. Intra-amniotic administration of various concentrations of teff extract improved brush border membrane functionality through increases in villus architecture, surface area, and goblet cell expansion and related mucin production. Consequently, this contributed to increased relative expression of various duodenal enzymes responsible for mineral absorption and transport, and increased levels of hepatic Fe and Zn concentration, although serum concentrations remained unchanged. Although we did not observe significant alterations in the taxonomy of the cecal microbiota, various relevant bacterial metabolic pathways, such as fatty acid synthesis, were upregulated, which may demonstrate that teff administration positively influences the metagenome of the cecal microbiota, thus maximizing the solubilization and absorption of micronutrients in the gut. Given these findings, teff appears to represent a promising staple food crop and should be further evaluated in both long-term animal and controlled human efficacy trials.

Supplementary Materials: The following are available online at http://www.mdpi.com/2072-6643/12/10/3020/s1.

Author Contributions: Conceptualization, E.T.; methodology, N.K. and J.C; and E.T.; formal analysis, O.K., A.E., N.K., and E.T.; investigation, J.C., N.K., and E.T.; resources, E.T.; data curation, N.K., S.R., J.C., and E.T.; writing—original draft preparation, J.C. and S.R.; writing—review and editing, S.R. and E.T.; supervision, E.T.; funding acquisition, E.T. All authors have read and agreed to the published version of the manuscript.

Funding: This research received no external funding.

Acknowledgments: The authors wish to thank Hercia Martino and Barbara Silva (Department of Nutrition and Health, Federal University of Viçosa, Viçosa, Minas Gerais, Brazil) for conducting the fiber analysis. We also thank Ted Thannhauser and Tara Fish (Robert W. Holley Center for Agriculture and Health, Ithaca NY) for conducting the polyphenols analysis.

Conflicts of Interest: The authors declare no conflict of interest.

References

1. Abebe, Z.; Takele, W.W.; Anlay, D.Z.; Ekubagewargies, D.T.; Getaneh, Z.; Abebe, M.; Melku, M. Prevalence of anemia and its associated factors among children in Ethiopia: A protocol for systematic review and meta-analysis. *EJIFCC* **2018**, *29*, 138–145. [CrossRef] [PubMed]
2. Gebreegziabher, T.; Stoecker, B.J. Iron deficiency was not the major cause of anemia in rural women of reproductive age in Sidama zone, southern Ethiopia: A cross-sectional study. *PLoS ONE* **2017**, *12*, e0184742. [CrossRef] [PubMed]
3. World Bank. *World Development Report 2019: The Changing Nature of Work.*; License: Creative Commons Attribution CC BY 3.0 IGO; World Bank: Washington, DC, USA, 2019. [CrossRef]
4. Satheesh, N.; Fanta, S.W. Review on structural, nutritional and anti-nutritional composition of Teff (*Eragrostis tef*) in comparison with Quinoa (*Chenopodium quinoa* Willd.). *Cogent Food Agric.* **2018**, *4*. [CrossRef]
5. Umeta, M.; West, C.E.; Fufa, H. Content of zinc, iron, calcium and their absorption inhibitors in foods commonly consumed in Ethiopia. *J. Food Compos. Anal.* **2005**, *18*, 803–817. [CrossRef]
6. Tako, E.; Glahn, R.P.; Knez, M.; Stangoulis, J.C. The effect of wheat prebiotics on the gut bacterial population and iron status of iron deficient broiler chickens. *Nutr. J.* **2014**, *13*, 58. [CrossRef]
7. Baye, K. *Teff: Nutrient Composition and Health Benefits*; The International Food Policy Research Institute: Washington, DC, USA, 2014.
8. Baye, K.; Mouquet-Rivier, C.; Icard-Vernière, C.; Picq, C.; Guyot, J.P. Changes in mineral absorption inhibitors consequent to fermentation of Ethiopian injera: Implications for predicted iron bioavailability and bioaccessibility. *Int. J. Food Sci. Technol.* **2014**, *49*, 174–180. [CrossRef]
9. Harika, R.; Faber, M.; Samuel, F.; Mulugeta, A.; Kimiywe, J.; Eilander, A. Are low intakes and deficiencies in iron, vitamin A, zinc, and iodine of public health concern in Ethiopian, Kenyan, Nigerian, and South African children and adolescents? *Food Nutr. Bull.* **2017**, *38*, 405–427. [CrossRef]
10. Preidis, G.A. Targeting the human microbiome with antibiotics, probiotics, and prebiotics: Gastroenterology enters the metagenomics era. *Gastroenterology* **2009**, *136*, 2015–2031. [CrossRef]
11. Dias, D.M.; Kolba, N.; Hart, J.J.; Ma, M.; Sha, S.T.; Lakshmanan, N.; Nutti, M.R.; Martino, H.S.D.; Glahn, R.P.; Tako, E. Soluble extracts from carioca beans (*Phaseolus vulgaris* L.) affect the gut microbiota and iron related brush border membrane protein expression in vivo (*Gallus gallus*). *Food Res. Int.* **2019**, *123*, 172–180. [CrossRef]

12. Hou, T.; Tako, E. The in ovo feeding administration (*Gallus Gallus*)—An emerging in vivo approach to assess bioactive compounds with potential nutritional benefits. *Nutrients* **2018**, *10*, 418. [CrossRef]
13. Wang, X.; Kolba, N.; Liang, J.; Tako, E. Alterations in gut microflora populations and brush border functionality following intra-amniotic administration (*Gallus gallus*) of wheat bran prebiotic extracts. *Food Funct.* **2019**, *10*, 4834–4843. [CrossRef] [PubMed]
14. Pacifici, S.; Song, J.; Zhang, C.; Wang, Q.; Glahn, R.P.; Kolba, N.; Tako, E. Intra amniotic administration of raffinose and stachyose affects the intestinal brush border functionality and alters gut microflora populations. *Nutrients* **2017**, *9*, 304. [CrossRef] [PubMed]
15. Hartono, K.; Reed, S.; Ankrah, N.A.; Glahn, R.P.; Tako, E. Alterations in gut microflora populations and brush border functionality following intra-amniotic daidzein administration. *RSC Adv.* **2014**, *5*, 6407–6412. [CrossRef]
16. Yeung, C.K.; Glahn, R.E.; Welch, R.M.; Miller, D.D. Prebiotics and iron bioavailability—Is there a connection? *J. Food Sci.* **2005**, *70*, 88–92. [CrossRef]
17. Rocchetti, G.; Lucini, L.; Giuberti, G.; Bhumireddy, S.R.; Mandal, R.; Trevisan, M.; Wishart, D.S. Transformation of polyphenols found in pigmented gluten-free flours during in vitro large intestinal fermentation. *Food Chem.* **2019**, *298*, 125068. [CrossRef]
18. Gebremariam, M.M.; Zarnkow, M.; Becker, T. Teff (*Eragrostis tef*) as a raw material for malting, brewing and manufacturing of gluten-free foods and beverages: A review. *J. Food Sci. Technol.* **2014**, *51*, 2881–2895. [CrossRef]
19. Reed, S.; Knez, M.; Uzan, A.; Stangoulis, J.C.R.; Glahn, R.P.; Koren, O.; Tako, E. Alterations in the gut (*Gallus gallus*) microbiota following the consumption of zinc biofortified wheat (*Triticum aestivum*)-based diet. *J. Agric. Food Chem.* **2018**, *66*, 6291–6299. [CrossRef]
20. Tako, E.; Rutzke, M.A.; Glahn, R.P. Using the domestic chicken (*Gallus gallus*) as an in vivo model for iron bioavailability. *Poultry Science* **2010**, *89*, 514–521. [CrossRef]
21. Reed, S.; Qin, X.; Ran-Ressler, R.; Brenna, J.T.; Glahn, R.P.; Tako, E. Dietary zinc deficiency affects blood linoleic acid: Dihomo-ihlinolenic acid (LA:DGLA) ratio; a sensitive physiological marker of zinc status in vivo (*Gallus gallus*). *Nutrients* **2014**, *6*, 1164. [CrossRef]
22. Wiesinger, J.A.; Glahn, R.P.; Cichy, K.A.; Kolba, N.; Hart, J.J.; Tako, E. An in vivo (*Gallus gallus*) feeding trial demonstrating the enhanced iron bioavailability properties of the fast cooking manteca yellow bean (*Phaseolus vulgaris* L.). *Nutrients* **2019**, *11*, 1768. [CrossRef]
23. Da Silva, B.P.; Kolba, N.; Stampini Duarte Martino, H.; Hart, J.; Tako, E. Soluble extracts from chia seed (*Salvia hispanica* L.) affect brush border membrane functionality, morphology and intestinal bacterial populations in vivo (*Gallus gallus*). *Nutrients* **2019**, *11*, 2457. [CrossRef] [PubMed]
24. Faith, D.P. Conservation evaluation and phylogenetic diversity. *Biol. Conserv.* **1992**, *61*, 1–10. [CrossRef]
25. Langille, M.G.I.; Zaneveld, J.; Caporaso, J.G.; McDonald, D.; Knights, D.; Reyes, J.A.; Clemente, J.C.; Burkepile, D.E.; Vega Thurber, R.L.; Knight, R.; et al. Predictive functional profiling of microbial communities using 16S rRNA marker gene sequences. *Nat. Biotechnol.* **2013**, *31*, 814–821. [CrossRef]
26. Segata, N.; Izard, J.; Waldron, L.; Gevers, D.; Miropolsky, L.; Garrett, W.S.; Huttenhower, C. Metagenomic biomarker discovery and explanation. *Genome Biol.* **2011**, *12*, R60. [CrossRef] [PubMed]
27. Fan, S.; Yosef, S.; Pandya-Lorch, R. *Agriculture for Improved Nutrition: Seizing the Momentum*; CABI: Boston, MA, USA, 2019.
28. Petry, N.; Egli, I.; Zeder, C.; Walczyk, T.; Hurrell, R. Polyphenols and phytic acid contribute to the low iron bioavailability from common beans in young women. *J. Nutr.* **2010**, *140*, 1977–1982. [CrossRef] [PubMed]
29. Petry, N.; Egli, I.; Gahutu, J.B.; Tugirimana, P.L.; Boy, E.; Hurrell, R. Phytic acid concentration influences iron bioavailability from biofortified beans in Rwandese women with low iron status. *J. Nutr.* **2014**, *144*, 1681–1687. [CrossRef]
30. Bouis, H.E.; Saltzman, A. Improving nutrition through biofortification: A review of evidence from HarvestPlus, 2003 through 2016. *Glob. Food Sec.* **2017**, *12*, 49–58. [CrossRef] [PubMed]
31. Knez, M.; Stangoulis, J.C.R.; Glibetic, M.; Tako, E. The linoleic acid: Dihomo-γ-linolenic acid ratio (LA:DGLA)—An emerging biomarker of Zn status. *Nutrients* **2017**, *9*, 825. [CrossRef]
32. Hou, T.; Kolba, N.; Glahn, R.P.; Tako, E. Intra-amniotic administration (*Gallus gallus*) of Cicer arietinum and Lens culinaris prebiotics extracts and duck egg white peptides affects calcium status and intestinal functionality. *Nutrients* **2017**, *9*, 785. [CrossRef]

33. Smirnov, A.; Tako, E.; Ferket, P.R.; Uni, Z. Mucin gene expression and mucin content in the chicken intestinal goblet cells are affected by in ovo feeding of carbohydrates. *Poult. Sci.* **2006**, *85*, 669–673. [CrossRef]
34. Sobolewska, A.; Elminowska-Wenda, G.; Bogucka, J.; Dankowiakowska, A.; Kułakowska, A.; Szczerba, A.; Stadnicka, K.; Szpinda, M.; Bednarczyk, M. The influence of in ovo injection with the prebiotic DiNovo®on the development of histomorphological parameters of the duodenum, body mass and productivity in large-scale poultry production conditions. *J. Anim. Sci. Biotechnol.* **2017**, *8*, 45. [CrossRef] [PubMed]
35. Zhao, J.; Liu, P.; Wu, Y.; Guo, P.; Liu, L.; Ma, N.; Levesque, C.; Chen, Y.; Zhao, J.; Zhang, J.; et al. Dietary fiber increases butyrate-producing bacteria and improves the growth performance of weaned piglets. *J. Agric. Food Chem.* **2018**, *66*, 7995–8004. [CrossRef] [PubMed]
36. Chen, H.; Wang, W.; Degroote, J.; Possemiers, S.; Chen, D.; De Smet, S.; Michiels, J. Arabinoxylan in wheat is more responsible than cellulose for promoting intestinal barrier function in weaned male piglets. *J. Nutr.* **2015**, *145*, 51–58. [CrossRef] [PubMed]

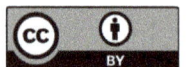

© 2020 by the authors. Licensee MDPI, Basel, Switzerland. This article is an open access article distributed under the terms and conditions of the Creative Commons Attribution (CC BY) license (http://creativecommons.org/licenses/by/4.0/).

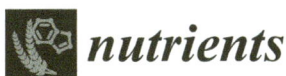

Article

Diet, Perceived Intestinal Well-Being and Compositions of Fecal Microbiota and Short Chain Fatty Acids in Oat-Using Subjects with Celiac Disease or Gluten Sensitivity

Lotta Nylund [1], Salla Hakkola [1], Leo Lahti [2], Seppo Salminen [3], Marko Kalliomäki [4,5], Baoru Yang [1] and Kaisa M. Linderborg [1,*]

[1] Food Chemistry and Food Development, Department of Biochemistry, University of Turku, 20520 Turku, Finland; lotta.nylund@utu.fi (L.N.); samahak@utu.fi (S.H.); baoru.yang@utu.fi (B.Y.)
[2] Department of Future Technologies, University of Turku, 20520 Turku, Finland; leo.lahti@utu.fi
[3] Functional Foods Forum, University of Turku, 20520 Turku, Finland; seppo.salminen@utu.fi
[4] Department of Pediatrics, University of Turku, 20500 Turku, Finland; marko.kalliomaki@utu.fi
[5] Department of Pediatrics and Adolescent Medicine, Turku University Hospital, 20521 Turku, Finland
* Correspondence: kaisa.linderborg@utu.fi

Received: 12 August 2020; Accepted: 20 August 2020; Published: 25 August 2020

Abstract: A gluten-free diet may result in high fat and low fiber intake and thus lead to unbalanced microbiota. This study characterized fecal microbiota profiles by 16S MiSeq sequencing among oat-using healthy adult subjects ($n = 14$) or adult subjects with celiac disease (CeD) ($n = 19$) or non-celiac gluten sensitivity (NCGS) ($n = 10$). Selected microbial metabolites, self-reported 4d food diaries and perceived gut symptoms were compared. Subjects with NCGS experienced the highest amount of gut symptoms and received more energy from fat and less from carbohydrates than healthy and CeD subjects. Oat consumption resulted in reaching the lower limit of the recommended fiber intake. Frequent consumption of gluten-free pure oats did not result in microbiota dysbiosis in subjects with CeD or NCGS. Thus, the high number of gut symptoms in NCGS subjects was not linked to the microbiota. The proportion of fecal acetate was higher in healthy when compared to NCGS subjects, which may be linked to a higher abundance of *Bifidobacterium* in the control group compared to NCGS and CeD subjects. Propionate, butyrate and ammonia production and β-glucuronidase activity were comparable among the study groups. The results suggest that pure oats have great potential as the basis of a gluten-free diet and warrant further studies in minor microbiota disorders.

Keywords: oats; celiac disease; non-celiac gluten sensitivity; intestinal microbiota; gluten-free; SCFAs

1. Introduction

Gluten-related disorders form an umbrella for all conditions related to gluten ingestion. These include, most importantly, celiac disease (CeD) and non-celiac gluten sensitivity (NCGS). The prevalence of these disorders has increased over the past 50 years, which makes them emerging health problems worldwide. Celiac disease is a chronic, systemic autoimmune disorder caused by gluten proteins in genetically susceptible individuals. In addition to CeD patients, NCGS subjects also require treatment with a gluten-free diet (GFD). These individuals develop adverse reactions such as gastrointestinal and extra-intestinal symptoms after exposure to gluten [1,2]. A life-long exclusion of gluten from the diet is currently the only effective treatment in alleviating the symptoms of these disorders. The adherence to a GFD and the following recovery from mucosal damage can be assumed to improve the nutritional status of the CeD patients observed at diagnosis. However, a long-term, strict GFD may be challenging to maintain due to social and economic burdens. Even when maintained,

GFD may be restricted and nutritionally suboptimal, since many gluten-free products have high fat and sugar but low fiber content. Such a diet predisposes patients to constipation, obesity and cardiovascular diseases [3–5].

The use of nutritious and fiber-rich whole-grain oats would diversify the GFD and improve the palatability, texture and fiber-content of the diet. Pure oats are being grown and produced following strict agricultural practices to minimize the contamination with other cereals. In Finland, oats are a major ingredient in the traditional daily diet and since the year 2000, pure oats have been considered suitable for the gluten-free diet [6]. Nowadays, oat products are widely used among Finnish celiac disease patients [7]. Although the inclusion of oats on GFD is recommended in Nordic countries, it is still not globally applied, possibly due to the debate regarding the safety of oats for CeD patients [8,9].

The intestinal microbiota primes the immune system and provides enzymes that expand the metabolic capacity of the host. The conversion of dietary components, such as dietary fiber, that escape the digestion of the host enzymes, support also the growth of microbes themselves. Intestinal microbiota and its metabolites play a major role in defining the antigen milieu of enterocytes, since they are able to interfere with the cells of the intestinal epithelium and modulate the signaling pathways through specific receptors [10]. It is assumed that a decreased microbiota diversity and relative abundances of specific bacterial taxa may lead to functional imbalance where the mutualistic relationship between the host and his microbes is disturbed. Indeed, deviations in the microbiota community structure have been associated with several local and systemic diseases, possibly contributing to the pathogenesis and/or clinical manifestation of these diseases (reviewed in [11]). In addition, GFD as such has been associated with potentially harmful alterations in microbiota, such as decreased microbiota richness, decreased amounts of bifidobacteria, lactobacilli as well as *Faecalibacterium prausnitzii* and increased amounts of *Proteobacteria* [12,13]. However, currently, the majority of the studies published on the fecal microbiota of celiac disease patients have been conducted with pediatric patients or by using conventional methods with limited throughput (reviewed in [14]).

To our understanding, the present study is one of the first on the gastrointestinal well-being and intestinal microbiota of persons with NCGS and within the few evaluating the intestinal microbiota of adult oat-using CeD subjects. The aim of this study was to evaluate the effect of oat consumption on the dietary status and gut well-being among adult subjects with gluten-related disorders who consume oat products on daily basis compared to healthy, oat consuming controls by using fecal microbiota signatures and its metabolites (short-chain fatty acids (SCFAs), ammoniacal nitrogen and β-glucuronidase activity) as biomarkers.

2. Materials and Methods

2.1. Subjects and Study Design

Celiac disease patients on a remission state (on a GFD at least 1 year), subjects with non-celiac gluten sensitivity (self-reported symptoms occurring after consuming a gluten-containing diet and adherence to a GFD for least 1 year) and healthy controls were recruited to the study. We decided not to test our NCGS subjects according to the Salerno criteria involving a separate gluten challenge trial for reasons discussed in later chapters [15]. The total number of the subjects recruited was 74, of which 49 completed the whole study period. After analyzing the food diary data, 6 subjects from NCGS group were excluded due to the consumption of gluten-containing food products. Thus, samples from celiac disease (CeD) patients (n = 19), non-celiac gluten sensitive subjects (n = 10) and healthy subjects (n = 14) were available for the further analyses. Based on food frequency questionnaire (FFQ) and 4d food diaries, all study subjects reported consumption of oat products daily. Demographic characteristics of study groups are presented in Table 1. Study subjects were recruited to the study from Turku region, Finland during the period August 2017–April 2018. Exclusion criteria were BMI below 18 or above 30, antibiotic treatment within the previous 6 months, use of any medication with gastrointestinal effects (e.g., laxatives or proton pump inhibitors) and blood donation or participation to another clinical study within a month. Before the study entry, the volunteers were interviewed to assess the eligibility of the study. The subjects were ascertained to be in good health by means of self-reporting and normal results in screening blood tests (total blood count, fasting glucose and liver, kidney and thyroid functions, wheatspecific immunoglobulin E (IgE), total immunoglobulin A (IgA) and IgA antibodies to tissue transglutaminase (tTGAbA)). After the screening tests, the study subjects were enrolled in the study and were instructed to keep gut symptom diaries for 30 days. Study subjects consumed their habitual diet throughout the study period and were asked to fulfill food diaries during the last four days of the study. In addition, volunteers were asked to fulfill an FFQ of their dietary habits. Based on the FFQ, The Index of Diet Quality was calculated as explained in detail by Leppälä et al. [16] to assess the adherence to a health-promoting diet. Fecal samples for the microbiota, SCFAs, β-glucuronidase and ammoniacal nitrogen analyses were collected on the last day of the study period. The study protocol was approved by the Ethics Committee of the Hospital District of Southwest Finland (Identifier: ETMK:42/1801/2016) and subjects were enrolled in the study after written informed consent was obtained. The study was registered at ClinicalTrials.gov (Identifier: NCT02761785).

Table 1. Basic characteristics and dietary intake of study subjects.

GROUP	CeD (n = 19)	NCGS (n = 10)	CTRL (n = 14)	p-Value
Subjects (n)	19	10	14	n.s.
Male/Female [1]	4/15	1/9	6/9	n.s.
Age (year) [2]	51 (24, 65) [a]	34 (22, 61) [b]	34 (24, 63) [b]	0.020
BMI (kg/m^2)	24.6 (3.2)	23.0 (2.6)	24.4 (2.6)	n.s.
Proteins (E %)	17.1 (3.6)	16.5 (3.4)	15.8 (3.1)	n.s.
Carbohydrates (E %)	41.9 (4.9) [a,b]	40.3 (6.1) [a]	45.8 (4.8) [b]	0.045
Fat (E %)	36.4 (5.7) [a,b]	41.0 (6.2) [a]	34.7 (4.6) [b]	0.025
Dietary fiber (g)	25.5 (9.1)	27.6 (7.7)	26.0 (7.4)	n.s.
Saccharose (g)	46.2 (19.3)	40.8 (12.3)	52.5 (23.0)	n.s.
Diet Quality Index	10.9 (1.7)	10.2 (2.2)	10.3 (1.5)	n.s.

Dietary data are presented as an average of 4d intake based on food diaries. Values are mean (SD), unless otherwise stated. CeD subjects with celiac disease, NCGS non-celiac gluten sensitivity, CTRL healthy controls. [1] Pearson Chi-Square. Others One-way ANOVA. [2] median (min, max) Values with different letters differ from one another in each row.

2.2. Dietary Intake Using Food Diaries

Subjects were given written and oral instructions on filling the food diaries during the four days preceding the last study visit (including at least 1 weekend day). Kitchen scales were provided to ensure accuracy. Mean daily intakes of energy and macronutrients were calculated by using computerized software (AivoDiet 2.0.2.3; Aivo, Turku, Finland) utilizing the food composition database provided by the Finnish National Institute for Health and Welfare [17].

The quality of overall diet was assessed by FFQ validated for the evaluation of diet quality index [16]. The questionnaire contains 18 questions regarding the frequency and amount of consumption of food products during the preceding week. The quality of the diet was defined as poor when index points were less than 10 out of the maximum 15 points and good when points were 10 or more.

2.3. Gut Symptom Diaries

For the 30 day report of perceived gut symptoms, the study subjects were asked to mark down the type of the symptom (upper abdominal pain, lower abdominal pain, cramping, bloating, flatulence, bowel movement, diarrhea or constipation), the severity of the symptom in a scale of 1 to 3 (one meaning mild pain, two being moderate pain and three being intense pain), and the duration of the symptom. The diary was divided into time slots of three hours, except night time, which was marked as six hours slot (from midnight until 6 a.m.).

2.4. Fecal Samples and DNA Extraction

Fecal samples were frozen immediately after collection (20 °C) and stored at −70 °C once arrived in the research laboratory which was typically during the defecation day. Microbial DNA was extracted from fecal samples using the repeated bead—beating with KingFisher®—method as described in detailed previously [18]. The quality and quantity of the received DNA were measured by using a Nanodrop 1000 spectrophotometer (Thermo Scientific, Wilmington, DE). The quality of the DNA was good in all samples (OD 260/280 ratio ≥ 1.8).

2.5. 16S Library Preparation

The library preparation was started from 12.5 ng of total DNA. For NGS (Next-Generation Sequencing) library preparation, the recommended protocol for preparing 16S ribosomal RNA gene amplicons for the Illumina MiSeq system was used (Illumina 2013). The suggested universal bacterial primers were utilized for amplifying the V3 and V4 hypervariable regions of the bacterial 16S rRNA gene with polymerase chain reaction (PCR) using the KAPA Hifi HotStart Ready Mix (Roche Diagnostics Deutschland, Mannheim, Germany). PCR products were purified, and dual indices and Illumina sequencing adapters were attached using the Nextera XT index kit, Illumina. Finally, the libraries were purified once more with AMPure XP beads, Agencourt. The high quality of libraries was ensured using Advanced Analytical Fragment Analyzer and the concentrations of the libraries were quantified with Qubit® Fluorometric Quantitation (Life Technologies, Invitrogen division, Darmstadt, Germany). In a second PCR sample-specific "barcode"—primers and adapter sequences were attached. Up to 96 libraries were normalized and pooled for an Illumina MiSeq sequencing run using the MiSeq Reagent Kit version (v.) 3 with marginally overlapping 300 base pairs (bp) paired-end reads.

2.6. 16S rDNA Sequencing

The libraries were normalized and pooled for the automated cluster preparation, which was carried out by Illumina MiSeq instrument. Phix control library was added to the sequencing pool to balance the sequencing run. The libraries were sequenced in a single 2 × 300 bp run with Illumina MiSeq instrument using v3 sequencing chemistry. The sequencing run used paired-end sequencing chemistry with 8 bp dual index run.

2.7. Short Chain Fatty Acids Assay

The amounts of fecal short-chain fatty acids (SCFAs) were measured by solid-phase microextraction coupled to gas chromatography and mass spectrometry (SPME-GC-MS) to evaluate the microbial metabolic activity. Fecal samples (0.1 g) were weighted and suspended into 5 mL of deionized water by vortexing. 1.5 mL of fecal suspension was added into 10 mL vial with 0.5 g of NaH_2PO_4 [19]. Acetic acid, propanoic acid and butyric acid (Sigma-Aldrich, WGK Germany) were used as external standards in order to control the daily variation of instrument and sample preparation. The SPME fiber used was 75 μm CAR/PDMS, Fused Silica (Supelco, Bellefonte, PA, USA). The SPME-GC-MS analysis was carried out with Thermo Trace 1310—TSQ 8000 Evo equipped with an autosampler (Thermo Scientific, Wilmington, DE, USA). Compounds were separated by Supelco fused silica capillary column SPB-624, (30 m × 0.25 mm × 1.4 μm) under a carrier gas (helium) 1 mL/min with a splitless mode. The oven temperature program was as follows: 40 °C hold for 2 min and then 5 °C/min rise until 200 °C, hold for 10 min. A voltage of 70 eV was set in the EI. The system was operated using Xcalibur 4.0 (Thermo Scientific, Wilmington, DE, USA). Compounds were identified by the NIST library [20] and quantified by comparison to external standards. To optimize the SPME analysis, five commercial fibers were screened: 50/30 μm DVB/CAR/PDMS, 65 μm PDMS/DVB Stableflex, 65 μm PDMS/DVB Fused Silica, 100 μm PDMS and 75 μm CAR/PDMS. 75 μm CAR/PDMS was evaluated by comparison of SCFA standard runs as the most suitable for SCFA detection and chosen for the analysis.

2.8. β-Glucuronidase and Ammoniacal Nitrogen Assays

The activity of β-glucuronidase enzyme and the amount of ammoniacal nitrogen were measured from fecal samples to evaluate differences in these potentially harmful microbial metabolic activities. Ammoniacal nitrogen assay was carried out by an indophenol blue method reported in detail elsewhere [21]. Briefly, 0.1 g of wet fecal sample was diluted with 5 mL of deionized water, shaken for 60 min, and centrifuged at 3000× g for 3 min. Ammoniacal nitrogen concentration was measured from supernatant based on absorbance measured at 630 nm (Hidex Sense microplate reader, Hidex Oy, Turku, Finland). β-glucuronidase assay was carried out by the protocol of Shen [22]. Briefly, 0.1 g of wet fecal sample was diluted with 5 mL of deionized water and shaken for 60 min. 0.1 mL of diluted sample was added into Eppendorf tube® with 0.4 mL of 2 mM p-nitrophenyl-β-D-glucuronide solution (Sigma Aldrich, WGK Germany). Suspensions were incubated in anaerobic conditions at 37 °C for 60 min, followed by addition of 0.5 mL of 0.5 M NaOH. This suspension was centrifuged at 3200× g for 10 min and absorbance was measured on 405 nm (Hidex Sense microplate reader, Hidex Oy, Turku, Finland).

2.9. Statistical and Data Analyses

Statistical analyses of food diary and microbial metabolites data were carried out using IBM SPSS Statistics 25 software. Normal distribution of data was tested with Shapiro–Wilks test and ANOVA with contrast test were used to determine the statistical differences between study groups.

In the preprocessing of the MiSeq sequencing reads, the workflow proposed by [23] was adapted. In summary, the reads were trimmed from the left at 25 bp and 10 bp for the forward and reverse reads, respectively; and from right at 245 bp and 230 bp based on manual inspection of the read quality summaries. The sequence variant table was constructed from the reads with DADA2 [24] based on DADA2-formatted training FASTA files that were derived from the Ribosomal Database Project's Training Set 16 and the 11.5 release of the RDP database [25]. The chimeras were removed. The phylogenetic tree was constructed with the DECIPHER [26] and phangorn R packages. The preprocessed data were converted into a phyloseq R object [27], and aggregated to the genus level with the microbiome R package (function aggregate_taxa). The full details are available in the source code that is openly deposited at Zenodo.

The Principal Coordinates Analysis (PCoA) was done for compositional data based on Bray–Curtis dissimilarity. Alpha diversity (Shannon index) was estimated with the *microbiome* [28] and *vegan* [29] R packages. For standard data manipulation and visualization, the *tidyverse* and *ggplot2* R packages were used, respectively. Beta diversity was done with PERMANOVA using the vegan R package and 999 permutations. The analyses were done with genus-level clr-transformed abundance tables unless otherwise mentioned. The group-level comparisons for individual genera were done with DESeq2.

3. Results

3.1. Dietary Intake and the Quality of Diet

Based on the food diary data (4 days), NCGS subjects received a higher proportion of their energy (E %) from fat and lower proportion (E %) from carbohydrates when compared to healthy controls ($p = 0.025$ and $p = 0.045$, respectively) (Table 1). Additionally, the gluten-sensitive subjects tended to get more energy than celiac disease patients when adjusted per body weight (kcal/kg of body weight, $p = 0.09$, data not shown). The mean intake of dietary fiber was at the lower end of the recommendation level in the three groups (Table 1). The dietary quality assessed by the validated index of diet quality questionnaire was considered good in most of the study subjects, average diet quality indices being higher than 10 in most of the study subjects (Table 1).

3.2. Gut Symptom Diaries

The highest amounts of gut symptoms per subject was reported by the NCGS groups subjects (61.4) when compared to CeD and healthy controls (39.1 and 19.7, respectively) ($p = 0.045$). In all study groups, the most often reported symptoms were flatulence, bloating and lower abdominal pain.

3.3. Intestinal Microbiota Signatures

The total microbiota profiles were comparable between CeD, NCGS and healthy controls (Figure 1). No statistically significant differences were observed in microbiota richness (Figure 2) or diversity (data not shown) between the study groups. Phylum-level microbial abundances were characterized by a high inter-individual variation and no statistically significant differences were observed between the study groups (Figure 3). However, the abundance of *Bifidobacterium* tended to be higher in the control group compared to CeD and NCGS ($p = 0.067$), (Figure 4).

3.4. Microbial Metabolic Activity

In CeD subjects, the amount of SCFAs was comparable to other groups (Table 2). However, the relative amount of acetate (% of total SCFAs) was higher in the control group compared to the NCGS group ($p = 0.03$). No statistically significant differences were observed in the proportions of propionate or butyrate between the groups. In addition, the amounts of ammoniacal nitrogen and β-glucuronidase activity were comparable between the study groups (Table 2).

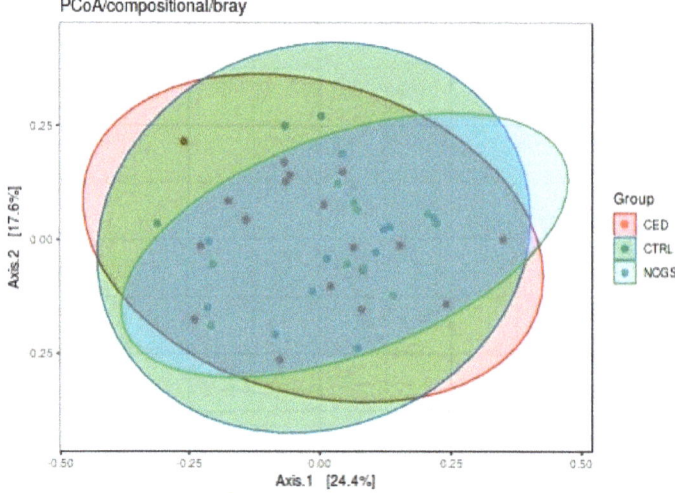

Figure 1. Total microbiota profiles of study subjects were comparable between the groups as assessed by Principal Component Analysis (PCoA). CED celiac disease ($n = 19$), NCGS non-celiac gluten sensitivity ($n = 10$) and CTRL healthy controls ($n = 14$).

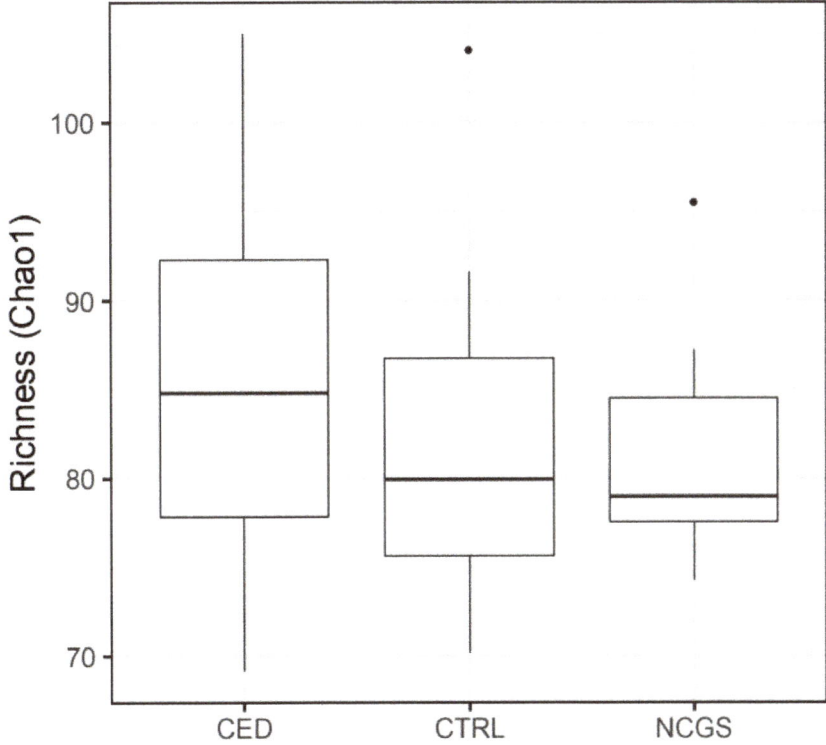

Figure 2. Microbiota richness was comparable in subjects with celiac disease (CED) ($n = 19$), non-celiac gluten sensitivity (NCGS) ($n = 10$) and healthy controls (CTRL) ($n = 14$). The box extends from 25th percentile to 75th percentile, with a line at median.

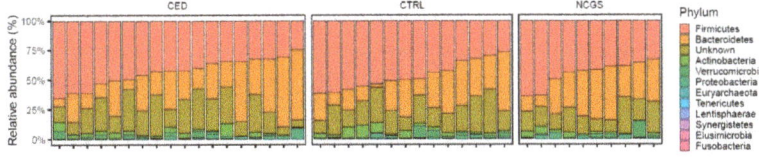

Figure 3. Relative abundances of bacterial phyla (% of total reads) in subjects with celiac disease (CED) ($n = 19$), healthy controls (CTRL) ($n = 14$) and subjects with non-celiac gluten sensitivity (NCGS) ($n = 10$). No statistically significant differences were observed between the study groups.

Table 2. Production of short-chain fatty acids (SCFAs), ammonia and the activity of β-glucuronidase in subjects with celiac disease (CeD), non-celiac gluten sensitivity (NCGS) and healthy controls (CTRL).

	CeD ($n = 19$)		NCGS ($n = 10$)		CTRL ($n = 14$)	
	Concentration	% of Total SCFA	Concentration	% of Total SCFA	Concentration	% of Total SCFA
Fecal acetic acid (µg)	2144 (1228)	63 [a,b]	2149 (1205)	59 [a]	2789 (1473)	71 [b]
Fecal propionic acid (µg)	806 (607)	23	948 (451)	28	698 (521)	19
Fecal butyric acid (µg)	337 (128)	14	456 (258)	13	424 (327)	10
Total SCFA (µg)	3287 (1786)		3553 (1680)		3912 (2072)	
Fecal ammonia (µmol)	18.0 (6.5)		18.5 (4.8)		15.7 (7.2)	
Fecal β-glucuronidase (U)	30.0 (15.0)		25.9 (15.0)		29.9 (18.0)	

Concentrations are presented per g of fecal wet weight. Values are presented as mean (SD). Values with different letters differ from one another in each row.

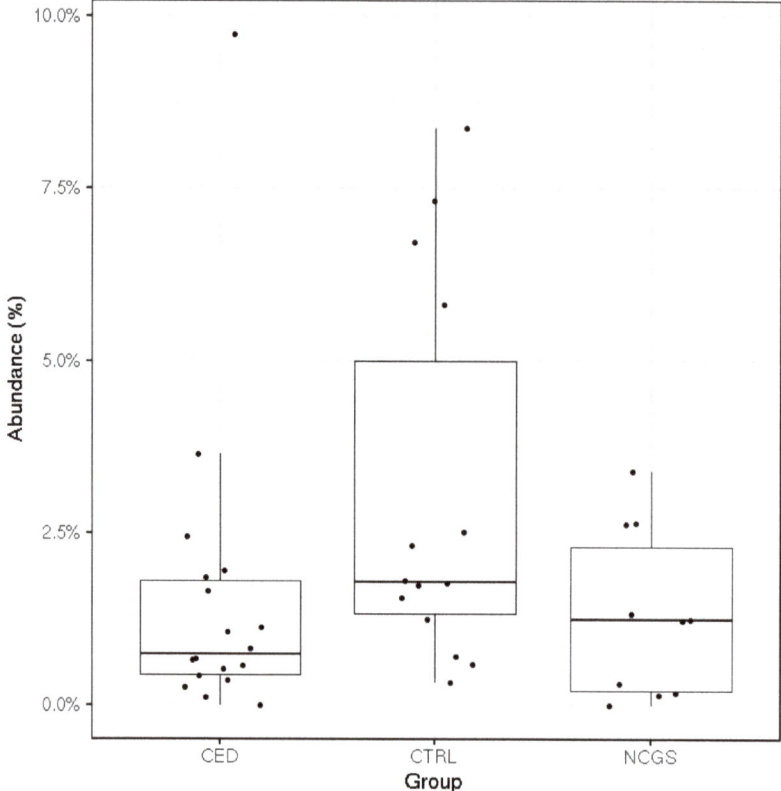

Figure 4. The mean relative abundance of *Bifidobacterium* in subjects with celiac disease (CED) (*n* = 19), healthy controls (CTRL) (*n* = 14) and subjects with non-celiac gluten sensitivity (NCGS) (*n* = 10). The difference between the three was borderline significant (p = 0.067; Kruskal–Wallis test).

4. Discussion

Currently, the only treatment for celiac disease and other gluten-related disorders is a life-long adherence to a GFD. Due to the shortage of whole-grain products in the diet, GFD often results in inadequate intake of nutrients and dietary fiber [30,31] while in our study the average intake of dietary fiber intake was at the lower end of recommendation in all three groups, and did not differ between them. The difference may result from the fact that our subjects consumed oat products as a part of their habitual diet. Pure oats suitable for the gluten-free diet are grown, milled and handled without contamination by other cereals. Recently, it was suggested that the current confounding clinical findings on the safety of oat consumption in CeD subjects [32] could be caused by contaminated oats assessed as "pure" [8]. Indeed, a decade ago, gluten cross-contamination was shown to exist in oat supply chains in Europe, the United States and Canada [33]. Yet, our results suggest a great potential for pure oats as a source of fiber to GFD.

While persons diagnosed with CeD receive professional dietary advice in Finland (The Finnish Medical Society Duodecim 2018), many NCGS subjects are self-educated in GFD. In our study, the dietary composition of CeD subjects was comparable with healthy controls while subjects with NCGS obtained more energy from fat (>40 E %) and less energy from carbohydrates when compared to healthy controls. In addition, the food diaries in this study revealed that a large number of volunteers initially assigned to the NCGS group (6/16) consumed gluten, most often from rye or barley. This may be an indication that they are not aware of the composition of GFD. According to a recent survey study of Potter et al. [34], 24% of responded Australians avoided gluten completely or partially, while 14% had self-reported non celiac wheat sensitivity and 1% had celiac disease. Others avoided gluten for "general health" or as a treatment of abdominal pain, without being diagnosed with CeD or NCGS. The authors considered that gluten avoidance may be due to the current well-being trend and that NCGS may overlap with other gastrointestinal disorders [34]. Additionally, we observed that the NCGS group reported more gut symptoms per subjects when compared to CeD and healthy controls ($p = 0.045$). This finding is in line with a recent study by Tovoli et al. [35], where a significant proportion (66%) of gluten-sensitive subjects, diagnosed according to Salerno criteria, reported intestinal symptoms even years after the beginning of GFD. Compared to CeD patients following the same diet, subjects with NCGS reported a higher amount of symptoms (33%). Additionally, Skodje et al. (2019) reported a high number of gastrointestinal complaints among subjects with self-reported NCGS on a GFD.

The existence of NCGS as a condition has been recently challenged and intake of other non-gluten wheat components such as fructans [36] and amylase–trypsin inhibitors have been suggested to lie behind the symptoms instead of gluten as such [37]. Even a term change from NCGS to non-celiac wheat sensitivity has been suggested [38]. Still, NCGS has its defenders among consumers and researchers. The Salerno criteria [15] have been proposed for standardization of the diagnosis of NCGS. Criteria based investigation involves reporting of symptoms during 6 weeks on gluten-containing diet followed by 6 weeks of GFD and a further 1 week of test period containing GFD supplemented with either gluten test meals or placebo, 1-week washout and another test period in a cross-over manner. For the status of NCGS, 30% variation of symptoms between GFD and gluten containing diet periods is required. Such a gluten challenge was not imposed on the NCGS subjects in our trial due to limited resources and burden on the volunteers to participate on multiple clinical investigations. More so, our aim of this study was not to investigate which proportion of our self-reported NCGS volunteers would fulfil the Salerno criteria nor to limit our volunteers only to those getting gastrointestinal problems in the gluten challenge but to include subjects who self-reported their need for gluten-free diet despite lack of diagnosis for CeD or wheat allergy. Instead, the subjects were screened for negative celiac serology, specific immunoglobulin E (IgE) and wheat allergy. Generally, CeD patients are screened to ensure the remission state of their disease and NCGS patients to exclude the celiac disease before landing on NCGS diagnosis. However, once the GFD is initiated, testing for celiac disease is no longer accurate, which may lead to false-negative results in the case of self-diagnosed NCGS patients.

Previously, the majority of the studies analyzing the fecal microbiota of celiac disease patients have been conducted with pediatric patients or by using conventional methods with limited throughput [14]. The most often reported hallmarks of CeD microbiota have been increased abundances of Gram-negative bacteria, such as *Proteobacteria* and *Bacteroidetes* and reduced abundances of *Bifidobacterium* spp. and *Lactobacillus* spp. [14]. Similar changes have been also reported in studies examining the microbiota of healthy subjects after 1 month on GFD [12,13]. Moreover, some studies have reported persistent microbiota dysbiosis in CeD subjects in remission and on a GFD [39–41]. Of these studies [12,13,39–41], only Wacklin et al. (2014) report that the subjects consumed oats. Likewise, the studies reviewed by Marasco et al. (2016) concerning the microbiota composition of CeD patients or subjects following GFD, do not report oat consumption of the subjects, apart from the mentioned study of Wacklin et al. (2014). Our study on pure-oat consuming CeD subjects did not detect any signs of microbiota dysbiosis typically observed in CeD subjects with active disease nor detected any major GFD related changes in microbiota on NCGS or CeD subjects. The mean abundance of *Bifidobacterium* was higher in the control group compared to CeD and NCGS subjects but the difference was only marginally significant ($p = 0.067$). One of the CeD subjects had a high level of *Bifidobacterium* (9.7%). The abundance is within the typical range of variation for this genus, although it was unexpected to observe in the CeD group which has been associated with a reduced level of *Bifidobacterium*. This, combined with the moderate sample size of our study, may partially explain the only marginally significant difference between the groups. Therefore, our results do not support the hypothesis that a significant intestinal microbiota dysbiosis would be the reason for the increased gastrointestinal symptoms reported by the NCGS group. The obtained results of microbiota composition agree with another Finnish study, where the CeD status of children who had consumed pure oats for 2 years was evaluated [42]. Small intestinal biopsies of these children showed normal histology and they had normal serological markers. Follow-up was continued for 7 years and all the markers remained normal during this period, suggesting that oats were well tolerated [42].

SCFAs are an important energy source for enterocytes and have been associated with several health-promoting effects including antipathogenic effects [43,44]. Their production varies among the individual microbiota compositions and by the type and amount of carbohydrates consumed [45]. We found that the relative amount of acetate (% of total SCFAs) was higher in the control group compared to NCGS group ($p = 0.03$), which may be linked to the higher abundance of *Bifidobacterium* in the control group compared to CeD and NCGS groups ($p = 0.067$) [46]. Proportions of propionate or butyrate did not differ between the groups. Thus, the intestinal microbiota of oat-using CeD and NCGS subjects was capable of producing similar amounts of propionate and butyrate than that of healthy controls. Previously, clinical studies assessing the SCFA levels have focused mainly on healthy adults [47–49], whereas adult celiac disease patients in remission have not been studied so far. Di Cagno et al. [50] analyzed volatile compounds from fecal samples of treated CeD children by SPME-GC-MS. The samples showed lower levels of SCFAs, such as butyric, isocaproic, and propanoic acids, when compared to healthy controls. However, the dietary habits of their subjects were not reported. It should be noted that SCFAs are rapidly absorbed in the colon and thus the fecal SCFA reflects losses rather than the amount of production in situ [43]. However, access to the proximal colon to quantify SCFA production rates is invasive and not possible in most study settings. Therefore, measurement of the fecal SCFAs is currently the only feasible way to estimate the production of compounds by gut microbiota. In this study, the interindividual variation of free-living human volunteers was large, but within the range observed previously [47–49]. The variation could possibly have been influenced by restrictions on the other parts of the diet than oats, but such were not applied in this study.

β-glucuronidase enzymes expressed by the intestinal microbiota mediate the reactivation of molecules important in human health and disease. For example, microbial glucuronidases regenerate toxic carcinogens whose increased activities in the GI tract have been associated with a higher incidence of gastrointestinal diseases such as colon cancer, Crohn's disease and colitis as well as to high-fat diets [51]. In rodent studies, high consumption of dietary fiber has been associated with decreased activity of β-glucuronidase [22,52]. In addition, a clinical crossover trial with 28 overweight male subjects demonstrated significantly decreased β-glucuronidase activity after consumption of wholegrain wheat and rye, when compared to low fiber control diet [53]. Our results show that CeD and NCGS subjects, who consume oat products on a daily basis, have similar β-glucuronidase activity levels than healthy controls.

No differences were seen in the ammonia production among the study groups. Ammoniacal nitrogen is a microbial end product produced by the deamination of amino acids. It is harmful to the host in high amounts, and previously the consumption of dietary fiber has been detected to decrease its production [53–55]. A study comparing the impact of diet on in vitro fermentation properties of whole grain flours and brans from corn, oats, rye and wheat reported significantly reduced ammonia concentrations after fermentation of oats and rye when compared to corn or wheat [54]. In general, ammonia concentrations of all groups studied were in line with previous results measured from healthy adults [47,56–60].

The strengths of this study were accurate analyses of fecal microbiota composition and metabolites of adult CeD and NCGS subjects, which has only received limited attention. A unique strength of the study was also the comparison of biological data to perceived symptoms by utilizing the gut symptom diaries. Moreover, the reliability of the results increased/enhanced the understanding of individual dietary habits of study subjects by analyzing 4d-food diaries as well as food frequency questionnaires assessing the overall quality of the study subject's diet. Additionally, the suitability of the study subjects was ensured by a detailed interview and screening at the recruitment to this study. The lack of non-oat-using CeD subjects can be considered as a limitation of this study since the inclusion of these subjects would have enabled a more accurate evaluation of the effect of the oat consumption on microbial biomarkers in celiac disease. However, the recruitment of non-oat using CeD subjects for the current study proved to be impossible. In Finland, the consumption of oats has been allowed for adult CeD subjects since 1997 and for pediatric patients since 2000 [6,61], and currently, most of the Finnish CeD subjects consume oats as part of their GFD [6,61].

To conclude, this study evaluated the influence of daily pure oat consumption on perceived and measured gut well-being in adult subjects with celiac disease and with subjects with non-celiac gluten sensitivity compared to healthy volunteers. No microbiota dysbiosis was detected among CeD nor NCGS subjects. However, further studies with metagenomic approaches should be conducted to assess the potential differences in microbiota composition and function in celiac patients consuming oats. The results of this study suggest that pure oats in a gluten-free diet represent a good alternative. We also demonstrate the need for further studies in NCGS subjects focusing on diet and microbiota interactions, and nutrition counseling to identify the causes of perceived gut symptoms.

Author Contributions: Conceptualization, K.M.L. and B.Y.; Methodology, L.N., S.H., S.S. and K.M.L.; Formal Analysis, L.N., S.H. and L.L.; Investigation, L.N., S.H., and L.L.; Resources, M.K., S.S., B.Y. and K.M.L.; Data Curation, L.N., S.H. and K.M.L.; Writing—Original Draft Preparation, L.N., S.H. and K.M.L.; Writing—Review & Editing, L.N., S.H., L.L., S.S., M.K., B.Y. and K.M.L.; Visualization, L.N., L.L., S.H. and K.M.L.; Supervision, K.M.L.; Project Administration, K.M.L.; Funding Acquisition, B.Y. and K.M.L. All authors have read and agreed to the published version of the manuscript.

Funding: This work was funded by Business Finland as part of the OATyourGUT project (grant number 5469/31/2016) co-funded by Finnish food companies and University of Turku, by Magnus Ehrnrooth Foundation (personal grant for SH) and by Academy of Finland (grant number 295741). The sequencing of the microbiological DNA was partially supported by Finnish Functional Genomics Centre, University of Turku, Åbo Akademi and Biocenter Finland.

Acknowledgments: All the volunteers who participated in this study are warmly acknowledged. Study nurse Sanna Himanen is acknowledged for the technical assistance in the screening blood tests. Annelie Damerau is thanked for technical advice in the SPME-GC-MS analyses. Annika Metsämarttila is acknowledged for discussions in the initial project planning phase.

Conflicts of Interest: The authors declare no conflict of interest.

Data Availability Statement: The cohort datasets generated and/or analyzed during the current study are not publicly available due to confidentiality, to protect the cohort participants' identity. The microbiota dataset analyzed in the current study is available from the corresponding author on reasonable request.

References

1. Sapone, A.; Lammers, K.M.; Casolaro, V.; Cammarota, M.; Giuliano, M.T.; De Rosa, M.; Stefanile, R.; Mazzarella, G.; Tolone, C.; Russo, M.I. Divergence of gut permeability and mucosal immune gene expression in two gluten-associated conditions: Celiac disease and gluten sensitivity. *BMC Med.* **2011**, *9*, 23. [CrossRef] [PubMed]
2. Carroccio, A.; Mansueto, P.; Iacono, G.; Soresi, M.; D'Alcamo, A.; Cavataio, F.; Brusca, I.; Florena, A.M.; Ambrosiano, G.; Seidita, A.; et al. Non-Celiac Wheat Sensitivity Diagnosed by Double-Blind Placebo-Controlled Challenge: Exploring a New Clinical Entity. *Am. J. Gastroenterol.* **2012**, *107*, 1898–1906. [CrossRef]
3. Lee, A.R.; Ng, D.L.; Dave, E.; Ciaccio, E.J.; Green, P.H.R. The effect of substituting alternative grains in the diet on the nutritional profile of the gluten-free diet. *J. Hum. Nutr. Diet.* **2009**, *22*, 359–363. [CrossRef] [PubMed]
4. Vici, G.; Belli, L.; Biondi, M.; Polzonetti, V. Gluten free diet and nutrient deficiencies: A review. *Clin. Nutr.* **2016**, *35*, 1236–1241. [CrossRef]
5. Melini, V.; Melini, F. Gluten-Free Diet: Gaps and Needs for a Healthier Diet. *Nutrients* **2019**, *11*, 170. [CrossRef] [PubMed]
6. Peräaho, M.; Collin, P.; Kaukinen, K.; Kekkonen, L.; Miettinen, S.; Mäki, M. Oats can diversify a gluten-free diet in celiac disease and dermatitis herpetiformis. *J. Am. Diet. Assoc.* **2004**, *104*, 1148–1150. [CrossRef]

7. Aaltonen, K.; Laurikka, P.; Huhtala, H.; Mäki, M.; Kaukinen, K.; Kurpp, K. The long-term con-sumption of oats in celiac disease patients is safe: A large cross-sectional study. *Nutrients* **2017**, *9*, 611. [CrossRef]
8. Fritz, R.D.; Chen, Y. Oat safety for celiac disease patients: Theoretical analysis correlates adverse symptoms in clinical studies to contaminated study oats. *Nutr. Res.* **2018**, *60*, 54–67. [CrossRef]
9. Pinto-Sanchez, M.I.; Calo, N.S.C.; Leffler, D.A.; Verdú, E.F.; Green, P.; Bercik, P.; Ford, A.C.; Murray, J.A.; Armstrong, D.; Semrad, C.; et al. Safety of Adding Oats to a Gluten-Free Diet for Patients With Celiac Disease: Systematic Review and Meta-analysis of Clinical and Observational Studies. *Gastroenterology* **2017**, *153*, 395–409. [CrossRef]
10. Walker, W.A. Initial Intestinal Colonization in the Human Infant and Immune Homeostasis. *Ann. Nutr. Metab.* **2013**, *63*, 8–15. [CrossRef]
11. Bonder, M.J.; Tigchelaar, E.F.; Cai, X.; Trynka, G.; Cenit, M.C.; Hrdlickova, B.; Zhong, H.; Vatanen, T.; Gevers, D.; Wijmenga, C.; et al. The influence of a short-term gluten-free diet on the human gut microbiome. *Genome Med.* **2016**, *8*, 45. [CrossRef] [PubMed]
12. De Palma, G.; Nadal, I.; Collado, M.C.; Sanz, Y. Effects of a gluten-free diet on gut microbiota and immune function in healthy adult human subjects. *Br. J. Nutr.* **2009**, *102*, 1154–1160. [CrossRef] [PubMed]
13. Marasco, G.; Di Biase, A.R.; Schiumerini, R.; Eusebi, L.H.; Iughetti, L.; Ravaioli, F.; Scaioli, E.; Colecchia, A.; Festi, D. Gut Microbiota and Celiac Disease. *Dig. Dis. Sci.* **2016**, *61*, 1461–1472. [CrossRef] [PubMed]
14. Lin, L.; Zhang, J.-Q. Role of intestinal microbiota and metabolites on gut homeostasis and human diseases. *BMC Immunol.* **2017**, *18*, 2. [CrossRef]
15. Catassi, C.; Elli, L.; Bonaz, B.; Bouma, G.; Carroccio, A.; Castillejo, G.; Cellier, C.; Cristofori, F.; De Magistris, L.; Dolinsek, J.; et al. Diagnosis of Non-Celiac Gluten Sensitivity (NCGS): The Salerno Experts' Criteria. *Nutrients* **2015**, *7*, 4966–4977. [CrossRef]
16. Leppälä, J.; Lagström, H.; Kaljonen, A.; Laitinen, K. Construction and evaluation of a self-contained index for assessment of diet quality. *Scand. J. Public Health* **2010**, *38*, 794–802. [CrossRef]
17. Finnish Food Composition Database. National Institute for Health and Welfare, Nutrition Unit Fineli. Available online: https://fineli.fi/fineli/en/index? (accessed on 20 June 2018).
18. Nylund, L.; Heilig, H.G.; Salminen, S.; De Vos, W.M.; Satokari, R. Semi-automated extraction of microbial DNA from feces for qPCR and phylogenetic microarray analysis. *J. Microbiol. Methods* **2010**, *83*, 231–235. [CrossRef]
19. Fiorini, D.; Pacetti, D.; Gabbianelli, R.; Gabrielli, S.; Ballini, R. A salting out system for improving the efficiency of the headspace solid-phase microextraction of short and medium chain free fatty acids. *J. Chromatogr. A* **2015**, *1409*, 282–287. [CrossRef]
20. Nist Chemistry Webbook. National Institute of Standards and Technology. Available online: https://webbook.nist.gov/chemistry/ (accessed on 27 September 2018).
21. Koroleff, F. Direct spectrophotometric determination of ammonia in precipitation. *Tellus* **1966**, *18*, 562–565. [CrossRef]
22. Shen, R.L.; Dang, X.Y.; Dong, J.L.; Hu, X.Z. Effects of oat beta-glucan and barley beta-glucan on fecal characteristics, intestinal microflora, and intestinal bacterial metabolites in rats. *J. Agric. Food Chem.* **2012**, *60*, 11301–11308. [CrossRef]
23. Callahan, B.J.; Sankaran, K.; Fukuyama, J.A.; McMurdie, P.J.; Holmes, S.P. Bioconductor workflow for microbiome data analysis: From raw reads to community analyses. *F1000Research* **2016**, *5*, 1492. [CrossRef] [PubMed]
24. Callahan, B.J.; McMurdie, P.J.; Rosen, M.J.; Han, A.W.; Johnson, A.J.; Holmes, S. DADA2: High-resolution sample inference from Illumina amplicon data. *Nat. Methods* **2016**, *13*, 581–583. [CrossRef] [PubMed]
25. RDP Taxonomic Training Data Formatted for DADA2 (RDP Trainset 16/Release 11.5). Available online: https://zenodo.org/record/801828#.X0CLyjURWUl (accessed on 1 October 2018).
26. Wright, E.S. DECIPHER: Harnessing local sequence context to improve protein multiple sequence alignment. *BMC Bioinform.* **2015**, *16*, 322. [CrossRef] [PubMed]
27. McMurdie, P.J.; Holmes, S. phyloseq: An R Package for Reproducible Interactive Analysis and Graphics of Microbiome Census Data. *PLoS ONE* **2013**, *8*, e61217. [CrossRef] [PubMed]
28. Lahti, L.; Shetty, S. Introduction to the Microbiome R Package Version 2.1.26. Available online: https://microbiome.github.io/microbiome/ (accessed on 1 October 2018).

29. Oksanen, J.; Blanchet, F.G.; Friendly, M. Community Ecology Package. R Package Version 2.5-6. Available online: https://CRAN.R-project.org/package=vegan (accessed on 1 October 2018).
30. Hallert, C.; Grant, C.; Grehn, S.; Granno, C.; Hulten, S.; Midhagen, G.; Strom, M.; Svensson, H.; Valdimason, T. Evidence of poor vitamin status in coeliac patients on a gluten-free diet for 10 years. *Aliment. Pharmacol. Ther.* **2002**, *16*, 1333–1339. [CrossRef]
31. Thompson, T.; Dennis, M.; Higgins, L.A.; Lee, A.R.; Sharrett, M.K. Gluten-free diet survey: Are Americans with coeliac disease consuming recommended amounts of fibre, iron, calcium and grain foods? *J. Hum. Nutr. Diet.* **2005**, *18*, 163–169. [CrossRef]
32. De Souza, M.C.P.; Deschênes, M.-E.; Laurencelle, S.; Godet, P.; Roy, C.C.; Djilali-Saiah, I. Pure Oats as Part of the Canadian Gluten-Free Diet in Celiac Disease: The Need to Revisit the Issue. *Can. J. Gastroenterol. Hepatol.* **2016**, *2016*, 1–8. [CrossRef]
33. Hernando, A.; Mujico, J.R.; Mena, M.C.; Lombardía, M.; Méndez, E. Measurement of wheat gluten and barley hordeins in contaminated oats from Europe, the United States and Canada by Sandwich R5 ELISA. *Eur. J. Gastroenterol. Hepatol.* **2008**, *20*, 545–554. [CrossRef]
34. Potter, M.D.E.; Jones, M.P.; Walker, M.M.; Koloski, N.A.; Keely, S.; Holtmann, G.; Talley, A. Incidence and prevalence of self-reported non-coeliac wheat sensitivity and gluten avoidance in Australia. *Med. J. Aust.* **2020**, *212*, 126–131. [CrossRef]
35. Tovoli, F.; Granito, A.; Negrini, G.; Guidetti, E.; Faggiano, C.; Bolondi, L. Long term effects of gluten-free diet in non-celiac wheat sensitivity. *Clin. Nutr.* **2019**, *38*, 357–363. [CrossRef]
36. Skodje, G.I.; Sarna, V.K.; Minelle, I.H.; Rolfsen, K.L.; Muir, J.G.; Gibson, P.R.; Veierød, M.B.; Henriksen, C.; Lundin, K.E. Fructan, Rather Than Gluten, Induces Symptoms in Patients With Self-Reported Non-Celiac Gluten Sensitivity. *Gastroenterology* **2018**, *154*, 529–539. [CrossRef] [PubMed]
37. Reig-Otero, Y.; Mañes, J.; Manyes, L. Amylase–Trypsin Inhibitors in Wheat and Other Cereals as Potential Activators of the Effects of Nonceliac Gluten Sensitivity. *J. Med. Food* **2018**, *21*, 207–214. [CrossRef] [PubMed]
38. Dale, H.F.; Biesiekierski, J.R.; Lied, G.A. Non-coeliac gluten sensitivity and the spectrum of gluten-related disorders: An updated overview. *Nutr. Res. Rev.* **2018**, *32*, 28–37. [CrossRef] [PubMed]
39. Viitasalo, L.; Kurppa, K.; Ashorn, M.; Saavalainen, P.; Huhtala, H.; Ashorn, S.; Mäki, M.; Ilus, T.; Kaukinen, K.; Iltanen, S. Microbial Biomarkers in Patients with Nonresponsive Celiac Disease. *Dig. Dis. Sci.* **2018**, *63*, 3434–3441. [CrossRef] [PubMed]
40. Wacklin, P.; Laurikka, P.; Lindfors, K.; Collin, P.; Salmi, T.; Lähdeaho, M.L.; Saavalainen, P.; Mäki, M.; Matto, J.; Kurppa, K. Altered duodenal microbiota composition in celiac disease patients suffering from persistent symptoms on a long-term gluten-free diet. *Am. J. Gastroenterol.* **2014**, *109*, 1933–1941. [CrossRef]
41. Collado, M.C.; Donat, E.; Ribes-Koninckx, C.; Calabuig, M.; Sanz, Y. Specific duodenal and faecal bacterial groups associated with paediatric coeliac disease. *J. Clin. Pathol.* **2008**, *62*, 264–269. [CrossRef]
42. Holm, K.; Maki, M.; Vuolteenaho, N.; Mustalahti, K.; Ashorn, M.; Ruuska, T.; Kaukinen, K. Oats in the treatment of childhood coeliac disease: A 2-year controlled trial and a long-term clinical follow-up study. *Aliment. Pharmacol. Ther.* **2006**, *23*, 1463–1472. [CrossRef]
43. Louis, P.; Hold, G.L.; Flint, H.J. The gut microbiota, bacterial metabolites andcolorectal cancer. *Nat. Rev. Microbiol.* **2014**, *12*, 661–672. [CrossRef]
44. O'Keefe, S.J.D. Diet, microorganisms and their metabolites, and colon cancer. *Nat. Rev. Gastroenterol. Hepatol.* **2016**, *13*, 691–706. [CrossRef]
45. Pylkas, A.M.; Juneja, L.R.; Slavin, J.L. Comparison of Different Fibers for In Vitro Production of Short Chain Fatty Acids by Intestinal Microflora. *J. Med. Food* **2005**, *8*, 113–116. [CrossRef]
46. Fukuda, S.; Toh, H.; Hase, K.; Oshima, K.; Nakanishi, Y.; Yoshimura, K.; Tobe, T.; Clarke, J.M.; Topping, D.L.; Suzuki, T.; et al. Bifidobacteria can protect from enteropathogenic infection through production of acetate. *Nature* **2011**, *469*, 543–547. [CrossRef] [PubMed]
47. McOrist, A.L.; Miller, R.B.; Bird, A.R.; Keogh, J.B.; Noakes, M.; Topping, D.L.; Conlon, M.A. Fecal butyrate levels vary widely among individuals but are usually increased by a diet high in re-sistant starch. *J. Nutr.* **2011**, *141*, 883–889. [CrossRef] [PubMed]
48. Garcia-Villalba, R.; Gimenez-Bastida, J.A.; Garcia-Conesa, M.T.; Tomas-Barberan, F.A.; Espin, J.C.; Larrosa, M. Alternative method for gas chromatography-mass spectrometry analysis of short-chain fatty acids in faecal samples. *J. Sep. Sci.* **2012**, *35*, 1906–1913. [CrossRef] [PubMed]

49. Delgado, S.; Ruas-Madiedo, P.; Suárez, A.; Mayo, B. Interindividual Differences in Microbial Counts and Biochemical-Associated Variables in the Feces of Healthy Spanish Adults. *Dig. Dis. Sci.* **2006**, *51*, 737–743. [CrossRef]
50. Di Cagno, R.; De Angelis, M.; De Pasquale, I.; Ndagijimana, M.; Vernocchi, P.; Ricciuti, P.; Gagliardi, F.; Laghi, L.; Crecchio, C.; Guerzoni, M.E.; et al. Duodenal and faecal microbiota of celiac children: Molecular, phenotype and metabolome characterization. *BMC Microbiol.* **2011**, *11*, 219. [CrossRef]
51. Pellock, S.J.; Redinbo, M.R. Glucuronides in the gut: Sugar-driven symbioses between microbe and host. *J. Boil. Chem.* **2017**, *292*, 8569–8576. [CrossRef]
52. Freeman, H.J. Effects of differing purified cellulose, pectin, and hemicellulose fiber diets on fecal enzymes in 1,2-dimethylhydrazine-induced rat colon carcinogenesis. *Cancer Res.* **1986**, *46*, 5529–5532.
53. McIntosh, G.; Noakes, M.; Royle, P.J.; Foster, P.R. Whole-grain rye and wheat foods and markers of bowel health in overweight middle-aged men. *Am. J. Clin. Nutr.* **2003**, *77*, 967–974. [CrossRef]
54. Brahma, S.; Martinez, I.; Walter, J.; Clarke, J.; Gonzalez, T.; Menon, R.; Rose, D.J. Impact of die-tary pattern of the fecal donor on in vitro fermentation properties of whole grains and brans. *J. Funct. Foods* **2017**, *29*, 281–289. [CrossRef]
55. Lupton, J.R.; Marchant, L.J. Independent effects of fiber and protein on colonic luminal am-monia concentration. *J. Nutr.* **1989**, *119*, 235–241. [CrossRef]
56. Nemoto, H.; Kataoka, K.; Ishikawa, H.; Ikata, K.; Arimochi, H.; Iwasaki, T.; Ohnishi, Y.; Kuwahara, T.; Yasutomo, K. Reduced Diversity and Imbalance of Fecal Microbiota in Patients with Ulcerative Colitis. *Dig. Dis. Sci.* **2012**, *57*, 2955–2964. [CrossRef] [PubMed]
57. Shinohara, K.; Ohashi, Y.; Kawasumi, K.; Terada, A.; Fujisawa, T. Effect of apple intake on fecal microbiota and metabolites in humans. *Anaerobe* **2010**, *16*, 510–515. [CrossRef] [PubMed]
58. Clarke, J.M.; Topping, D.L.; Christophersen, C.T.; Bird, A.R.; Lange, K.; Saunders, I.; Cobiac, L. Butyrate esterified to starch is released in the human gastrointestinal tract. *Am. J. Clin. Nutr.* **2011**, *94*, 1276–1283. [CrossRef] [PubMed]
59. Slavin, J.; Feirtag, J. Chicory inulin does not increase stool weight or speed up intestinal transit time in healthy male subjects. *Food Funct.* **2011**, *2*, 72–77. [CrossRef] [PubMed]
60. Tiihonen, K.; Ouwehand, A.C.; Rautonen, N. Effect of overweight on gastrointestinal micro-biology and immunology: Correlation with blood biomarkers. *Br. J. Nutr.* **2010**, *103*, 1070–1078. [CrossRef] [PubMed]
61. Kaukinen, K.; Collin, P.; Huhtala, H.; Mäki, M. Long-Term Consumption of Oats in Adult Celiac Disease Patients. *Nutrients* **2013**, *5*, 4380–4389. [CrossRef]

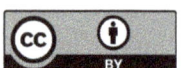

© 2020 by the authors. Licensee MDPI, Basel, Switzerland. This article is an open access article distributed under the terms and conditions of the Creative Commons Attribution (CC BY) license (http://creativecommons.org/licenses/by/4.0/).

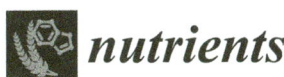

Article

Low Phytate Peas (*Pisum sativum* L.) Improve Iron Status, Gut Microbiome, and Brush Border Membrane Functionality In Vivo (*Gallus gallus*)

Tom Warkentin [1], Nikolai Kolba [2,†] and Elad Tako [2,*,†]

[1] Crop Development Centre, Department of Plant Sciences, University of Saskatchewan, 51 Campus Dr., Saskatoon, SK S7N 5A8, Canada; tom.warkentin@usask.ca
[2] USDA-ARS, Robert W. Holley Center for Agriculture and Health, Cornell University, Ithaca, NY 14853, USA; nk598@cornell.edu
* Correspondence: et79@cornell.edu
† Current Affiliation: Department of Food Science, Cornell University, Stocking Hall, Ithaca, NY 14853-7201, USA.

Received: 5 August 2020; Accepted: 20 August 2020; Published: 24 August 2020

Abstract: The inclusion of pulses in traditional wheat-based food products is increasing as the food industry and consumers are recognizing the nutritional benefits due to the high protein, antioxidant activity, and good source of dietary fiber of pulses. Iron deficiency is a significant global health challenge, affecting approximately 30% of the world's population. Dietary iron deficiency is the foremost cause of anemia, a condition that harms cognitive development and increases maternal and infant mortality. This study intended to demonstrate the potential efficacy of low-phytate biofortified pea varieties on dietary iron (Fe) bioavailability, as well as on intestinal microbiome, energetic status, and brush border membrane (BBM) functionality in vivo (*Gallus gallus*). We hypothesized that the low-phytate biofortified peas would significantly improve Fe bioavailability, BBM functionality, and the prevalence of beneficial bacterial populations. A six-week efficacy feeding ($n = 12$) was conducted to compare four low-phytate biofortified pea diets with control pea diet (CDC Bronco), as well as a no-pea diet. During the feeding trial, hemoglobin (Hb), body-Hb Fe, feed intake, and body weight were monitored. Upon the completion of the study, hepatic Fe and ferritin, pectoral glycogen, duodenal gene expression, and cecum bacterial population analyses were conducted. The results indicated that certain low-phytate pea varieties provided greater Fe bioavailability and moderately improved Fe status, while they also had significant effects on gut microbiota and duodenal brush border membrane functionality. Our findings provide further evidence that the low-phytate pea varieties appear to improve Fe physiological status and gut microbiota in vivo, and they highlight the likelihood that this strategy can further improve the efficacy and safety of the crop biofortification and mineral bioavailability approach.

Keywords: pea; phytate; iron; bioavailability; bio active compound; in vivo; *Gallus gallus*; brush border membrane; microbiome

1. Introduction

Micronutrient malnutrition affects more than half of the global population, primarily in developing regions [1,2]. Iron (Fe), zinc (Zn), and vitamin A deficiencies are prominent health constraints worldwide [3]. In low-income countries, plants are the significant source of food. In crude cereal and legume foods, the low bioavailability of Fe and Zn leads to metabolic disorders that are associated with these nutritional factors. Hence, increasing the nutritional value of such types of dietary ingredients will contribute to the nutritional status of the target population. Mineral, phosphorous, and phytate content is much higher in bran than whole grain [4–6].

Field pea (*Pisum sativum* L.) is a main pulse crop grown for human consumption as a source of protein, carbohydrates, minerals, and bioactive plant-origin bioactive compounds, contributing to better metabolic health. In 2014, the global production of peas was 11.2 million tons [7]. The main component of pea is starch, which includes two polymers of D-glucose: amylose and amylopectin [8,9]. Because of the alterations in physiochemical characteristics between pulses and cereal starches, starch from pulses can deliver some specific features to food systems as high gelation temperature, resistance to shear thinning, increased elasticity, and high concentration of resistant starch [10].

In addition, field peas include bioactive compounds such as oligosaccharides, polyphenols, and phytate [11]. Water-soluble carbohydrates in peas comprise mostly disaccharides and oligosaccharides. The raffinose group of oligosaccharides (RFOs) is the most targeted in pea research. These factors include galactose molecules (linked by α-D-1, 6-glycosidic bonds) attached to sucrose [12]. Humans lack the essential enzymes that are essential to break down these RFOs, and this results in these oligosaccharides being digested by intestinal bacterial populations via fermentation, leading to elevated short-chain fatty acid production [13]. Furthermore, a recent study indicated that intra-amniotic administration of raffinose upregulated the expression of brush border membrane (BBM) functional proteins, downregulated the expression of Fe-related proteins (indicating improvement of dietary iron bioavailability), and elevated villus surface area. Furthermore, raffinose increased the richness and composition of probiotic populations, and it reduced that of pathogenic bacterial species. Overall, raffinose improved microbial population, dietary Fe bioavailability, and BBM functionality in vivo [14].

The main phenolic compounds found in peas comprise condensed tannins, flavonoids, and phenolic acids [15]. These phenolic compounds are found specifically in the seed coat and are biosynthesized via the phenylpropanoid pathway, with condensed tannin molecules being responsible for the seed-coat coloring [16]. In dark-colored hulls, tannin and flavonoid compounds are the majority of phenolic compounds; however, in seeds with clear hulls, phenolic acids are the main compounds [17]. Polyphenols in the seed coat present antioxidant and anti-mutagenic activity, shielding the seed from oxidative stress [18]. In field conditions, these compounds also deliver chemical resistance against pathogens and insect pests during the growing process of the plant [19]. Polyphenols in peas appear mostly as insoluble or bound forms, covalently bonded to structural components of the cell wall such as cellulose, hemicellulose, lignin, and pectin [20,21]. The polyphenolic composition of peas is predominantly interesting with respect to metabolic health, given their alleged protective properties against oxidative stress [15,22]. According to Campos-Vega [11] and Rochfort [23], isoflavone polyphenols are linked with biological pathways in the lessening of osteoporosis and cardiovascular disease, the deterrence of cancer, and treating symptoms related to menopause. Phenolic compounds also display anti-nutritional effects, and related research showed a decrease in the bioavailability of proteins triggered by phenolic compounds [24]. Phytate functions as a storage for phosphate and minerals in seeds that can be recovered during germination process [25]. Phytate was recognized as an anti-nutrient due to its ability to chelate with multivalent ions, specifically Zn, Ca, and Fe, inhibiting the body's capability to absorb dietary minerals by limiting their bioavailability [24]. There is increasing interest in utilizing pulses in wheat-based products with blends [26]. The demand for gluten-free products led to investigation of the nutritional characteristics of baked products from pulses like chickpea and lentil [27], as well as peas [28]. The rheological properties of pea flour, including the gelation properties of starch, may be considered when exploring the potential application of pea flour in baked goods. Recent uses for pulses could increase the demand for pulses with specific nutritional and rheological properties, which will increase the need to investigate the components affecting the nutritional and functional properties of pulses. It was previously demonstrated that low-phytate pea lines had higher Fe bioavailability than regular or standard pea [29]; in addition, pea varieties which were low-phytate combined with relatively higher carotenoid concentration in some cases resulted in a further increase in Fe bioavailability in vitro [30].

Biofortified staple foods are an effective instrument through which to address micronutrient deficiencies worldwide, with emphasis on Fe and Zn, in numerous target populations [1,31–35].

The in vivo (*Gallus gallus*) model was established as an excellent model to assess dietary Fe and Zn bioavailability [33–39]. Hence, the objective of the current study was to evaluate the ability of low-phytate pea varieties in the context of a complete meal to improve Fe bioavailability and absorption, physiological status, intestinal BBM functionality, and intestinal microbial populations in vivo (*Gallus gallus*). We suggest the further use of in vivo screening model to guide future studies aimed to investigate biofortified staple food crops, as this method will allow proceeding to human efficacy studies with superior confidence and success.

2. Materials and Methods

2.1. Plants Materials—University of Saskatchewan Pea Varieties

The pea varieties evaluated in this research arose from the Crop Development Center, University of Saskatchewan (Canada) pea breeding program (Figure 1). Low-phytate line 1-2347-144 was derived from cultivar CDC Bronco [39,40] through chemical mutagenesis [41]. Varieties 4802-8-46Y-L, 4802-8-60G-L, and 4802-8-87Y-L resulted from the cross 1-2347-144/CDC 2235-4 made in 2011. CDC 2235-4 was later registered as CDC Raezer [42]. Variety 4803-4-78G-L resulted from the cross 1-150-81/CDC 2336-1 made in 2011. Line 1-150-81 is a second low-phytate line derived from CDC Bronco [41]. CDC 2336-1 was later registered as CDC Limerick [43]. The varieties from crosses 4802 and 4803 were previously described [30].

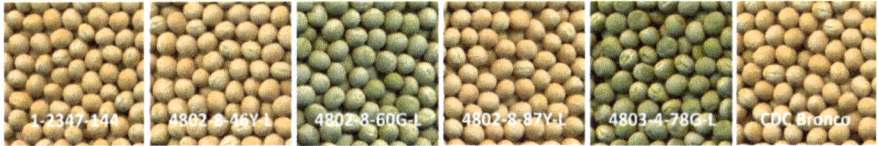

Figure 1. High-resolution photographs depicting six varieties used to evaluate the iron bioavailability of the Saskatchewan peas. To compare the differences in seed sizes, all photographs were taken to scale under standardized lighting conditions.

2.2. Growing Conditions and Post-Harvest Handling

All six pea varieties that were used in this experiment were grown at the Sutherland farm, located 10 km east of Saskatoon (Canada), with planting in May 2017 and harvest in August 2017. The harvested samples were stored in a non-heated warehouse, with temperature ranging between 15 and 20 °C based on the season, until shipment to Ithaca for dietary processing.

2.3. Ingredient Preparation and Diet Composition

For this study, raw pea seeds were rinsed and cleaned thoroughly in distilled water to remove dust, debris, and non-edible material. Peas were pre-soaked in distilled water (1:6 *w/w*) for 12 h at room temperature prior to cooking. Peas were cooked in boiling distilled water in stainless-steel steam kettles. Cooked peas were then stored at −20 °C for 24 h prior to freeze-drying (VirTis Research Equipment, Gardiner, NY, USA). Basmati rice and wheat were purchased from a local food store located in Ithaca, New York, USA. Our rationale with regard to the inclusion of basmati rice, wheat, and carrots in the tested pea-based diets was to approximately simulate the ingredients of a pea-based meal in India, which is one of the key consumers of pea, and where dietary Fe deficiency is a major health concern. Cooked rice was stored at −20 °C for 24 h before freeze-drying. Cooked/air-dried carrots were purchased from North Bay Trading Co. (Brule, WI, USA). Dried ingredients were milled into a course powder using a Waring Commercial® CB15 stainless-steel blender (Torrington, CT, USA). Other dietary ingredients included chicken Vitamin Mixture (#330002) and chicken Mineral Mix (#230000, no added iron) (Dyets Inc., Bethlehem, PA, USA), DL-methionine, and choline chloride (Sigma-Aldrich, St. Louis, MO, USA). The compositions of the experimental diets are shown in Table 1

2.4. Iron Analysis

Iron analysis was conducted as previously described [14,33,36,38,39]. For the analysis, a 500-mg sample of dietary ingredient, a 500-mg sample of pea-based diets, or a 100-mg sample of tissue (wet weight) was analyzed.

2.5. Phytate Analysis

Phytate (phytic acid) determination was conducted as previously described [14,33–39]. For the analysis, a 500-mg sample of dietary ingredients and a 500-mg of pea-based diets were analyzed, according to a phosphorous kit (K-PHYT; Megazyme International, Ireland).

2.6. Protein and Fiber Analysis

Analysis was conducted as previously described [36,43–45].

2.7. Animals and Feeding Trial Design

Cornish-cross fertile broiler eggs were delivered from a commercial hatchery (Moyer's Chicks, Quakertown, PA, USA). The eggs were incubated under ideal conditions at the Cornell University Animal Science poultry farm incubator. Upon hatch (hatchability = 98%), hatchlings were arbitrarily divided into seven treatment groups (n = 15) (Table 1), with ad libitum access to food and water (Fe concentration < 0.4 µg/L). Chicks were kept in a total confinement building (two animals per 1-m^2 metal cage) under controlled temperature and humidity with 16 h of light. Cages were equipped with an automatic watering system and a manual self-feeder. Feed intakes were documented daily, and, as of day of hatch, body weights were documented weekly. Animal protocols were approved by the Cornell University Institutional Animal Care and Use Committee (protocol number 2007-0129).

2.7.1. Blood Collection, Hemoglobin, and Physiological Fe Status Parameters

Blood samples were collected and hemoglobin (Hb) assays were conducted according to the Hb kit manufacturer's instructions (BioAssay Systems, Hayward, CA, USA). Total body hemoglobin Fe (Hb-Fe), a parameter of iron absorption, was calculated from Hb concentrations and blood volume according to specific body weight (85 mL per kg of body weight) [33–36,39,46].

Hemoglobin maintenance efficiency (HME) was calculated as the cumulative difference in total body Hb Fe from the start of the study, divided by total dietary Fe intake. [33–36,39,46].

Upon the conclusion of the study (42 days), animals were euthanized by CO_2 exposure and blood, small intestine, cecum, and liver samples were collected. Tissue samples were instantly frozen in liquid nitrogen and stored at −80 °C in a freezer until analyzed.

2.7.2. Liver Iron and Ferritin

The quantifications of liver Fe and ferritin were conducted as previously described [46–48].

2.7.3. Isolation of Total RNA from Duodenum

Total RNA extraction was conducted as previously described [14,33–39,46,49], according to the manufacturer's protocol (RNeasy Mini Kit, Qiagen Inc., Valencia, CA, USA).

2.7.4. Real-Time Polymerase Chain Reaction (RT-PCR)

The complementary DNA (cDNA) reaction was conducted as previously described (BioRad C1000 touch thermocycler using the Improm-II Reverse Transcriptase Kit, Promega Corp., Madison, WI, USA) [37–39].

Table 1. Composition of the experimental pea-based diets [1].

Ingredient [1]	Iron (µg/g) [2]	Dietary Formulation (g/kg)						
		1-2347-144	4803-4-78G-L	4802-8-46Y-L	4802-8-60G-L	4802-8-87Y-L	CDC Bronco	No Pea
1-2347-144	37.687 ± 0.106 [a]	500	–	–	–	–	–	–
4803-4-78G-L	42.512 ± 0.388 [b]	–	500	–	–	–	–	–
4802-8-46Y-L	41.277 ± 0.258 [c]	–	–	500	–	–	–	–
4802-8-60G-L	38.020 ± 0.275 [d]	–	–	–	500	–	–	–
4802-8-87Y-L	39.539 ± 0.285 [d]	–	–	–	–	500	–	–
CDC Bronco	39.850 ± 0.283 [d]	–	–	–	–	–	500	–
No pea	–	–	–	–	–	–	–	400
Wheat (whole)	43.863 ± 0.320	150	150	150	150	150	150	400
Basmati rice	4.367 ± 0.028	150	150	150	150	150	150	50
Carrots	25.717 ± 4.762	50	50	50	50	50	50	50
Milk powder	1.742 ± 0.103	50	50	50	50	50	50	70
Vitamin/mineral premix [3]	0.00 ± 0.0	70	70	70	70	70	70	30
Oil	0.00 ± 0.0	30	30	30	30	30	30	2.5
DL-Methionine	0.00 ± 0.0	2.5	2.5	2.5	2.5	2.5	2.5	0.75
Choline chloride	0.00 ± 0.0	0.75	0.75	0.75	0.75	0.75	0.75	1000
Total composition (g)		1000	1000	1000	1000	1000	1000	
Pea Only Analysis [4]								
Phytate concentration (mg/g)		3.96 ± 0.04 [d]	3.74 ± 0.05 [e]	4.38 ± 0.01 [c]	4.76 ± 0.04 [b]	3.84 ± 0.05 [de]	5.82 ± 0.01 [a]	–
Phytate–iron molar ratio		8.90 [c]	7.44 [e]	8.98 [c]	10.59 [b]	8.21 [d]	12.36 [a]	–
Dietary Analysis [4]								
Iron concentration (µg/g)		35.717 ± 0.378 [b]	39.473 ± 1.089 [a]	36.017 ± 0.370 [b]	36.274 ± 0.302 [b]	38.087 ± 0.448 [ab]	37.208 ± 0.157 [ab]	27.603 ± 1.754 [c]
Phytate concentration (mg/g)		1.57 ± 0.01 [e]	2.30 ± 0.32 [c]	2.62 ± 0.04 [c]	2.34 ± 0.32 [c]	3.03 ± 0.10 [b]	3.32 ± 0.08 [a]	1.88 ± 0.14 [d]
Phytate–iron molar ratio		3.71 [d]	4.93 [cd]	5.52 [bc]	5.46 [bc]	6.73 [ab]	7.55 [a]	5.75 [bc]

[1] Food constituents were cooked, drained, and lyophilized before milling and for chemical analysis. [2] Values are means ± SEM ($n = 5$). [3] Vitamin and mineral premix: #330,002 Chick vitamin mixture; #230,000 Salt mix (no iron) for chick diet (Dyets Inc., Bethlehem, PA, USA). [4] Values are means ± SEM of five replicates for each of the pea-based diets. [a–e] Treatment groups not indicated by the same letter are significantly different ($p \leq 0.05$).

2.7.5. Primer Design for Duodenal Gene Expression

Primers sequences were designed and selected using the Real-Time Primer Design Tool software (IDT DNA, Coralvilla, IA, USA). The *Gallus gallus* primers (forward/reverse) that were used in this study are indicated in Table 2.

Table 2. Sequences of primers used in this study.

Gene [1]	Forward Primer (5′–3′)	Reverse Primer (5′–3′)	Length (bp)	GI ID
DMT-1	TTGATTCAGAGCCTCCCATTAG	GCGAGGAGTAGGCTTGTATTT	101	206597489
Ferroportin	CTCAGCAATCACTGGCATCA	ACTGGGCAACTCCAGAAATAAG	98	61098365
DcytB	CATGTGCATTCTCTTCCAAAGTC	CTCCTTGGTGACCGCATTAT	103	20380692
ZnT1	GGTAACAGAGCTGCCTTAACT	GGTAACAGAGCTGCCTTAACT	105	54109718
AP	CGTCAGCCAGTTTGACTATGTA	CTCTCAAAGAAGCTGAGGATGG	138	45382360
SGLT-1	GCATCCTTACTCTGTGGTACTG	TATCCGCACATCACACATCC	106	8346783
SI	CCAGCAATGCCAGCATATTG	CGGTTTCTCCTTACCACTTCTT	95	2246388
18S rRNA	GCAAGACGAACTAAAGCGAAAG	TCGGAACTACGACGGTATCT	100	7262899

[1] DMT-1, divalent metal transporter-1; DcytB, duodenal cytochrome b; ZnT1, zinc transporter 1; AP, amino peptidase; SGLT-1, sodium-glucose transporter-1; SI, sucrose isomaltase; 18S rRNA, 18S ribosomal RNA subunit.

2.7.6. Real-Time qPCR Design

Isolated cDNA was used for the reaction (Cat. #1725274, Hercules, CA, USA) as previously indicated [36–39].

2.7.7. Collection of Microbial Samples and DNA Isolation of Intestinal Contents

The cecum was removed and stored at −80°C until analyzed. Microbial DNA isolation was conducted as previously described [36–38].

2.7.8. Primer Design and PCR Amplification of Bacterial 16S rRNA

Primers for *Bifidobacterium*, *Lactobacillus*, *Escherichia coli*, and *Clostridium* were used in accordance with previously published data [46].

2.7.9. Glycogen Analysis

At the conclusion of the study (day 42), the pectoral muscle (200 mg) was removed, and glycogen contents were determined as previously described [50–52].

2.8. Statistical Analysis

Statistical analyses were conducted using IBM SPSS Statistics 25 (IBM Analytics, Armonk, NY, USA). Measured parameters were found to have a normal distribution and equal variance, and they were acceptable for ANOVA. Mean separations for measured parameters were determined using ANOVA with the model including dietary treatment (seven levels) as the fixed effect, followed by a Duncan post hoc test. Differences with p-values ≤0.05 were considered statistically significant.

3. Results

3.1. Seed Iron and Phytate Concentrations in Experimental Peas Varieties

Iron concentrations of dietary ingredients are shown in Table 1. Differences in seed Fe contents in the pea varieties were significant ($p \leq 0.05$), ranging from 37 µg/g in 1-2347-144 to 42 µg/g in 4803-4-78G-L (Table 1). Phytate concentrations and molar ratios of dietary ingredients of the pea-based diets are indicated in Table 1. Significant ($p \leq 0.05$) differences in phytate concentrations were measured between peas varieties, from 3.7 mg/g in 4803-4-78G-L to 5.82 mg/g in CDC Bronco (Table 1). Phytate-to-Fe molar ratios varied significantly ($p \leq 0.05$), from a ratio of 7.4 in 4803-4-78G-L to a ratio of 12.4 in CDC Bronco (Table 1).

3.2. Protein and Fiber Contents

Table 3 indicates the total crude protein content in experimental tested pea varieties, with significant differences ($p \leq 0.05$) between pea varieties, ranging from 22.5 g/100 g in CDC Bronco to 26.75 g/100 g in 4803-4-78G-L. Concentrations of insoluble, soluble, and total fiber for experimental peas are shown in Table 3, with significant differences ($p \leq 0.05$) in each of the fiber fractions between experimental peas. The lowest concentrations of the insoluble, soluble, and total fiber were detected in the 4803-4-78G-L pea variety. Significantly ($p \leq 0.05$) higher concentrations of all three fiber fractions were measured in 1-2347-144. As a reference, the total protein content in the control diet (no pea) was measured at 10.72 g/100 g ± 0.16 g/100 g of total protein.

Table 3. Protein and fiber concentrations (g/100 g) of tested peas varieties [1].

Variety	Insoluble Fiber	Soluble Fiber	Total Fiber	Total Protein
1-2347-144	22.37 ± 1.26 [a]	1.31 ± 0.18 [a]	23.68 ± 1.43 [a]	22.69 ± 0.06 [d]
4803-4-78G-L	16.49 ± 1.32 [c]	0.94 ± 0.39 [a]	17.43 ± 1.71 [c]	26.75 ± 0.35 [a]
4802-8-46Y-L	19.52 ± 1.10 [abc]	1.08 ± 0.06 [a]	20.60 ± 1.05 [abc]	23.22 ± 0.31 [c]
4802-8-60G-L	20.20 ± 1.87 [ab]	1.12 ± 0.30 [a]	21.32 ± 2.17 [abc]	22.94 ± 0.09 [cd]
4802-8-87Y-L	17.94 ± 0.12 [bc]	1.13 ± 0.26 [a]	19.07 ± 0.14 [bc]	24.78 ± 0.13 [b]
CDC Bronco	20.66 ± 1.93 [ab]	1.30 ± 0.16 [a]	21.97 ± 1.77 [ab]	22.50 ± 0.90 [d]

[1] Values are means ± standard error of the mean (SEM) (n = 3 replicates). [a–d] Treatment groups not indicated by the same letter are significantly different ($p \leq 0.05$).

3.3. Iron–Phytate Analysis of Pea Based Diets

The final composition of the six pea-based diets and no-pea diet are shown in Table 3. Iron concentrations amongst the pea-based diets were significantly different ($p \leq 0.05$). Diets formulated from 4802-8-87Y-L and 4803-4-78G-L had the highest iron concentrations (38 µg/g and 39 µg/g, respectively) relative to the control diet (no-pea diet) (27 µg/g). Final phytate concentrations also varied between experimental diets ranging from 1.57 mg/g in 1-2347-144 to 2.66 mg/g in the no-pea diet. Significant ($p \leq 0.05$) differences in phytate–Fe molar ratios were observed between the pea-based diets, ranging from 3.79 mg/g in 1-2347-144 to 8.66 mg/g in CDC Bronco (Table 1).

3.4. In Vivo Assay (Gallus gallus Feeding Trial)

3.4.1. Growth Rates, Hemoglobin (Hb), Total Body Hemoglobin Fe (Hb-Fe), and Hemoglobin Maintenance Efficiency (HME)

Feed intakes and Fe intakes were higher ($p < 0.05$) in all pea-based dietary treatment groups relative to the no-pea dietary treatment group (Tables 4 and 5).

Table 4. Experimental cumulative feed intake [1].

	Feed Intake (g)					
Pea Diet	Day 7	Day 14	Day 21	Day 28	Day 35	Day 42
1-2347-144	329.6 ± 26.7 [a]	699.2 ± 55.4 [a]	1210.9 ± 120.7 [a]	1773.1 ± 105.8 [a]	2511.2 ± 86.4 [a]	3272.1 ± 115.6 [a]
4803-4-78G-L	331.1 ± 21.2 [a]	706.7 ± 50.6 [a]	1229.6 ± 95.6 [a]	1579.6 ± 328.0 [a]	2370.9 ± 348.9 [a]	3266.8 ± 340.3 [a]
4802-8-46Y-L	390.8 ± 11.6 [a]	797.7 ± 58.5 [a]	1420.9 ± 134.6 [a]	2051.6 ± 180.1 [a]	2822.3 ± 230.4 [a]	3691.3 ± 225.5 [a]
4802-8-60G-L	351.6 ± 7.8 [a]	729.8 ± 17.8 [a]	1283.5 ± 30.3 [a]	1898.6 ± 5.8 [a]	2698.8 ± 13.1 [a]	3644.7 ± 35.7 [a]
4802-8-87Y-L	370.4 ± 17.1 [a]	742.0 ± 74.2 [a]	1312.2 ± 158.6 [a]	1934.7 ± 167.2 [a]	2781.9 ± 182.2 [a]	3769.6 ± 186.9 [a]
CDC Bronco	353.3 ± 12.2 [a]	735.1 ± 28.9 [a]	1299.4 ± 73.6 [a]	1901.0 ± 56.6 [a]	2664.4 ± 49.8 [a]	3530.4 ± 60.9 [a]
No pea	224.6 ± 29.1 [b]	293.9 ± 28.8 [b]	428.3 ± 48.2 [b]	609.5 ± 66.3 [b]	799.5 ± 105.2 [b]	930.6 ± 133.1 [b]

[1] Values are means ± SEM (n = 15 animals per treatment group). [a,b] Treatment groups not indicated by the same letter are significantly different ($p \leq 0.05$).

Table 5. Experimental cumulative iron intake [1].

Pea Diet	Iron Intake (mg)					
	Day 7	Day 14	Day 21	Day 28	Day 35	Day 42
1-2347-144	11.77 ± 0.95 [b]	24.97 ± 1.98 [a]	43.25 ± 4.31 [a]	63.33 ± 3.78 [a]	89.69 ± 3.09 [a]	116.87 ± 4.13 [b]
4803-4-78G-L	13.07 ± 0.84 [ab]	27.89 ± 2.00 [a]	48.53 ± 3.78 [a]	62.35 ± 12.95 [a]	93.59 ± 13.77 [a]	128.95 ± 13.43 [ab]
4802-8-46Y-L	14.07 ± 0.42 [a]	28.73 ± 2.11 [a]	51.18 ± 4.85 [a]	73.89 ± 6.49 [a]	101.65 ± 8.30 [a]	132.95 ± 8.13 [ab]
4802-8-60G-L	12.75 ± 0.28 [ab]	26.47 ± 0.65 [a]	46.56 ± 1.10 [a]	68.87 ± 0.21 [a]	97.89 ± 0.48 [a]	132.21 ± 1.29 [ab]
4802-8-87Y-L	14.11 ± 0.65 [a]	28.26 ± 2.83 [a]	49.98 ± 6.04 [a]	73.69 ± 6.37 [a]	105.96 ± 6.94 [a]	143.57 ± 7.12 [a]
CDC Bronco	13.14 ± 0.46 [a]	27.35 ± 1.07 [a]	48.35 ± 2.74 [a]	70.73 ± 2.11 [a]	99.14 ± 1.85 [a]	131.36 ± 2.27 [ab]
No pea	6.20 ± 0.80 [c]	8.11 ± 0.80 [b]	11.82 ± 1.33 [b]	16.82 ± 1.83 [b]	22.07 ± 2.18 [b]	25.69 ± 3.67 [c]

[1] Values are means ± SEM (n = 15 animals per treatment group). [a–c] Treatment groups not indicated by the same letter are significantly different ($p \leq 0.05$).

Also, as from day 35 of the study, body weights were consistently higher ($p < 0.05$) in several of the low phytate pea based dietary groups (4803-4-78G-L, and 4802-8-87Y-L), relative to the CDC Bronco and no-pea dietary groups (Table 6). Hemoglobin (Hb) values did not differ between treatment groups; however, significant differences in total body Hb-Fe, a physiological biomarker of Fe bioavailability and status, were detected as of week five of the study (Table 7), demonstrating an improvement in Fe status in the 4802-8-87Y-L group, relative to CDC Bronco and no-pea diet groups. In addition, the standard pea variety treatment group (CDC Bronco) had a lower HME ($p < 0.05$) at each time point when compared to the group receiving the lower-phytate pea-based diets (groups 1-2347-144, 4803-4-78G-L), indicating a higher dietary Fe bioavailability and increased absorbable Fe (Table 8).

Table 6. Experimental body weights [1].

Pea Diet	Body Weights (kg)					
	Day 7	Day 14	Day 21	Day 28	Day 35	Day 42
1-2347-144	0.133 ± 0.004 [a]	0.327 ± 0.010 [a]	0.547 ± 0.009 [a]	0.904 ± 0.031 [b]	1.326 ± 0.082 [bc]	1.820 ± 0.130 [b]
4803-4-78G-L	0.137 ± 0.006 [a]	0.334 ± 0.013 [a]	0.576 ± 0.022 [a]	0.997 ± 0.037 [ab]	1.447 ± 0.058 [ab]	2.040 ± 0.100 [ab]
4802-8-46Y-L	0.137 ± 0.011 [a]	0.337 ± 0.025 [a]	0.578 ± 0.043 [a]	0.994 ± 0.067 [ab]	1.384 ± 0.085 [bc]	1.880 ± 0.110 [ab]
4802-8-60G-L	0.136 ± 0.005 [a]	0.334 ± 0.026 [a]	0.563 ± 0.044 [a]	0.974 ± 0.050 [ab]	1.393 ± 0.076 [bc]	1.930 ± 0.110 [ab]
4802-8-87Y-L	0.131 ± 0.006 [a]	0.322 ± 0.016 [a]	0.561 ± 0.037 [a]	1.024 ± 0.049 [a]	1.536 ± 0.059 [a]	2.140 ± 0.070 [a]
CDC Bronco	0.131 ± 0.002 [a]	0.317 ± 0.006 [a]	0.541 ± 0.008 [a]	0.922 ± 0.019 [b]	1.300 ± 0.006 [c]	1.840 ± 0.020 [b]
No pea	0.072 ± 0.003 [b]	0.090 ± 0.005 [b]	0.118 ± 0.006 [b]	0.161 ± 0.009 [c]	0.201 ± 0.011 [d]	0.240 ± 0.010 [c]

[1] Values are means ± SEM (n = 15 animals per treatment group). [a–d] Treatment groups not indicated by the same letter are significantly different ($p \leq 0.05$). Body weights averaged 38 g at the start of the experiment.

Table 7. Experimental total body hemoglobin iron (Hb-Fe) [1].

Pea Diet	Hb-Fe (mg)			
	Day 7	Day 21	Day 35	Day 42
1-2347-144	4.981 ± 0.152 [a]	20.845 ± 0.339 [a]	55.186 ± 3.392 [bc]	97.790 ± 7.150 [b]
4803-4-78G-L	5.496 ± 0.245 [a]	23.452 ± 0.914 [a]	56.839 ± 2.276 [ab]	107.280 ± 5.140 [ab]
4802-8-46Y-L	5.539 ± 0.444 [a]	22.967 ± 1.727 [a]	51.886 ± 3.200 [bc]	96.610 ± 5.600 [ab]
4802-8-60G-L	5.301 ± 0.207 [a]	21.814 ± 1.668 [a]	48.939 ± 2.659 [bc]	96.980 ± 5.480 [ab]
4802-8-87Y-L	4.730 ± 0.223 [a]	19.886 ± 1.314 [a]	57.088 ± 2.198 [a]	116.910 ± 3.590 [a]
CDC Bronco	4.177 ± 0.062 [a]	17.249 ± 0.268 [a]	45.414 ± 0.209 [c]	100.450 ± 1.250 [b]
No pea	2.354 ± 0.090 [b]	4.048 ± 0.206 [b]	6.447 ± 0.348 [d]	9.480 ± 0.550 [c]

[1] Values are means ± SEM (n = 15 animals per treatment group). [a–d] Treatment groups not indicated by the same letter are significantly different ($p \leq 0.05$). Total body hemoglobin iron averaged 0.65 milligrams at the start of the experiment.

Table 8. Experimental hemoglobin maintenance efficacy (HME) [1].

Pea Diet	HME (%)		
	Day 21	Day 35	Day 42
1-2347-144	37.44 ± 3.81 [a]	56.21 ± 4.66 [a]	80.58 ± 8.13 [a]
4803-4-78G-L	39.82 ± 3.85 [a]	57.37 ± 8.61 [a]	78.90 ± 7.61 [a]
4802-8-46Y-L	34.35 ± 2.52 [ab]	45.72 ± 0.79 [ab]	70.18 ± 0.23 [ab]
4802-8-60G-L	37.29 ± 4.09 [a]	44.56 ± 2.31 [ab]	71.66 ± 4.45 [ab]
4802-8-87Y-L	32.22 ± 2.51 [ab]	49.66 ± 2.29 [ab]	61.10 ± 1.26 [b]
CDC Bronco	27.24 ± 1.85 [b]	41.63 ± 0.96 [b]	62.92 ± 1.40 [b]
No pea	14.57 ± 1.33 [c]	19.04 ± 2.18 [c]	28.53 ± 3.03 [c]

[1] Values are means ± SEM ($n = 15$ animals per treatment group). [a–c] Treatment groups not indicated by the same letter are significantly different ($p \leq 0.05$).

3.4.2. Hepatic Iron and Ferritin Concentrations

The contents of liver iron and ferritin (day 42) are shown in Table 9. Significant ($p \leq 0.05$) differences in liver iron were detected among the seven treatment groups with concentrations ranging from 73 µg/g in the group receiving the 4803-4-78G-L diet to 96 µg/g in the 1-2347-144 diet. Significant ($p \leq 0.05$) differences in liver ferritin concentrations were also measured between the seven dietary treatment groups (Table 9).

Table 9. Hepatic iron and ferritin protein concentrations [1].

Pea Diet	Liver Iron (µg/g)	Liver Ferritin (AU)
1-2347-144	96.49 ± 6.52 [a]	1.078 ± 0.014 [a]
4803-4-78G-L	73.30 ± 7.58 [b]	1.084 ± 0.015 [a]
4802-8-46Y-L	77.61 ± 17.72 [b]	1.063 ± 0.009 [a]
4802-8-60G-L	87.46 ± 4.98 [ab]	1.050 ± 0.005 [a]
4802-8-87Y-L	71.88 ± 4.79 [b]	0.469 ± 0.160 [b]
CDC Bronco	91.34 ± 9.79 [ab]	0.257 ± 0.017 [c]
No pea	75.71 ± 6.29 [b]	0.280 ± 0.007 [c]

[1] Values are means ± SEM ($n = 12$ animals per treatment group). [a–c] Treatment groups not indicated by the same letter are significantly different ($p \leq 0.05$). Total iron concentrations were measured as micrograms per gram of liver tissue (wet weight). Liver ferritin concentrations were measured as arbitrary units of liver tissue (wet weight).

3.4.3. Serum Iron Concentrations

Significant differences ($p \leq 0.05$) in serum iron concentrations were detected on day 21 and 35 of the study. On day 21, the lowest concentration of serum iron was 1.526 µg/µL in the no-pea dietary group, while the highest concentration was in the 4802-8-87Y-L pea-based dietary group (2.812 µg/µL). On day 35, the lowest concentration of serum iron was 1.488 µg/µL (no-pea dietary group), while the highest concentration was detected in the 4803-4-78G-L dietary group (2.633 µg/µL) (Table 10).

Table 10. Serum iron concentrations [1].

Pea Diet	Serum Iron (µg/µL)			
	Day 7	Day 21	Day 35	Day 42
1-2347-144	2.089 ± 0.161 [a]	1.682 ± 0.120 [b]	2.226 ± 0.243 [ab]	2.116 ± 0.183 [a]
4803-4-78G-L	1.604 ± 0.108 [a]	2.322 ± 0.198 [ab]	2.633 ± 0.451 [a]	2.104 ± 0.280 [a]
4802-8-46Y-L	3.029 ± 0.636 [a]	2.596 ± 0.700 [ab]	1.795 ± 0.225 [b]	2.349 ± 0.289 [a]
4802-8-60G-L	2.383 ± 0.282 [a]	2.058 ± 0.170 [b]	1.583 ± 0.106 [b]	2.240 ± 0.218 [a]
4802-8-87Y-L	2.767 ± 0.774 [a]	2.812 ± 0.425 [a]	1.578 ± 0.144 [b]	2.132 ± 0.178 [a]
CDC Bronco	1.936 ± 0.237 [a]	1.829 ± 0.223 [b]	1.670 ± 0.190 [b]	2.292 ± 0.224 [a]
No pea	2.248 ± 0.490 [a]	1.526 ± 0.215 [ab]	1.488 ± 0.088 [b]	2.105 ± 0.187 [a]

[1] Values are means ± SEM ($n = 12$ animals per treatment group). [a,b] Treatment groups not indicated by the same letter are significantly different ($p \leq 0.05$).

3.4.4. Glycogen Concentrations in Pectoral Muscle

As an indicator of energetic status [52,53], pectoral muscle glycogen concentrations were measured on days 21 and 42 of the study (Table 11). No significant differences were detected on day 21; however, significant differences ($p \leq 0.05$) were measured on day 42 in the abundance of glycogen stored in pectoral muscles. The highest values of glycogen were in the 4802-8-60G-L pea-based dietary group, and the lowest concentration of glycogen was in the no-pea dietary group.

Table 11. Pectoral muscle glycogen concentrations (AU) [1].

Pea Diet	Day 21	Day 42
1-2347-144	0.020 ± 0.012 [a]	0.044 ± 0.010 [ab]
4803-4-78G-L	0.023 ± 0.012 [a]	0.037 ± 0.006 [b]
4802-8-46Y-L	0.040 ± 0.011 [a]	0.041 ± 0.026 [ab]
4802-8-60G-L	0.031 ± 0.008 [a]	0.055 ± 0.011 [a]
4802-8-87Y-L	0.024 ± 0.007 [a]	0.053 ± 0.005 [a]
CDC Bronco	0.029 ± 0.034 [a]	0.034 ± 0.003 [a]
No pea	0.023 ± 0.004 [a]	0.033 ± 0.008 [b]

[1] Values are means ± SEM (n = 5 animals per treatment group). [a,b] Treatment groups not indicated by the same letter are significantly different ($p \leq 0.05$). Glycogen concentrations were measured as milligrams per milliliter of pectoral tissue (wet weight).

3.4.5. Duodenal Gene Expression

The duodenal gene expression of iron- and zinc-related proteins, as well as BBM functional proteins, is shown in Figure 2. Significant ($p \leq 0.05$) differences in the expression of DcytB and ferroportin were identified, with no significant differences in divalent metal transporter-1 (DMT1) expression between treatment groups.

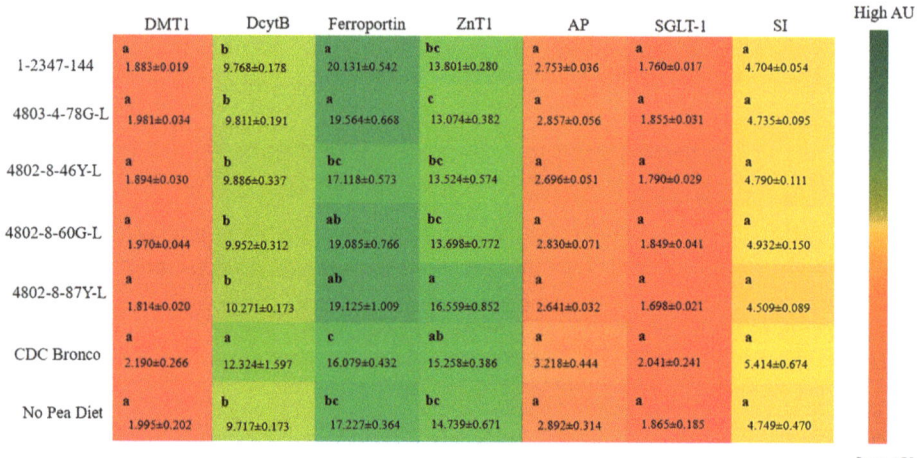

Figure 2. Gene expression of iron proteins in the duodenum after six weeks of consuming pea-based diets. Values are means ± SEM (n = 10 per treatment group). [a–c] Treatment groups not indicated by the same letter are significantly different (p < 0.05). DMT-1, divalent metal transporter-1; DcytB, duodenal cytochrome b; ZnT1, zinc transporter 1; AP, amino peptidase; SGLT-1, sodium-glucose transporter 1; SI, sucrose isomaltase.

3.4.6. Cecum Content Bacterial Populations Analysis

As shown in Figure 3, the relative abundance of *Bifidobacterium* was significantly higher (p < 0.05) in the 4802-8-87Y-L and CDC Bronco groups relative to all other treatment groups. Furthermore, the abundance of *Lactobacillus* was significantly higher ($p < 0.05$) in the 1-2347-144 and 4803-4-78G-L groups relative to all other treatment groups.

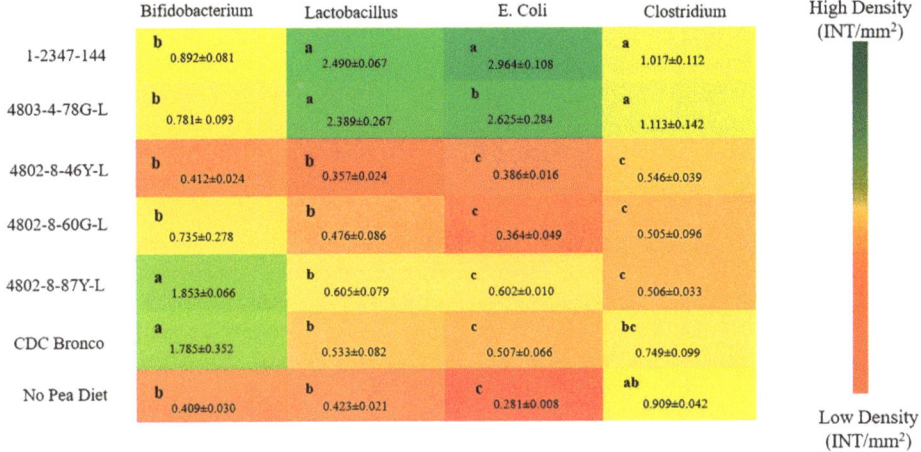

Figure 3. Genus- and species-level bacterial populations (AU) from cecal contents after six weeks of consuming pea-based diets. Values are means ± SEM ($n = 10$ per treatment group). [a–c] Treatment groups not indicated by the same letter are significantly different ($p < 0.05$).

4. Discussion

The objective of the current study was to investigate the effects of low-phytate peas, in the context of a complete meal, on Fe bioavailability, absorption, physiological status, intestinal BBM functionality, and gastrointestinal microbial populations in vivo (*Gallus gallus*).

In studies of biofortification, the process via which the nutritional quality of food crops is improved through agronomic practices, conventional plant breeding, or modern biotechnology [2], it is necessary and advantageous to utilize in vivo screening tools that are capable of assessing biofortified varieties of staple crops, as well as in relation to the diet in which they are consumed [1,33,36,38,39,46,54–56]. The present study, for the first time, presents a demonstration of how the *Gallus gallus* model of Fe (and Zn) bioavailability could be useful in the design of the current study aimed at assessing the potential nutritional benefit of lower-phytate versus standard peas. The chosen dietary composition was specifically formulated in accordance to a potential target population (Indian/Bangladeshi pea-based dal meal), similar to previous in vivo studies aimed at assessing dietary Fe bioavailability in beans [35,55] and wheat [38] (Table 1). Overall, our data agree with previously published knowledge [1,39,49,55], demonstrating that this in vivo screening approach is effective in the evaluation process of nutritional qualities of the low-phytate pea varieties. Furthermore, the data suggested that lower-phytate pea-based diets were able to moderately improve Fe physiological status in vivo.

Peas are a common staple food crop consumed worldwide, primarily in India, China, Russia, Ethiopia, and Bangladesh. Global dry pea production increased from 9.9 million tons in 2012 to 16.2 million tons in 2017 [7]. Currently, the leading producers are Canada, Russia, China, Ukraine, and India. In Canada, a leading producer and exporter of dry peas, pea was grown on 1.6 million ha in western Canada (Saskatchewan, Alberta, and Manitoba) in 2017, indicating a significant alteration in cropping practices from the 300 ha reported in 1967. Pea was the major alternative crop as farmers shifted toward a more diversified crop production. Pea varieties (yellow and green cotyledon) are grown, with an average of 80% production in yellow cotyledon varieties. The five-year (2013–2017) average pea yield in western Canada is 2.6 tons/ha (38 bu/ac) [57]. As for their nutritional value, it was previously demonstrated that pea seeds are high in protein, carbohydrates, fiber, B vitamins, and minerals (potassium, magnesium, calcium, iron), and they are considered an inexpensive source of energy-dense, nutrient-rich food [58–60]. In addition, pea seeds are low in fat and cholesterol-free. Because of these nutritional benefits, worldwide pea utilization is expected to continue to grow.

Plant seeds, such as pea, contain a high concentration of phosphorus. However, about 60–80% of the total phosphorus in seeds is stored in the form of phytate, a mixed-cation salt of phytic acid [59]. This introduces a nutritional challenge, as negatively charged sites of phytic acid bind and form salts with K^+, Mg^{2+}, Ca^{2+}, Mn^{2+}, Zn^{2+}, or Fe^{3+} [61]. Phytate causes multiple difficulties, as non-ruminant animals including pig, poultry, fish, and humans, are unable to digest phytate due to lack of a phytase enzyme [61]; as a result, important micronutrients (as Zn^{2+} and Fe^{3+}) bound to phytate are also excreted and not absorbed, potentially leading to micronutrient deficiencies [62]. Recently, the development of cultivars with low-phytate content became an effective approach to potentially reducing nutritional concerns ascending from the consumption of phytate-rich grains. Low-phytate varieties were chemically persuaded in maize (*Zea mays* L.) [63], soybean (*Glycine max* (L.) Merr.) [64], barley (*Hordeum vulgare* L.) [63,65], rice (*Oryza sativa* L.) [66], wheat (*Triticum aestivum* L.) [67], bean (*Phaseolus vulgaris* L.) [68], and pea [41]. The concentration of phytate phosphorus is significantly reduced in the mutants with an associated increase in available phosphorus. Wilcox et al. [65] reported an 80% reduction in phytate phosphorus content in a low-phytate soybean mutant, as compared with its nonmutant sibling, and this reduction was matched by an equal increase in inorganic phosphorus.

It was previously demonstrated that low-phytate crops increase the bioavailability of phosphorus and several important nutritional cations, including Fe. These crops could assist in increasing the health of a large proportion of the global population, which is dietary Fe-deficient, primarily in target regions where dietary peas are consumed regularly. For example, in a previous study focused on the nutritional evaluation of low-phytate pea diets in vivo, it was demonstrated that animals fed the low-phosphorus diets had lower weight gain and feed intake ($p < 0.01$) than those fed the higher phosphorus level. Bone strength was higher ($p < 0.01$) for animals fed diets based on low-phytate pea than for those fed diets based on normal pea or soybean meal. The authors concluded that increasing the availability of the phosphorus in peas could mean that less inorganic phosphorus would be required in order to meet the nutritional requirements of broilers [59].

In the context of the current study, the results indicated that, despite Hb levels not being significantly higher in the lower-phytate pea groups, significant differences in total body Hb-Fe, the physiological Fe status biomarker [33–36,39,46,55], were observed (Table 8), representing an enhancement in Fe status in the 4802-8-87Y-L dietary group, relative to CDC Bronco and the no-pea dietary group. In addition, the standard pea variety (CDC Bronco) treatment group had a lower HME ($p < 0.05$) ratio compared to the group receiving the lower-phytate pea-based diets (groups 1-2347-144, 4803-4-78G-L) (Table 8), indicating improved dietary Fe bioavailability and increased absorbable Fe [36,46,54]. The CDC Bronco diet presented a higher PA–Fe ratio compared to the all low-phytate pea-based diets (Table 1), which was associated with increased dietary Fe bioavailability in these pea-based diets [69–71]. These results agree with preceding experiments intended to assess Fe bioavailability in Fe-biofortified legumes, such as black beans [72], red mottled beans [33], Carioca beans [36], and pearl millet [73], as well as in the context of a complete diet. Thus, several intrinsic factors, including phytates, may influence the bioavailability of Fe from these pea varieties and other crops [56,74–76], potentially limiting their nutritional benefit.

Previous research suggested that increased Fe content alone in biofortified crops may not be adequate to produce a significant physiological improvement in Fe status and in Fe-deficient populations [36,55,76]. In the current study, it appears that, although Fe contents of all tested pea varieties were similar, the consumption of lower-phytate peas was able to moderately improve Fe status and storage, as further suggested by the hepatic ferritin contents of lower-phytate groups relative to CDC Bronco and no-pea diets. Furthermore, the duodenal brush border membrane (BBM) gene expression of ferroportin (FPN) was significantly upregulated, while DcytB was downregulated in the groups receiving the lower-phytate pea-based diets, relative to the CDC Bronco dietary group

($p < 0.05$, Figure 2). However, no significant alterations in the expression of BBM functional proteins were detected amongst treatment groups. Previous studies showed a downregulation of the gene expression of Fe-related BBM proteins (DMT-1, FPN, and Dcytb) in Fe-biofortified diets compared to the Fe-standard diets [36,46,55]. Ferroportin is the Fe exporter that transfers Fe across the enterocyte's basolateral membrane [77]. Hence, since the lower-phytate pea-based dietary groups had a higher expression of FPN, more Fe could be transported from the enterocyte into the blood and target tissue; therefore, this mechanism indicates the potential increased amount of absorbable Fe and, hence, the total body Hb-Fe increased in some of the low phytate groups compared to the CDC Bronco and no-pea dietary groups.

Similar to humans and most animals, the *Gallus gallus* model harbors a complex and active intestinal microbiota [78], significantly and directly influenced by host genetics, environment, and diet [79]. There is a significant resemblance at the phylum level between the gut microbiota of *Gallus gallus* and humans, with Bacteroidetes, Firmicutes, Proteobacteria, and Actinobacteria representing the dominant bacterial phyla in both [80]. In this study, a genus- and species-level bacterial population delineation among the low-phytate, standard (CDC Bronco), and no-pea dietary groups was observed. Results indicated that the abundance of *Bifidobacterium* was significantly higher ($p < 0.05$) in the 4802-8-87Y-L and CDC Bronco groups relative to all other treatment groups. Furthermore, the abundance of *Lactobacillus* was significantly higher ($p < 0.05$) in the 1-2347-144 and 4803-4-78G-L treatment groups relative to all other treatment groups (Figure 3). These results suggest that the above lower-phytate pea-based diets may potentially improve the host overall gut health by promoting the abundance of beneficial bacterial populations. Moreover, some of the low-phytate pea varieties (as 1-2347-144) presented a higher ($p < 0.05$) total fiber content (soluble and insoluble) compared to the standard CDC Bronco pea (Table 3). It was previously demonstrated that soluble fiber can increase villi height by elevating intestinal cell proliferation [81]. In the current study, some of the low-phytate pea dietary groups (such as 4803-4-78G-L, 4802-8-46Y-L, and 4802-8-87Y-L) presented higher ($p < 0.05$) protein content compared to the standard CDC Bronco pea (Table 3), where a higher dietary protein content was shown to increase villi height and intestinal cell proliferation [82]. Furthermore, indigested dietary proteins and fibers are fermented in the lower intestine, and this action produces short-chain fatty acids (SCFAs), such as acetate, propionate, and butyrate. Production of SCFAs affects metabolism and gastrointestinal health [83]. Acetate and propionate are energy substrates for peripheral tissues, and butyrate is referentially used as an energy source by colonocytes [84,85].

In summary, the current study focused on the performance of low-phytate pea varieties in chicken diets. Phytate phosphorus concentration was reduced by approximately 40% in these varieties. The low-phytate pea variety-based diets were able to moderately improve the Fe status in vivo, suggesting that low-phytate field pea has the potential to improve Fe bioavailability in human diets, particularly in the Indian subcontinent, as one of the major importing regions for Canadian peas, and a region where dietary Fe deficiency is a major health concern. Furthermore, as the abolition of micronutrient malnutrition remains a widespread global health problem in developing countries, the current study suggests that increasing micronutrient intake in food through food-based approaches is a sustainable method for the potential prevention of micronutrient deficiencies. Biofortification offers a long-term, sustainable, food-based solution for a world population, and breeding programs may aim to improve grain Zn and Fe concentrations; however, as previously suggested, improving Fe or Zn content may not necessarily result in the desired outcome (i.e., breeding toward increased mineral content may also lead to increased potential dietary inhibitors) and, hence, may not be as effective. In low-income countries, breeding for mineral solidity may remain the only agricultural involvement available to improve the nutritional content of staple crops, and, as suggested in the current study, the genetic improvement of staple food crops, specifically the development of low-phytate pea verities, resulted in improved nutritional quality and dietary Fe bioavailability, including in a complete diet context.

Additionally, as previously demonstrated, the current study presents a cost-effective approach designed to assess the effectiveness of biofortified pea varieties in vivo, as these varieties were developed with an aim to reduce the inhibitory effect of dietary phytate on Fe bioavailability. Therefore, our findings suggest that the use of lower-phytate biofortified peas may be an effective and sustainable approach to decreasing the global abundance of Fe deficiency, with added improvements in intestinal bacterial population structure and intestinal BBM functionality.

5. Conclusions

Nutritional approaches aimed to ease global Fe deficiency, such as Fe supplementation or fortification, are moderately successful at achieving optimal Fe status. This study showed how biofortified low-phytate pea affects dietary Fe bioavailability, physiological status, and the composition and metagenome of the gut microbiota and intestinal function. Animals (*Gallus gallus*) that consumed the low-phytate pea-based diets had increased abundance of beneficial bacteria, with associated surges in SCFA-producing bacteria with known phenolic catabolic capability, which resulted in an improvement in intestinal functionality. In addition, some of the low-phytate peas presented a higher protein content versus the standard CDC Bronco pea, which can possibly improve Fe bioavailability and intestinal functionality. Furthermore, parallel to preceding data, the current research suggests that a key aspect to include is the in vivo measurement of dietary Fe bioavailability in biofortified crop variety-based diets, as part of the plant breeding procedure.

Overall, our discoveries provide further evidence that, unlike other nutritional approaches to improving Fe status, the low-phytate pea varieties appear to improve Fe physiological status and gut microbiota in vivo, and they present an option for this strategy to further advance the efficacy and safety of crop biofortification and mineral bioavailability. We recommend the application of in vivo screening tools to guide studies aimed at developing and appraising Fe bioavailability in biofortified food crops, as well as their possible nutritional benefit. Based on the data presented in the current study, a human efficacy study will be conducted to compare the 4802-8-87YL (low phytate) and CDC Bronco (standard/normal phytate) varieties, along with a no-pea control.

Author Contributions: Data curation, T.W. and E.T.; formal analysis, N.K. and E.T.; investigation, T.W. and E.T.; methodology, N.K., T.W., and E.T.; resources, T.W. and E.T.; supervision, E.T.; writing—original draft, E.T.; writing—review and editing, T.W. and E.T. All authors have read and agreed to the published version of the manuscript.

Funding: This research received no external funding.

Acknowledgments: The authors wish to thank Martino and Silva (Department of Nutrition and Health, Federal University of Viçosa, Viçosa, Minas Gerais, Brazil) for conducting the protein and fiber analyses.

Conflicts of Interest: The authors declare no conflict of interest.

References

1. Bouis, H.; Hotz, C.; McClafferty, B.; Meenakshi, J.V.; Pfeiffer, W.H. Biofortification: A New Tool to Reduce Micronutrient Malnutrition. *Food Nutr. Bull.* **2011**, *32*, S31–S40. [CrossRef] [PubMed]
2. Welch, R.M. Biotechnology, biofortification, and global health. *Food Nutr. Bull.* **2005**, *26*, 419–421. [CrossRef] [PubMed]
3. Mayer, J.E.; Pfeiffer, W.H.; Beyer, P. Biofortified crops to alleviate micronutrient malnutrition. *Curr. Opin. Plant Biol.* **2008**, *11*, 166–170. [CrossRef] [PubMed]
4. Iskander, F.Y.; Morad, M.M. Multielement determination in wheat and bran. *J. Radioanal. Nucl. Chem.* **1986**, *105*, 151–156. [CrossRef]
5. Guttieri, M.J.; Bowen, D.; Dorsch, J.A.; Raboy, V.; Souza, E. Identification and characterization of low phytic acid wheat. *Crop Sci.* **2004**, *44*, 418–424. [CrossRef]
6. Steiner, T.; Mosenthin, R.; Zimmermann, B.; Greiner, R.; Roth, S. Distribution of phytase activity, total phosphorus and phytate phosphorus in legume seeds, cereals and cereal by-products as influenced by harvest year and cultivar. *Anim. Feed Sci. Technol.* **2007**, *133*, 320–334. [CrossRef]
7. FAOSTAT. Production. Crops. 2014. Available online: http://www.fao.org/faostat/en/#data/QC (accessed on 15 January 2019).

8. Hood-Niefer, S.D.; Warkentin, T.D.; Chibbar, R.N.; Vandenberg, A.; Tyler, R.T. Effect of genotype and environment on the concentrations of starch and protein in, and the physicochemical properties of starch from, field pea and fababean. *J. Sci. Food Agric.* **2011**, *92*, 141–150. [CrossRef]
9. Simsek, S.; Herken, E.N.; Ovando-Martinez, M. Chemical composition, nutritional value and in vitro starch digestibility of roasted chickpeas. *J. Sci. Food Agric.* **2016**, *96*, 2896–28905. [CrossRef]
10. Ambigaipalan, P.; Hoover, R.; Donner, E.; Liu, Q.; Jaiswal, S.; Chibbar, R.; Nantanga, K.; Seetharaman, K. Structure of faba bean, black bean and pinto bean starches at different levels of granule organization and their physicochemical properties. *Food Res. Int.* **2011**, *44*, 2962–2974. [CrossRef]
11. Campos-Vega, R.; Loarca-Piña, G.; Oomah, B.D. Minor components of pulses and their potential impact on human health. *Food Res. Int.* **2010**, *43*, 461–482. [CrossRef]
12. Berrios, J.D.J.; Morales, P.; Hurtado, M.C.; Mata, M.C.S. Carbohydrate composition of raw and extruded pulse flours. *Food Res. Int.* **2010**, *43*, 531–536. [CrossRef]
13. Adamidou, S.; Nengas, I.; Grigorakis, K.; Nikolopoulou, D.; Jauncey, K. Chemical Composition and Antinutritional Factors of Field Peas (*Pisum sativum*), Chickpeas (*Cicer arietinum*), and Faba Beans (*Vicia faba*) as Affected by Extrusion Preconditioning and Drying Temperatures. *Cereal Chem. J.* **2011**, *88*, 80–86. [CrossRef]
14. Pacifici, S.; Song, J.; Zhang, C.; Wang, Q.; Glahn, R.P.; Kolba, N.; Tako, E. Intra Amniotic Administration of Raffinose and Stachyose Affects the Intestinal Brush Border Functionality and Alters Gut Microflora Populations. *Nutrients* **2017**, *9*, 304. [CrossRef]
15. Zhang, L.; Garneau, M.G.; Majumdar, R.; Grant, J.; Tegeder, M. Improvement of pea biomass and seed productivity by simultaneous increase of phloem and embryo loading with amino acids. *Plant J.* **2014**, *81*, 134–146. [CrossRef] [PubMed]
16. Vogt, T. Phenylpropanoid Biosynthesis. *Mol. Plant* **2010**, *3*, 2–20. [CrossRef]
17. Troszyńska, A.; Ciska, E. Phenolic compounds of seed coats of white and coloured varieties of pea (*Pisum sativum* L.) and their total antioxidant activity. *Czech J. Food Sci.* **2011**, *20*, 15–22. [CrossRef]
18. Estrella, I.; Dueñas, M.; Hernández, T. Occurrence of phenolic compounds in the seed coat and the cotyledon of peas (*Pisum sativum* L.). *Eur. Food Res. Technol.* **2004**, *219*, 116–123. [CrossRef]
19. Zadernowski, R.; Pierzynowska-Korniak, G.; Ciepielewska, D.; Fornal, L. Chemical characteristics and biological functions of phenolic acids of buckwheat and lentil seeds. *Fagopyrum* **1992**, *12*, 27–35.
20. Acosta-Estrada, B.A.; Gutiérrez-Uribe, J.A.; Serna-Saldívar, S.O. Bound phenolics in foods, a review. *Food Chem.* **2014**, *152*, 46–55. [CrossRef]
21. Wong, D.W. Feruloyl esterase. *Appl. Biochem. Biotech.* **2006**, *133*, 87–112. [CrossRef]
22. Frei, B.; Higdon, J.V. Antioxidant Activity of Tea Polyphenols In Vivo: Evidence from Animal Studies. *J. Nutr.* **2003**, *133*, 3275S–3284S. [CrossRef] [PubMed]
23. Rochfort, S.; Panozzo, J.F. Phytochemicals for Health, the Role of Pulses. *J. Agric. Food Chem.* **2007**, *55*, 7981–7994. [CrossRef] [PubMed]
24. Champ, M.M. Non-nutrient bioactive substances of pulses. *Brit. J. Nutr.* **2002**, *88*, 307–319. [CrossRef] [PubMed]
25. Raboy, V. myo-Inositol-1,2,3,4,5,6-hexakisphosphate. *Phytochemistry* **2003**, *64*, 1033–1043. [CrossRef]
26. Portman, D.; Blanchard, C.; Maharjan, P.; McDonald, L.S.; Mawson, J.; Naiker, M.; Panozzo, J.F. Blending studies using wheat and lentil cotyledon flour-Effects on rheology and bread quality. *Cereal Chem. J.* **2018**, *95*, 849–860. [CrossRef]
27. Wu, T.; Taylor, C.; Nebl, T.; Ng, K.; Bennett, L.E. Effects of chemical composition and baking on in vitro digestibility of proteins in breads made from selected gluten-containing and gluten-free flours. *Food Chem.* **2017**, *233*, 514–524. [CrossRef]
28. Vici, G.; Belli, L.; Biondi, M.; Polzonetti, V. Gluten free diet and nutrient deficiencies: A review. *Clin. Nutr.* **2016**, *35*, 1236–1241. [CrossRef]
29. Liu, X.; Glahn, R.P.; Arganosa, G.C.; Warkentin, T.D. Iron Bioavailability in Low Phytate Pea. *Crop. Sci.* **2015**, *55*, 320–330. [CrossRef]
30. Bangar, P.; Arganosa, G.C.; Whiting, S.; Bett, K.E.; Warkentin, T.D. Effect of iron, phytate and carotenoid concentration on iron bioavailability in field pea seeds. *Crop Sci.* **2017**, *57*, 891–902. [CrossRef]

31. Blair, M.W.; González, L.F.; Kimani, P.M.; Butare, L. Genetic diversity, inter-gene pool introgression and nutritional quality of common beans (*Phaseolus vulgaris* L.) from Central Africa. *Theor. Appl. Genet.* **2010**, *121*, 237–248. [CrossRef]
32. Blair, M.W. Mineral Biofortification Strategies for Food Staples: The Example of Common Bean. *J. Agric. Food Chem.* **2013**, *61*, 8287–8294. [CrossRef] [PubMed]
33. Tako, E.; Blair, M.W.; Glahn, R.P. Biofortified red mottled beans (*Phaseolus vulgaris* L.) in a maize and bean diet provide more bioavailable iron than standard red mottled beans: Studies in poultry (*Gallus gallus*) and an in vitro digestion/Caco-2 model. *Nutr. J.* **2011**, *10*, 113. [CrossRef] [PubMed]
34. Tako, E.; Hoekenga, O.A.; Kochian, L.V.; Glahn, R.P. High bioavailablilty iron maize (*Zea mays* L.) developed through molecular breeding provides more absorbable iron in vitro (Caco-2 model) and in vivo (*Gallus gallus*). *Nutr. J.* **2013**, *12*, 3. [CrossRef] [PubMed]
35. Tako, E.; Rutzke, M.A.; Glahn, R.P. Using the domestic chicken (*Gallus gallus*) as an in vivo model for iron bioavailability. *Poult. Sci.* **2010**, *89*, 514–521. [CrossRef]
36. Dias, D.M.; Kolba, N.; Binyamin, D.; Ziv, O.; Regini Nutti, M.; Martino, H.S.D.; Koren, O.; Tako, E. Iron Biofortified Carioca Bean (*Phaseolus vulgaris* L.)-Based Brazilian Diet Delivers More Absorbable Iron and Affects the Gut Microbiota In Vivo (*Gallus gallus*). *Nutrients* **2018**, *13*, 1970. [CrossRef]
37. Reed, S.; Knez, M.; Uzan, A.; Stangoulis, J.C.R.; Glahn, R.P.; Koren, O.; Tako, E. Alterations in the Gut (*Gallus gallus*) Microbiota Following the Consumption of Zinc Biofortified Wheat (*Triticum aestivum*)-Based Diet. *J. Agric. Food Chem.* **2018**, *66*, 6291–6299. [CrossRef]
38. Knez, M.; Tako, E.; Glahn, R.P.; Kolba, N.; De Courcy-Ireland, E.; Stangoulis, J.C.R. Linoleic Acid: Dihomo-γ-Linolenic Acid Ratio Predicts the Efficacy of Zn-Biofortified Wheat in Chicken (*Gallus gallus*). *J. Agric. Food Chem.* **2018**, *66*, 1394–1400. [CrossRef]
39. Wiesinger, J.A.; Glahn, R.; Cichy, K.A.; Kolba, N.; Hart, J.; Tako, E. An In Vivo (*Gallus gallus*) Feeding Trial Demonstrating the Enhanced Iron Bioavailability Properties of the Fast Cooking Manteca Yellow Bean (*Phaseolus vulgaris* L.). *Nutrients* **2019**, *11*, 1768. [CrossRef]
40. Warkentin, T.; Vandenberg, A.; Banniza, S.; Slinkard, A. CDC Bronco field pea. *Can. J. Plant Sci.* **2005**, *85*, 649–650. [CrossRef]
41. Warkentin, T.D.; Delgerjav, O.; Arganosa, G.; Rehman, A.U.; Bett, K.E.; Anbessa, Y.; Rossnagel, B.; Raboy, V. Development and Characterization of Low-Phytate Pea. *Crop. Sci.* **2012**, *52*, 74–78. [CrossRef]
42. Warkentin, T.D.; Vandenberg, A.; Tar'An, B.; Banniza, S.; Arganosa, G.; Barlow, B.; Ife, S.; Horner, J.; De Silva, D.; Thompson, M.; et al. CDC Limerick green field pea. *Can. J. Plant Sci.* **2014**, *94*, 1547–1549. [CrossRef]
43. Warkentin, T.D.; Vandenberg, A.; Tar'An, B.; Banniza, S.; Arganosa, G.; Barlow, B.; Ife, S.; Horner, J.; De Silva, D.; Thompson, M.; et al. CDC Raezer green field pea. *Can. J. Plant Sci.* **2014**, *94*, 1535–1537. [CrossRef]
44. AOAC. *Appendix J: AOAC INTERNATIONAL Methods Committee Guidelines for Validation of Microbiological Methods for Food and Environmental Surfaces*; AOAC Off. Methods Anal.: Rockville, MD, USA, 2012; pp. 1–21.
45. Jones, D.B. *Factors for Converting Percentages of Nitrogen in Foods and Feeds into Percentages of Protein*; Department of Agriculture-circ.: Washington, DC, USA, 1941; p. 183.
46. Tako, E.; Bar, H.; Glahn, R.P. The Combined Application of the Caco-2 Cell Bioassay Coupled with In Vivo (*Gallus gallus*) Feeding Trial Represents an Effective Approach to Predicting Fe Bioavailability in Humans. *Nutrients* **2016**, *8*, 732. [CrossRef] [PubMed]
47. Mete, A.; Van Zeeland, Y.R.A.; Vaandrager, A.B.; Van Dijk, J.E.; Marx, J.J.M.; Dorrestein, G. Partial purification and characterization of ferritin from the liver and intestinal mucosa of chickens, turtledoves and mynahs. *Avian Pathol.* **2005**, *34*, 430–434. [CrossRef]
48. Passaniti, A.; Roth, T.F. Purification of chicken liver ferritin by two novel methods and structural comparison with horse spleen ferritin. *Biochem. J.* **1989**, *258*, 413–419. [CrossRef]
49. Tako, E.; Glahn, R.P.; Laparra, J.M.; Welch, R.M.; Lei, X.; Kelly, J.D.; Rutzke, M.A.; Miller, D.D. Iron and Zinc Bioavailabilies to Pigs from Red and White Beans (*Phaseolus vulgaris* L.) Are Similar. *J. Agric. Food Chem.* **2009**, *57*, 3134–3140. [CrossRef]
50. Kornasio, R.; Halevy, O.; Kedar, O.; Uni, Z. Effect of in ovo feeding and its interaction with timing of first feed on glycogen reserves, muscle growth, and body weight. *Poult. Sci.* **2011**, *90*, 1467–1477. [CrossRef]

51. Dreiling, C.E.; Brown, D.E.; Casale, L.; Kelly, L. Muscle glycogen: Composition of iodine binding and enzyme digestion assays and application to meat samples. *Meat Sci.* **1987**, *20*, 167–177. [CrossRef]
52. Uni, Z.; Ferket, P.R.; Tako, E.; Kedar, O. In ovo feeding improves energy status of late-term chicken embryos. *Poult. Sci.* **2005**, *84*, 764–770. [CrossRef]
53. Tako, E.; Ferket, P.; Uni, Z. Changes in chicken intestinal zinc exporter mRNA expression and small intestinal functionality following intra-amniotic zinc-methionine administration. *J. Nutr. Biochem.* **2005**, *16*, 339–346. [CrossRef]
54. Nestel, P.; Bouis, H.E.; Meenakshi, J.V.; Pfeiffer, W. Symposium: Food Fortification in Developing Countries. Biofortification of Staple Food Crops. *J. Nutr.* **2006**, *136*, 1064–1067. [CrossRef] [PubMed]
55. Tako, E.; Reed, S.; Anandaraman, A.; Beebe, S.E.; Hart, J.J.; Glahn, R.P. Studies of Cream Seeded Carioca Beans (*Phaseolus vulgaris* L.) from a Rwandan Efficacy Trial: In Vitro and In Vivo Screening Tools Reflect Human Studies and Predict Beneficial Results from Iron Biofortified Beans. *PLoS ONE* **2015**, *10*, e0138479. [CrossRef] [PubMed]
56. IBGE. Instituto Brasileiro de Geografia e Estatística, Coordenação de Trabalho e Rendimento. In *Pesquisa de Orçamentos Familiares: 2008–2009. Análise Do Consumo Alimentar Pessoal No Brasil*; IBGE: Rio de Janeiro, Brazil, 2011.
57. FAOSTAT. Food and Agriculture Organization of the United Nations, Statistics Division. Forestry Production and Trade. Available online: http://www.fao.org/faostat/en/#data/FO (accessed on 4 April 2019).
58. Wang, N.; Daun, J.K. Effect of variety and crude protein content on nutrients and certain antinutrients in field peas (*Pisum sativum*). *J. Sci. Food Agric.* **2004**, *84*, 1021–1029. [CrossRef]
59. Thacker, P.A.; Deep, A.; Petri, D.; Warkentin, T. Nutritional evaluation of low-phytate peas (*Pisum sativum* L.) for young broiler chicks. *Arch. Anim. Nutr.* **2013**, *67*, 1–14. [CrossRef]
60. Gupta, R.K.; Gangoliya, S.S.; Singh, N.K. Reduction of phytic acid and enhancement of bioavailable micronutrients in food grains. *J. Food Sci. Technol.* **2013**, *52*, 676–684. [CrossRef]
61. Lott, J.N.; Ockenden, I.; Raboy, V.; Batten, G.D. Phytic acid and phosphorus in crop seeds and fruits: A global estimate. *Seed Sci. Res.* **2000**, *10*, 11–33. [CrossRef]
62. Larson, S.; Young, K.A.; Cook, A.; Blake, T.K.; Raboy, V. Linkage mapping of two mutations that reduce phytic acid content of barley grain. *Theor. Appl. Genet.* **1998**, *97*, 141–146. [CrossRef]
63. Raboy, V.; Gerbasi, P.F.; Young, K.A.; Stoneberg, S.D.; Pickett, S.G.; Bauman, A.T.; Murthy, P.P.; Sheridan, W.F.; Ertl, D.S. Origin and Seed Phenotype of Maize low phytic acid 1-1 and low phytic acid 2-1. *Plant Physiol.* **2000**, *124*, 355–368. [CrossRef]
64. Wilcox, J.R.; Premachandra, G.S.; Young, K.A.; Raboy, V. Isolation of High Seed Inorganic P, Low-Phytate Soybean Mutants. *Crop. Sci.* **2000**, *40*, 1601–1605. [CrossRef]
65. Rasmussen, S.K.; Hatzack, F. Identification of two Low-Phytate Barley (*Hordeum Vulgare* L.) Grain Mutants by TLC and Genetic Analysis. *Hereditas* **2004**, *129*, 107–112. [CrossRef]
66. Larson, S.; Rutger, J.N.; Young, K.A.; Raboy, V. Isolation and Genetic Mapping of a Non-Lethal Rice (*Oryza sativa* L.) low phytic acid 1 Mutation. *Crop. Sci.* **2000**, *40*, 1397–1405. [CrossRef]
67. Guttieri, M.J.; Becker, C.; Souza, E.J. Application of Wheat Meal Solvent Retention Capacity Tests Within Soft Wheat Breeding Populations. *Cereal Chem. J.* **2004**, *81*, 261–266. [CrossRef]
68. Campion, B.; Perrone, D.; Galasso, I.; Bollini, R. Common bean (*Phaseolus vulgaris* L.) lines devoid of major lectin proteins. *Plant Breed.* **2009**, *128*, 199–204. [CrossRef]
69. Hurrell, R.F.; Juillerat, M.A.; Reddy, M.B.; Lynch, S.R.; Dassenko, S.A.; Cook, J.D. Soy protein, phytate, and iron absorption in humans. *Am. J. Clin. Nutr.* **1992**, *56*, 573–578. [CrossRef]
70. Anton, A.A.; Ross, K.A.; Beta, T.; Fulcher, R.G.; Arntfield, S.D. Effect of pre-dehulling treatments on some nutritional and physical properties of navy and pinto beans (*Phaseolus vulgaris* L.). *LWT* **2008**, *41*, 771–778. [CrossRef]
71. Petry, N.; Egli, I.; Campion, B.; Nielsen, E.; Hurrell, R. Genetic Reduction of Phytate in Common Bean (*Phaseolus vulgaris* L.) Seeds Increases Iron Absorption in Young Women. *J. Nutr.* **2013**, *143*, 1219–1224. [CrossRef]
72. Tako, E.; Beebe, S.; Reed, S.; Hart, J.J.; Glahn, R.P. Polyphenolic compounds appear to limit the nutritional benefit of biofortified higher iron black bean (*Phaseolus vulgaris* L.). *Nutr. J.* **2014**, *13*, 28. [CrossRef]
73. Tako, E.; Reed, S.; Budiman, J.; Hart, J.J.; Glahn, R.P. Higher iron pearl millet (*Pennisetum glaucum* L.) provides more absorbable iron that is limited by increased polyphenolic content. *Nutr. J.* **2015**, *14*, 11. [CrossRef]

74. Petry, N.; Egli, I.; Zeder, C.; Walczyk, T.; Hurrell, R. Polyphenols and Phytic Acid Contribute to the Low Iron Bioavailability from Common Beans in Young Women. *J. Nutr.* **2010**, *140*, 1977–1982. [CrossRef]
75. Petry, N.; Egli, I.; Gahutu, J.B.; Tugirimana, P.L.; Boy, E.; Hurrell, R. Phytic Acid Concentration Influences Iron Bioavailability from Biofortified Beans in Rwandese Women with Low Iron Status. *J. Nutr.* **2014**, *144*, 1681–1687. [CrossRef]
76. Hart, J.J.; Tako, E.; Glahn, R.P. Characterization of Polyphenol Effects on Inhibition and Promotion of Iron Uptake by Caco-2 Cells. *J. Agric. Food Chem.* **2017**, *65*, 3285–3294. [CrossRef] [PubMed]
77. Duda-Chodak, A.; Tarko, T.; Satora, P.; Sroka, P. Interaction of dietary compounds, especially polyphenols, with the intestinal microbiota: A review. *Eur. J. Nutr.* **2015**, *54*, 325–341. [CrossRef] [PubMed]
78. Zhu, X.Y.; Zhong, T.; Pandya, Y.; Joerger, R.D. 16S rRNA-Based Analysis of Microbiota from the Cecum of Broiler Chickens. *Appl. Environ. Microbiol.* **2002**, *68*, 124–137. [CrossRef] [PubMed]
79. Yegani, M.; Korver, D. Factors Affecting Intestinal Health in Poultry. *Poult. Sci.* **2008**, *87*, 2052–2063. [CrossRef] [PubMed]
80. Qin, J.; Li, R.; Raes, J.; Arumugam, M.; Burgdorf, K.S.; Manichanh, C.; Nielsen, T.; Pons, N.; Levenez, F.; Yamada, T.; et al. A human gut microbial gene catalogue established by metagenomic sequencing. *Nature* **2010**, *464*, 59–65. [CrossRef]
81. Adam, C.L.; Williams, P.A.; Garden, K.E.; Thomson, L.M.; Ross, A.W. Dose-dependent effcts of soluble dietary fibre (pectin) on food intake, adiposity, guy hypertrophy and gut satiety hormone secretion in rats. *PLoS ONE* **2015**, *10*, e0115438. [CrossRef]
82. Chen, X.; Song, P.; Fan, P.; He, T.; Jacobs, D.; Levesque, C.L.; Johnston, L.J.; Ji, L.; Ma, N.; Chen, Y.; et al. Moderate Dietary Protein Restriction Optimized Gut Microbiota and Mucosal Barrier in Growing Pig Model. *Front. Microbiol.* **2018**, *8*. [CrossRef]
83. Tan, J.; McKenzie, C.; Potamitis, M.; Thorburn, A.; Mackay, C.; Macia, L. The role of short-chain fatty acids in health and disease. *Adv. Immunol.* **2014**, *121*, 91–119.
84. Tremaroli, V.; Bäckhed, F. Functional interactions between the gut microbiota and host metabolism. *Nature* **2012**, *489*, 242–249. [CrossRef]
85. Backhed, F.; Ding, H.; Wang, T.; Hooper, L.V.; Koh, G.Y.; Nagy, A.; Semenkovich, C.F.; Gordon, J.I. The gut microbiota as an environmental factor that regulates fat storage. *Proc. Natl. Acad. Sci. USA* **2004**, *101*, 15718–15723. [CrossRef]

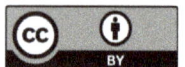

© 2020 by the authors. Licensee MDPI, Basel, Switzerland. This article is an open access article distributed under the terms and conditions of the Creative Commons Attribution (CC BY) license (http://creativecommons.org/licenses/by/4.0/).

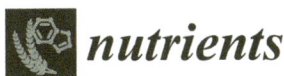

Article

A Novel Non-Digestible, Carrot-Derived Polysaccharide (cRG-I) Selectively Modulates the Human Gut Microbiota while Promoting Gut Barrier Integrity: An Integrated In Vitro Approach

Pieter Van den Abbeele [1], Lynn Verstrepen [1], Jonas Ghyselinck [1], Ruud Albers [2], Massimo Marzorati [1,3] and Annick Mercenier [2,*]

1. ProDigest BV, Technologiepark 82, 9052 Ghent, Belgium; Pieter.VandenAbbeele@prodigest.eu (P.V.d.A.); lynn.verstrepen@prodigest.eu (L.V.); Jonas.Ghyselinck@prodigest.eu (J.G.); massimo.marzorati@prodigest.eu (M.M.)
2. Nutrileads BV, Bronland 12-N, 6708WH Wageningen, The Netherlands; ruud.albers@nutrileads.com
3. Center of Microbial Ecology and Technology (CMET), Ghent University, Coupure Links 653, 9000 Ghent, Belgium
* Correspondence: annick.mercenier@nutrileads.com; Tel.: +31-683-697-288

Received: 30 May 2020; Accepted: 24 June 2020; Published: 29 June 2020

Abstract: Modulation of the gut microbiome as a means to improve human health has recently gained increasing interest. In this study, it was investigated whether cRG-I, a carrot-derived pectic polysaccharide, enriched in rhamnogalacturonan-I (RG-I) classifies as a potential prebiotic ingredient using novel in vitro models. First, digestion methods involving α-amylase/brush border enzymes demonstrated the non-digestibility of cRG-I by host-derived enzymes versus digestible (starch/maltose) and non-digestible controls (inulin). Then, a recently developed short-term (48 h) colonic incubation strategy was applied and revealed that cRG-I fermentation increased levels of health-promoting short-chain fatty acids (SCFA; mainly acetate and propionate) and lactate comparable but not identical to the reference prebiotic inulin. Upon upgrading this fermentation model by inclusion of a simulated mucosal environment while applying quantitative 16S-targeted Illumina sequencing, cRG-I was additionally shown to specifically stimulate operational taxonomic units (OTUs) related to health-associated species such as *Bifidobacterium longum*, *Bifidobacterium adolescentis*, *Bacteroides dorei*, *Bacteroides ovatus*, *Roseburia hominis*, *Faecalibacterium prausnitzii*, and *Eubacterium hallii*. Finally, in a novel model to assess host–microbe interactions (Caco-2/peripheral blood mononuclear cells (PBMC) co-culture) fermented cRG-I increased barrier integrity while decreasing markers for inflammation. In conclusion, by using novel in vitro models, cRG-I was identified as a promising prebiotic candidate to proceed to clinical studies.

Keywords: prebiotic; microbiome; SCFA; colon; bifidobacteria; pectin; rhamnogalacturonan; transepithelial electrical resistance (TEER)

1. Introduction

The colon contains a vast number of bacteria that largely impact human health. Next to preventing pathogen colonization through secretion of antimicrobial agents [1–3], the gut microbiota is involved in food processing, synthesis of essential vitamins and production of health-promoting short-chain fatty acids (SCFA), including acetate, propionate and butyrate [4], upon anaerobic fermentation of for instance dietary fibers [5]. While butyrate is an important energy source for colonocytes with anti-inflammatory and intestinal barrier-protecting effects, propionate exerts anti-lipogenic and cholesterol-lowering effects in the liver [6]. In addition, as with butyrate, propionate has been reported to exert anti-cancer effects in the colon [7,8]. Finally, acetate is used in the liver as a substrate for cholesterol and fatty acid synthesis [9,10]. In terms of composition, the human gut microbiome mainly consists of the *Firmicutes*, *Bacteroidetes*, *Actinobacteria*, *Proteobacteria*, *Fusobacteria*, and *Verrucomicrobia* phyla [11]. Despite having provided key insights, many studies have been limited to (descriptive) analysis of fecal samples as in situ samples from the site of fermentation are difficult to obtain. To allow in-depth research focusing on not only luminal, but also gut wall-associated mucosal microbes, a novel in vitro model (M-SHIME®; Mucosal Simulator of the Human Intestinal Microbial Ecosystem) was recently developed as a complementary in vitro tool [12]. In this model, the mucosal microbiota was enriched with butyrate-producing *Clostridium* cluster XIVa members, correlating with in vivo findings from biopsies [13–18].

Modulation of the human gut microbiome as a route to improve human health has gained a lot of interest over recent years. Prebiotics are defined as non-digestible food ingredients that selectively stimulate health-promoting bacteria [19]. A key feature of prebiotics is their resistance to upper gastro-intestinal digestion so that they reach the colon where they are fermented by the gut microbiome. To assess potential digestibility of polysaccharides, two complementary enzyme sources are to be considered, i.e., amylases [20] and brush border enzymes [21]. α-amylase is present in both saliva and pancreatic juice and can liberate maltose from starch [20]. Furthermore, sucrase-isomaltase and maltase-glycoamylase, collectively known as α-glucosidases, are complexes consisting of 4 enzymes that release glucose from oligosaccharides present at the intestinal brush border [21]. These host-derived enzymes jointly digest carbohydrates and hence their specificity determines whether carbohydrates reach the colon and can exert prebiotic effects. Although critical to the definition of potential prebiotic ingredients, studies confirming their indigestibility are scarce.

Fructans, such as fructooligosaccharides (FOS) and inulin are considered to be "gold standard" prebiotics, with human clinical trials supporting their beneficial effect in acute and chronic diseases such as obesity and type 2 diabetes (T2D), allergy, inflammatory bowel disease (IBD), Traveler's diarrhea and constipation (an overview is given in [19]). As many health-related species belong to the *Bifidobacteriaceae*, prebiotic potential has often been related to an increase of this family. There is however increasing understanding that prebiotics can be fermented by a wider range of gut microbes. Inulin can e.g., also be rapidly fermented by health-promoting *Bacteroidaceae* members, such as *Bacteroides caccae* [22,23]. Currently, there is growing interest to develop novel prebiotics. A specific class of candidates includes pectin-derived polysaccharides enriched in the branched part of pectin, i.e., the rhamnogalacturonan-I (RG-I) domains, which can be extracted from several food crops including carrot. The backbone of RG-I is a repeating unit of the disaccharide [-2)-α-L-rhamnose-(1,4)-α-D-galacturonic acid-(1] and RG-I side-chains consist of galactans (β-1,4-D-galactose (D-Gal) units) and/or arabinans (α-1,5-linked L-arabinofuranose (L-Araf) units with additional L-Araf side-chains), with varying length and composition [24]. Given their structural complexity, RG-I extracts would require fermentation by a consortium of gut microbes with complementary metabolic capabilities [25].

Gut microbial modulation is linked to human health with the concept of a "leaky gut" having gained attention, not only in the context of inflammatory bowel disease, but also in a wider range of psychological and metabolic disorders [26]. Increased intestinal epithelial permeability would allow translocation of bacterial cell wall components, metabolites, or even whole bacteria into the systemic circulation, hence contributing to inflammation and injury, not only in the gut but also in remote organs such as the liver and the brain. Host–microbe interaction studies are increasingly being performed to document this. As an example, microbial fermentation samples can be combined with a human co-culture model [27], including intestinal epithelial cells (Caco-2) and monocytes (THP-1) [28], which demonstrated the gut barrier protective effects together with immuno-modulatory capacity of several prebiotics, including arabinoxylo-oligosaccharides (AXOS) [29], inulin, FOS [30] and a dried yeast fermentate [31]. Despite its usefulness, this model has the limitation that monocytes are only one of the cell lineages involved in the immune response. Therefore, using a co-culture model including Caco-2 cells and peripheral blood mononuclear cells (PBMCs), containing lymphocytes (T-cells, B-cells, and NK-cells), monocytes and dendritic cells [32], could increase the in vivo relevance.

Therefore, the present study investigated whether a carrot-derived RG-I enriched extract (cRG-I) classifies as a potential prebiotic ingredient using a combination of novel in vitro models (Figure 1). First, potential digestion by amylase/brush border enzymes was investigated (Test 1). Then, a recently developed short-term colonic incubation strategy was applied [29] to assess the potential impact of cRG-I on microbial metabolic activity including inulin as a reference (Test 2). Subsequently, after upgrading the fermentation model by inclusion of a simulated mucosal microbiota [12], more in-depth fermentation tests were performed to characterize the prebiotic potential of two carrot RG-I formulations that differed in absence (cRG-I) or presence of low molecular weight carbohydrates (cRG-I+LMWC) (Test 3). To obtain detailed insights in modulation of microbial composition, a novel technique was used where flow cytometry was combined with 16S-targeted Illumina sequencing to obtain quantitative information at high phylogenetic resolution [33]. Finally, fermentation samples were screened for potential beneficial effects on gut barrier integrity and immune modulation in a newly optimized Caco-2/PBMC co-culture model (test 4).

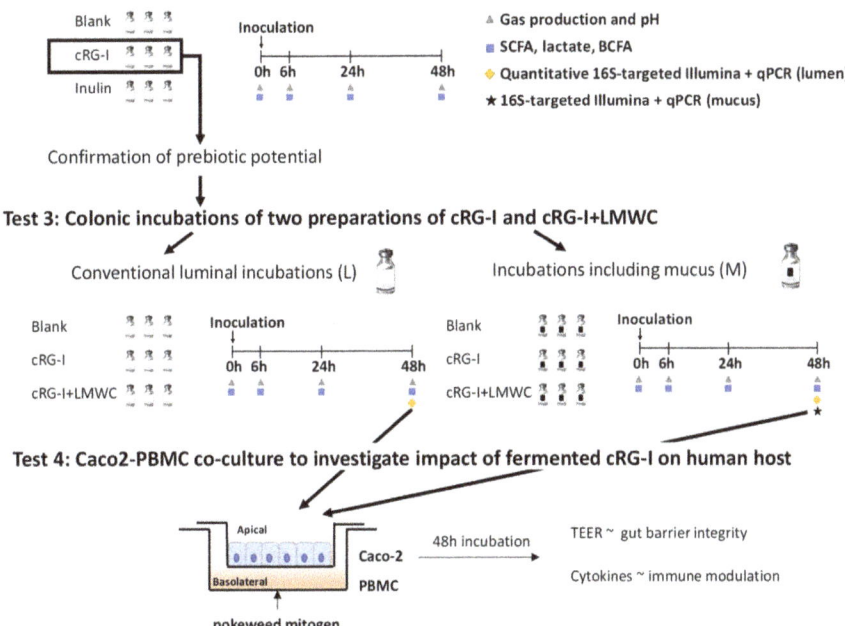

Figure 1. Schematic representation of the integrated in vitro approach to investigate the prebiotic potential of cRG-I (carrot-derived rhamnogalacturonan-I). First, potential digestion of cRG-I by amylase/brush border enzymes was investigated (Test 1). In Test 2, short-term colonic batch incubations were used to assess the prebiotic potential on microbial metabolic activity of cRG-I compared to inulin. In Test 3, the prebiotic potential of two formulations that differed in absence (cRG-I) or presence of low molecular weight carbohydrates (cRG-I+LMWC) was assessed in both conventional luminal incubations (L) and incubations including a mucosal compartment (M). Samples were collected to evaluate the effect of the test products on microbial activity, community composition and on intestinal permeability and immunity (Test 4, Caco-2/PBMC co-culture model).

2. Materials and Methods

2.1. Products

The two carrot RG-I preparations used in this study (cRG-I [34] and cRG-I+LMWC) were provided by NutriLeads (Wageningen, The Netherlands). Both are pectin-derived polysaccharides and cRG-I+LMWC differs from cRG-I by containing small size sugars, mainly mono- and disaccharides of galactose, glucose, and uronic acids. Pectin is a linear homogalacturonan (HG) interspaced with branched rhamnogalacturonan (RG) regions. HG consists of α-1,4-linked D-galacturonic acid (GalA) monomers while the RG-I backbone is a repeating unit of the disaccharide [-2)-α-L-rhamnose-1,4)-(α-D-galacturonic acid-(1]. The RG-I backbone is decorated with galactans (β-1,4-D-galactose (D-Gal) units) and/or arabinans (α-1,5-linked L-arabinofuranose (L-Araf) units [25]. Inulin (Orafti® HP, 100% inulin, 0% sweetness level, average DP ≥ 23) was generously provided by Beneo GmbH (Mannheim, Germany).

2.2. Digestion by Amylase and Brush Border Enzymes (Test 1)

Digestion with amylase was performed as described previously [20]. Briefly, cooked starch (positive control), inulin (negative control) and cRG-I were suspended in distilled water at 15 g/L. A stock solution of 1500U α-amylase/mL (10080, Sigma–Aldrich, Bornem, Belgium) was prepared and added to the substrates to simulate the small intestinal phase, while respecting the ratio of units of amylase versus amount of test product according to the Infogest consensus method (1300 units per gram test product [20]). Samples were incubated for 60′ at 37 °C. Furthermore, digestion with brush border enzymes was performed as previously described in [21]. Briefly, intestinal aceton powder from rat (Sigma–Aldrich, Bornem, Belgium) was dissolved in 0.9% NaCl solution, vortexed, and sonicated. 15 g/L stock solutions of inulin (negative control) and maltose (positive control) were prepared in sodium phosphate buffer (pH 7), while cRG-I was prepared in distilled water. 100 µL enzyme solution and 50 µL substrates were mixed with 100 µL phosphate buffer and incubated for 90′ at 37 °C. High Performance Anion Exchange Chromatography with Pulsed Amperometric Detection (HPAEC-PAD) was used to measure rhamnose, arabinose, galactose, fructose, glucose, maltose, and galacturonic acid in both digestion experiments. All tests were done in technical triplicate.

2.3. Short-Term Colonic Batch Incubations (Tests 2 and 3)

Short-term colonic incubations were performed as described in [29]. Briefly, freshly collected fecal material of a healthy human donor (f, 26) was collected and after preparation of an anaerobic fecal slurry inoculated at 10 vol% in a sugar-depleted nutritional medium containing 5.2 g/L K_2HPO_4, 16.3 g/L KH_2PO_4, 2.0 g/L $NaHCO_3$ (Chem-lab NV, Zedelgem, Belgium), 2.0 g/L Yeast Extract, 2.0 g/L pepton (Oxoid, Aalst, Belgium), 1.0 g/L mucin (Carl Roth, Karlsruhe, Germany), 0.5 g/L L-cystein and 2.0 mL/L Tween80 (Sigma–Aldrich, Bornem, Belgium). When mucin-coated carriers were added to the reactors during Test 3, 1.0 g/L mucin was omitted from the nutritional medium. Five mucin-coated carriers were added per reactor after being prepared according to Van den Abbeele et al. (2013) [12]. Test products were dosed at 5 g/L and reactors were anaerobically incubated at 37 °C for 48 h. All experiments were performed in technical triplicate.

2.4. Microbial Metabolic Activity (Tests 2 and 3)

Samples were collected upon 0 h, 6 h, 24 h, and 48 h of incubation from each colon reactor. Gas production was measure with a pressure meter (Hand-held pressure indicator CPH6200; Wika, Echt, The Netherlands) and pH measurements were performed with a Senseline pH meter F410 (ProSense, Oosterhout, The Netherlands). Total SCFA were determined as the sum of acetate, propionate, butyrate and branched-chain fatty acids (bCFA; isobutyrate, isovalerate and isocaproate) levels, and were measured as described previously [35]. Lactate production was assessed with a commercially available kit (R-Biopharm, Darmstadt, Germany), according to manufacturer's instructions.

2.5. Microbial Community Composition (Test 3)

After 48 h of incubation, samples from both lumen and mucus were collected for analysis of the microbial community composition through quantitative polymerase chain reaction (qPCR) and 16S-targeted Illumina sequencing. DNA was isolated as described in [36] from either 1 mL luminal samples or 0.1 g mucus samples. Subsequently, qPCR was performed on a QuantStudio 5 Real-Time PCR system (Applied Biosystems, Foster City, CA, USA). Each sample was run in technical triplicate and outliers with more than 1 C_T difference were omitted. The qPCRs were performed as described previously for the following groups: *Lactobacillus* spp. [37], *Bifidobacterium* spp. and *Eubacterium rectale/Clostridium coccoides* [38], *Akkermansia muciniphila* [39], *Bacteroidetes* [40], *Enterobacteriaceae* [41], *Faecalibacterium prausnitzii* [42], *Roseburia* and *Eubacterium hallii* [43]. In addition, microbiota profiling was performed using 16S-targeted Illumina sequencing analysis (LGC genomics GmbH, Berlin, Germany) as described in [44] to obtain proportional abundances (%) at different phylogenetic levels (phylum, family, and operational taxonomic unit (OTU) level). Briefly, library preparation and sequencing were performed on an Illumina MiSeq platform with v3 chemistry. The 16S rRNA gene V3-V4 hypervariable regions were amplified using primers 341F (5'-CCT ACG GGN GGC WGC AG-3') and 785Rmod (5'-GAC TAC HVG GGT ATC TAA KCC-3') [45]. As described in [46,47], the 16S-targeted sequencing analysis was adapted from the MiSeq protocol for read assembly and cleanup using the mothur software (v. 1.39.5) as follows: (1) reads were assembled into contigs, (2) alignment-based quality filtering was performed by alignment to the mothur-reconstructed SILVA SEED alignment (v. 123), (3) chimeras were removed, (4) taxonomy was assigned via a naïve Bayesian classifier [48] and RDP release 14 [49] and (5) contigs were clustered into OTUs at 97% sequence similarity. Sequences classified as Eukaryota, Archaea, Chloroplasts, Mitochondria, and non-classified sequences were also removed. For each OTU, representative sequences were selected as the most abundant sequence within that OTU. Finally, the obtained high-resolution proportional phylogenetic information (i.e., proportional abundances (%)) was combined with an accurate quantification of total bacterial cells via flowcytometry to obtain quantitative data at phylum, family, and OTU level. This was done by multiplying the proportional abundances with absolute cell numbers (cells/mL) obtained via flowcytometry. For flowcytometry analysis, 10-fold serial dilutions were prepared in Dulbecco's Phosphate-buffered Saline (DPBS) (Sigma–Aldrich, Bornem, Belgium) of all samples and stained with 0.01 mM SYTO24 (Life Technologies Europe, Merelbeke, Belgium) for 15' at 37 °C in the dark. Samples were analyzed on a BD Facsverse (BDBiosciences, Erembodegem, Belgium) using the high-flow-rate setting and bacteria were separated from medium debris and signal noise by applying a threshold level of 200 on the SYTO channel. Flowcytometry data were analyzed using FlowJo, version 10.5.2.

2.6. Caco-2/PBMC Co-Culture Model (Test 4)

Caco-2 cells (HTB-37; American Type Culture Collection) were cultured in Dulbecco's Modified Eagle Medium (DMEM) containing glucose and glutamine (Sigma–Aldrich, Bornem, Belgium) and supplemented with HEPES (4-(2-hydroxyethyl)-1-piperazineethanesulfonic acid) and 20% (v/v) heat-inactivated (HI) fetal bovine serum (FBS) (Gibco, Life Technologies Europe, Merelbeke, Belgium). PBMCs were isolated from buffy coats of healthy donors (Red Cross, Ghent, Belgium) using Lymphoprep^{TM} (STEMCELL technologies SARL, Grenoble, France). In brief, blood was collected and diluted (1/5, v/v) in DPBS without Ca/Mg (Sigma–Aldrich, Bornem, Belgium). Then, Lymphoprep^{TM} solution was added and samples were centrifuged at $1027\times g$ for 20' at room temperature (RT) to separate the mononuclear cells (MNCs) and red blood cells by density-gradient centrifugation. MNCs were collected and washed 3 times with ice-cold DPBS ($340\times g$, 7'). Aliquots of PBMCs were frozen in liquid nitrogen. Baseline IL-8 levels were determined by enzyme-linked immunosorbent assay (ELISA) (Invitrogen, Thermo Fisher Scientific, Merelbeke, Belgium) to eliminate donors with high basal cytokine levels. For experiments, Caco-2 cells were seeded on 24-well semipermeable inserts (0.4 µm pore size) at a density of 1×10^5 cells/insert and cultured for 14 days until a functional cell monolayer with a transepithelial electrical resistance (TEER) of more than 300 Ωcm^2 was obtained. PBMCs, stimulated with 2.5 µg/mL pokeweed mitogen (PWM) were added to the basolateral chamber at a concentration of 1×10^6 cells/well. PBMCs without PWM stimulation were included as negative control. At the same time, colonic suspensions (filter-sterilized (0.22 µm) and diluted 1/5 (v/v) in culture medium) or 5 mM sodium butyrate (NaB) (Sigma–Aldrich, Bornem, Belgium) were added to the Caco-2 cells at the apical side. Caco-2 cells were also treated with medium as negative control. Cells were incubated for 48 h at 37 °C in a humidified atmosphere of air/CO_2 (95:5, v/v). TEER was measured at start (0 h timepoint) and after 48 h of incubation using a Millicell ERS2 Voltohmmeter (EMD Millipore, Sigma–Aldrich, Bornem, Belgium). All 48 h values were normalized to their own 0 h value after subtraction of the empty insert value and are presented as percentage of initial value. In addition, basolateral supernatant was collected after 48 h of incubation for cytokine analysis. Human IFN-γ, IL-17A, IL-21, IL-22, IL-4, and IL-9 levels were determined by Luminex® multiplex (Procartaplex, Invitrogen, Thermo Fisher Scientific) and IL-10 levels were measured by ELISA (Invitrogen, Thermo Fisher Scientific), according to the manufacturers' instructions. All experiments were performed in triplicate.

2.7. Statistics

To evaluate differences in microbial metabolites (tests 2 and 3) and microbial community composition at phylum level between blank and treatment incubations (Test 3), a two-way analysis of variance (ANOVA) with Dunnett's multiple comparisons test was performed. Statistically significant differences between the blank and treatments are presented by (*, Δ0 h–6 h), ($, Δ6 h–24 h) or (#, Δ24 h–48 h). 1 sign = $p < 0.05$, 2 signs = $p < 0.01$, 3 signs = $p < 0.001$ and 4 signs = $p < 0.0001$. Statistical analysis was performed with the GraphPad Prism software (version 8.3.0, San Diego, USA). To evaluate differences in microbial community composition at family and OTU level between blank and treatment incubations (Test 3), a Student's t-test was performed (Excel Software). Differences were found significant if $p < 0.05$. To evaluate differences between PWM+ and PWM- or NaB in the Caco-2/PBMC co-culture assay (Test 4), an ordinary one-way ANOVA with Dunnett's multiple comparisons test was performed; while differences between blank and treatment incubations were assessed with an ordinary one-way ANOVA with Tukey's multiple comparisons test. Statistically significant differences are presented by (*). (*) = $p < 0.05$, (**) = $p < 0.01$, (***) = $p < 0.001$ and (****) = $p < 0.0001$. Statistical analysis was performed with the GraphPad Prism software (version 8.3.0, San Diego, USA).

3. Results

3.1. cRG-I is Resistant to Digestion in the Human Upper Gastro-Intestinal Tract (GIT) (Test 1)

One of the characteristics of a prebiotic is its non-digestibility by host enzymes upon passage along the upper GIT [19]. First, upon exposure to amylase, the positive control cooked starch was readily degraded into maltose, demonstrating its known digestibility (Figure 2A), while the negative control inulin and also cRG-I were not digested to any of the simple sugars measured. Likewise, maltose was digested by brush border enzymes into glucose (Figure 2B), in contrast to the negative control inulin and cRG-I. Therefore, cRG-I can be considered to be a polysaccharide that likely escapes upper GIT digestion in vivo thereby reaching the colon where it could be fermented by the gut microbiota.

3.2. Effect of cRG-I on Microbial Metabolic Activity in Short-Term Colonic Incubations (Test 2)

Short-term colonic incubations were performed to investigate the potential prebiotic effect of cRG-I on microbial activity, including inulin as a positive control. A first indication of cRG-I fermentation by the gut microbiota followed from the significant pH decrease and enhanced gas production during the first 6 h of incubation (Δ0–6 h) versus the blank (Figure 3A,B). These changes were even stronger compared to inulin. Between 6 h and 24 h, cRG-I significantly and strongly decreased pH while increasing gas production. pH decreases and gas production were more excessive for inulin. Finally, during the 24 h to 48 h time interval, relatively stable pH values and gas levels indicated substrate depletion.

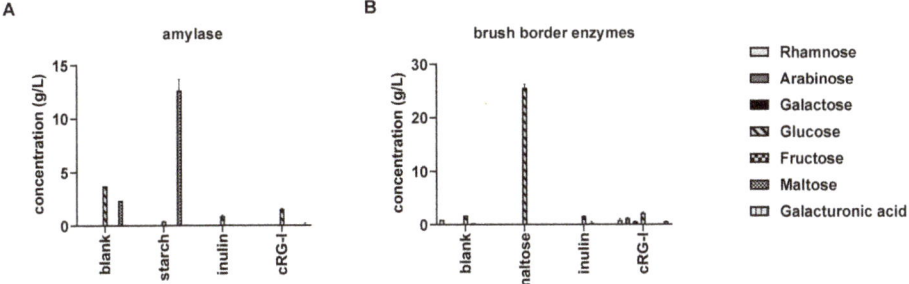

Figure 2. Digestion of cRG-I (carrot-derived rhamnogalacturonan-I) by amylase (**A**) and brush border enzymes (**B**) versus inulin, cooked starch, and maltose. Blank incubations containing all reagents in absence of a substrate were included. Average (± st. dev.) concentrations of different monosaccharides and maltose were measured by High Performance Anion Exchange Chromatography (HPAEC) ($n = 3$).

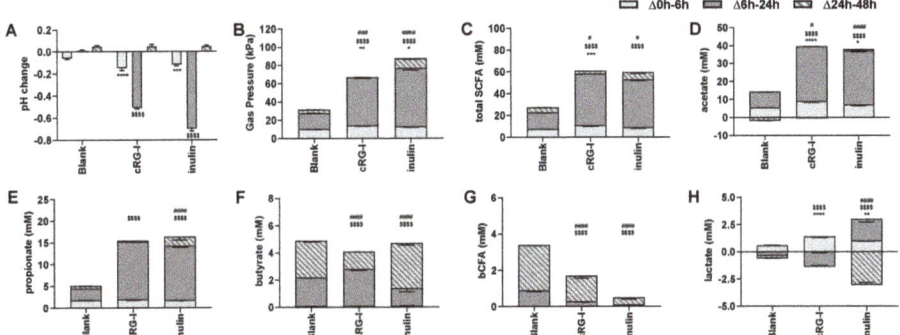

Figure 3. Effect of fermentation of cRG-I on microbial metabolic activity in short-term colonic incubations. Average changes (± st. dev.) in pH (**A**), gas production (**B**), total short-chain fatty acids (SCFA) (**C**), acetate (**D**), propionate (**E**), butyrate (**F**), branched CFA (bCFA) (**G**) and lactate (**H**) levels between 0 and 6 h (light gray), 6 h and 24 h (dark gray) and 24 h and 48 h (stripes) upon dosing cRG-I and inulin to the gut microbiota versus a blank incubation ($n = 3$). Statistically significant differences between blank and treatments for different time intervals are presented by * for Δ0 h–6 h, $ for Δ6 h–24 h or # for Δ24 h–48 h. (*, $, #) = $p < 0.05$, (**, $$, ##) = $p < 0.01$, (***, $$$, ###) = $p < 0.001$ and (****, $$$$, ####) = $p < 0.0001$.

Upon measuring lactate and SCFA production, acids responsible for aforementioned pH changes were elucidated. During the 0 h to 6 h time interval, cRG-I, but not inulin, significantly increased the production of total SCFA (Figure 3C) which resulted from more strongly elevated acetate levels (Figure 3D) next to significant raises in lactate production for cRG-I (Figure 3H). Furthermore, both treatments strongly augmented total SCFA production during the 6 h to 24 h time interval (merely due to increases in acetate and propionate (Figure 3D,E)), which were more profound for cRG-I compared to inulin. cRG-I, unlike inulin, also stimulated butyrate production during this interval (Figure 3F), which coincided with lactate consumption. Finally, during the 24 h to 48 h time interval, total SCFA production only increased upon treatment with inulin, which was related to increases of acetate, propionate, and butyrate levels, thus indicating slower fermentation of inulin versus cRG-I (Figure 3C–F). The stimulation of butyrate by inulin between 24–48 h correlated with the consumption of lactate during this time interval. Overall, lactate was entirely consumed at the end of the incubations, suggesting optimal conversion to propionate and/or butyrate [50]. Finally, bCFA result from protein fermentation by the gut microbiota [51,52], which is associated with detrimental health effects [51].

bCFA were mainly produced during the 6 h to 48 h time frame (Figure 3G), with both cRG-I and especially inulin significantly decreasing bCFA production.

3.3. Effect of cRG-I and cRG-I +LMWC on Microbial Metabolic Activity in Short-Term Colonic Incubations with or without a Mucosal Compartment (Test 3)

An in-depth characterization of the effects of cRG-I on microbial metabolic activity (Figure 4A–H) was performed by testing both cRG-I and a modified formulation containing small sugars (cRG-I +LMWC), dosed to colonic incubations including solely a luminal (L) or additionally also a mucosal (M) environment. In consistency with Test 2, cRG-I significantly decreased the pH during the first 6 h of incubation versus the blank due to enhanced acetate and lactate levels. Furthermore, the main fermentation occurred between 6 h and 24 h with strong increases in gas production and further decreases of pH due to stimulation of acetate, propionate, and to a lesser extent butyrate. The latter could again be linked to coinciding lactate consumption. Finally, the absence of marked changes of aforementioned parameters between 24 h and 48 h again indicated substrate depletion, while bCFA were significantly decreased thus illustrating the potential protective effects of cRG-I against toxic by-products of proteolytic fermentation.

cRG-I+LMWC exerted similar effects on microbial activity versus cRG-I with some minor differences. These included a more profound pH decrease for cRG-I+LMWC during the first 6 h of incubation due to enhanced acetate and lactate levels. Furthermore, acetate and propionate production between 6–24 h was less strongly increased with cRG-I+LMWC compared to cRG-I.

Overall, while no major differences were observed between incubations with or without mucosal environment, inclusion of mucus beads led to a tendency to higher gas production, with higher butyrate levels for the blank incubation, suggesting colonization of butyrate-producing bacteria on the mucin-coated carriers.

3.4. Effect of cRG-I and cRG-I +LMWC on Microbial Community Composition in Short-Term Colonic Incubations with or without a Mucosal Compartment (Test 3)

The data at phylum level are presented both as proportional (Figure 5A) and absolute values (Figure 5B). This demonstrated that for the luminal microbiota, quantitative data revealed greater insight in the true compositional changes since both cRG-I and cRG-I+LMWC largely increased total cell numbers. In contrast, due to the large variation in total cell numbers within identical replicates for the mucosal microbiota resulting in large variations of quantitative numbers, proportional abundances were preferred to draw conclusions on modulation of the mucosal microbiota. Therefore, abundances at the family level are presented as absolute data for the luminal microbiota, whereas they are presented as proportional values for the mucosal compartment (Table 1). Furthermore, proportional abundance of the 25 most abundant OTUs and 7 additional OTUs affected by at least one of the treatments are shown in Supplementary Table S1 to get insights at the highest phylogenetic resolution possible.

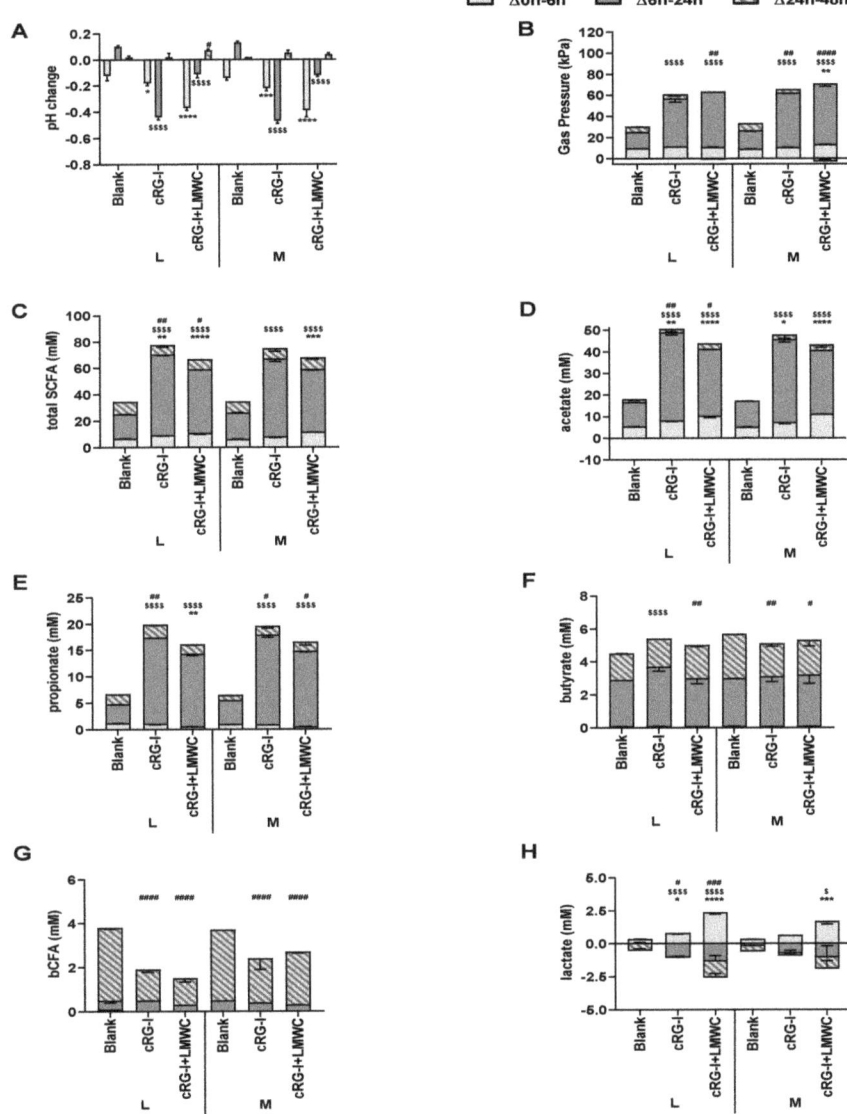

Figure 4. Effect of fermentation of cRG-I and cRG-I+LMWC on microbial metabolic activity in short-term colonic batch simulations in absence or presence of a mucosal compartment. Average changes (± st. dev.) in pH (A), gas production (B), total short-chain fatty acids (SCFA) (C), acetate (D), propionate (E), butyrate (F), branched CFA (bCFA) (G) and lactate (H) levels between 0 and 6 h (light gray), 6 h and 24 h (dark gray) and 24 h and 48 h (stripes) upon dosing cRG-I and cRG-I + LMWC to the gut microbiota versus a blank incubation ($n = 3$). Statistically significant differences between the blank and treatments for different time intervals are presented by * for Δ0 h–6 h, $ for Δ6 h–24 h or # for Δ24 h–48 h). (*, $, #) = $p < 0.05$, (**, $$, ##) = $p < 0.01$, (***, $$$, ###) = $p < 0.001$ and (****, $$$$, ####) = $p < 0.0001$. L = colonic incubations only simulating lumen; M = incubations simulating both lumen and mucus.

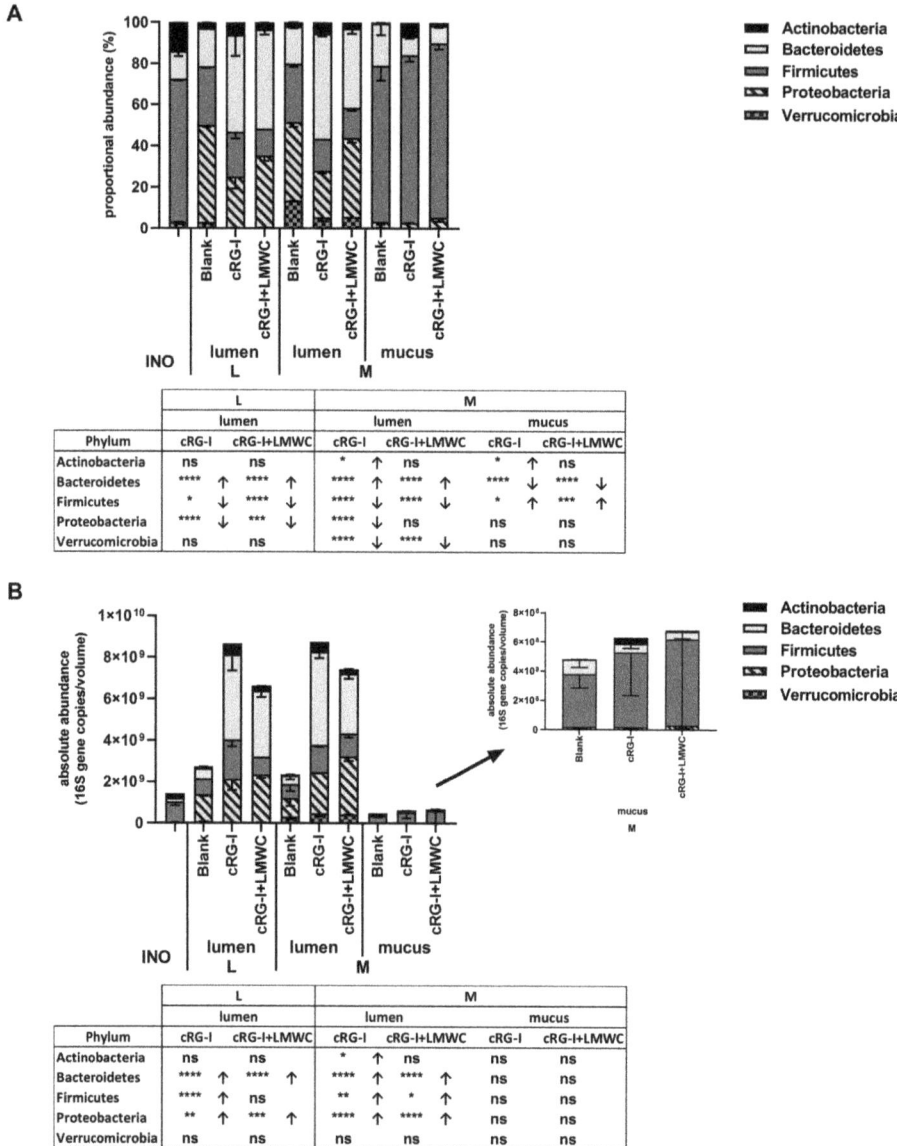

Figure 5. Effect of fermentation of cRG-I and cRG-I+LMWC on microbial community composition at phylum level in short-term colonic incubations in absence or presence of a mucosal compartment. Average (± st. dev.) proportional (%) (**A**) and absolute (16S gene copies/mL) (**B**) abundance of the different phyla in the original (diluted) inoculum (INO) and after 48 h of incubation upon dosing of cRG-I and cRG-I+LMWC versus a blank control (n = 3). Statistically significant differences between the blank and treatments are presented by *. (*) = $p < 0.05$, (**) = $p < 0.01$, (***) = $p < 0.001$ and (****) = $p < 0.0001$. L = colonic incubations only simulating lumen; M = incubations simulating both lumen and mucus.

Table 1. Effect of fermentation of cRG-I and cRG-I+LMWC on microbial composition at family level in short-term colonic incubations in absence or presence of a mucosal compartment. Average proportional (%) (mucus) and absolute (16S gene copies/mL) (lumen) abundance of the different bacterial families in the original (diluted) inoculum and after 48 h of incubation upon dosing cRG-I and cRG-I +LMWC versus a blank control ($n = 3$). Statistically significant differences between the blank and treatments are indicated in bold ($p < 0.05$). Upon reaching statistically significant differences, highest values are underlined. Values indicated in italicsy are strongly increased, although not significant. L = colonic incubations only simulating lumen; M = incubations simulating both lumen and mucus.

Phylum	Family	Inoculum	Absolute Abundance (16S Gene Copies/mL)						Proportional Abundance (%)		
			L			M			M		
			lumen			lumen			mucus		
			blank	cRG-I	cRG-I+LMWC	blank	cRG-I	cRG-I+LMWC	blank	cRG-I	cRG-I+LMWC
Actinobacteria	Bifidobacteriaceae	7.28	7.18	8.68	**8.28**	6.89	8.63	**8.26**	0.2%	6.4%	1.2%
	Coriobacteriaceae	8.22	6.60	6.39	6.88	6.25	6.36	6.80	0.0%	0.0%	0.0%
	Eggerthellaceae	6.56	**7.72**	**7.40**	**7.22**	7.49	7.29	7.09	0.1%	0.0%	0.0%
Bacteroidetes	Bacteroidaceae	7.94	8.63	**9.60**	**9.50**	8.52	**9.65**	**9.45**	20.1%	9.1%	8.5%
	Marinifilaceae	6.23	6.12	6.36	6.04	6.46	6.43	6.25	0.1%	0.0%	0.0%
	Muribaculaceae	6.10	7.02	6.73	**6.15**	6.78	6.56	6.03	0.1%	0.0%	0.0%
	Prevotellaceae	6.74	<LOQ	**7.04**	**6.04**	5.48	**6.55**	**6.15**	0.0%	0.0%	0.0%
	Rikenellaceae	7.94	6.85	7.02	6.60	6.57	6.83	6.68	0.1%	0.0%	0.1%
	Tannerellaceae	6.19	**7.70**	**7.35**	**7.05**	7.58	7.42	7.24	0.1%	0.0%	0.0%
Firmicutes	Christensenellaceae	7.58	7.06	7.14	6.66	6.82	6.94	6.75	0.0%	0.0%	0.0%
	Clostridiaceae cluster I	6.15	5.96	<LOQ	5.95	6.40	5.94	6.17	41.7%	2.1%	1.8%
	Erysipelotrichaceae	7.41	6.93	**7.32**	**7.33**	7.07	7.55	**7.81**	1.1%	1.0%	1.4%
	Clostridiaceae cluster XI	<LOQ	6.27	**6.58**	6.39	6.36	6.48	6.69	0.0%	0.0%	0.0%
	Clostridiaceae cluster XIII	6.43	6.45	6.14	<LOQ	**6.73**	6.16	**6.09**	0.0%	0.0%	0.0%
	Lachnospiraceae	8.59	8.65	**8.93**	8.57	8.51	8.73	8.58	28.3%	74.0%	79.1%
	Peptococcaceae	6.53	6.36	6.07	5.85	6.16	<LOQ	5.69	0.0%	0.0%	0.0%
	Peptostreptococcaceae	6.45	6.15	**6.70**	6.43	5.95	**7.16**	**7.30**	0.0%	0.0%	0.0%
	Ruminococcaceae	8.64	8.38	**8.83**	**8.30**	8.34	8.72	8.49	4.1%	3.0%	1.5%
	Streptococcaceae	6.37	<LOQ	**6.70**	**8.14**	5.26	5.80	**8.17**	0.1%	1.0%	*0.5%*
	Veillonellaceae	7.77	7.67	**8.45**	**8.01**	7.51	**8.31**	**8.16**	0.2%	0.2%	0.2%
Proteobacteria	Burkholderiaceae	5.18	6.78	6.83	6.32	6.74	6.60	6.41	0.0%	0.0%	0.0%
	Desulfovibrionaceae	6.19	6.26	**6.73**	**6.75**	6.15	**6.80**	**6.93**	0.0%	0.0%	0.0%
	Enterobacteriaceae	6.03	9.10	**9.32**	**9.35**	8.90	**9.29**	**9.45**	2.8%	2.8%	5.1%
Verrucomicrobia	Akkermansiaceae	7.63	7.91	7.55	7.71	8.46	8.67	8.64	0.6%	0.2%	0.4%

First, upon comparing the luminal and mucosal microbiota, it followed that the Firmicutes phylum was enriched in the mucosal compartment, while *Actinobacteria*, *Proteobacteria* and *Verrucomicrobia* were enriched in the lumen (Figure 5A), in accordance to what has been published for the M-SHIME® model [12]. At family level, the mucosal *Firmicutes* enrichment was due to a marked enrichment in *Clostridiaceae* cluster I and *Lachnospiraceae* (Table 1). At OTU level, this was reflected by an enrichment of OTU14 (related to *Clostridium butyricum*), OTU10 (related to *Clostridium tertium*), OTU8 (related to *Clostridium paraputrificum*), OTU12 (related to *Ruminococcus torques*), OTU3 (related to *Roseburia hominis*) and OTU19 (related to *Ruminococcus lactaris*) (Table S1). Furthermore, the decreased mucosal levels of *Actinobacteria*, *Proteobacteria* and *Verrucomicrobia* were solely related to a decreased mucosal colonization of members of the *Eggerthellaceae*, *Enterobacteriaceae*, and *Akkermansiaceae*. Another overall finding of the in vitro model was that the luminal microbiota of blank incubations in absence and presence of a mucosal environment were highly similar. The introduction of mucin beads only resulted in an enrichment of the luminal *Verrucomicrobia* levels (Figure 5A,B). At family level, this was due to an increased luminal abundance of *Akkermansiaceae* (+0.55 log copies/mL) (Table 1).

With respect to treatment effects in the lumen, cRG-I and cRG-I+LMWC both increased the absolute levels of *Actinobacteria*, *Bacteroidetes* and *Proteobacteria* compared to the blank (Figure 5B). Although the increase of *Actinobacteria* and *Bacteroidetes* was strongest for cRG-I, the increase in *Proteobacteria* was strongest for cRG-I+LMWC. cRG-I additionally increased luminal *Firmicutes* levels. The luminal increase in *Actinobacteria* by cRG-I was due to a significant increase of OTUs related to *Bifidobacterium longum* (OTU7) and *Bifidobacterium adolescentis* (OTU21) (Table S1), thus also strongly increasing *Bifidobacteriaceae* levels upon cRG-I treatment (Table 1). Furthermore, cRG-I also stimulated mucosal *Bifidobacteriaceae*, mostly due to the stimulation of the *Bifidobacterium longum*-related OTU7. The luminal *Bacteroidetes* increase upon treatment with both products was due to the stimulation of the *Bacteroidaceae* and *Prevotellaceae* families, with again the highest levels being reached for cRG-I. At OTU level, a wide spectrum of *Bacteroidaceae* members were stimulated upon dosing both cRG-I and cRG-I+LMWC, including OTUs related to *B. ovatus* (OTU22), *B. plebeius* (OTU6), *B. xylanisolvens* (OTU18) and especially *B. dorei* (OTU2). As a remark, a decrease in abundances of OTUs related to *B. caccae* (OTU13), *B. fragilis* (OTU11) and *B. uniformis* (OTU17) upon cRG-I and cRG-I+LMWC treatment was noted, but these decreases were less profound compared to observed increases in other OTUs. The increased abundance in *Proteobacteria* related to an enrichment of *Desulfovibrionaceae* and *Enterobacteriaceae*, which was most pronounced upon dosing of cRG-I+LMWC. Finally, the luminal increase in *Firmicutes* with cRG-I and cRG-I+LMWC was due to increased levels of *Erysipelotrichaceae*, *Peptostreptococcaceae*, *Streptococcacae*, *Ruminococcaceae*, and *Veillonellaceae*. The enrichment in *Streptococcacae* was most pronounced upon dosing cRG-I+LMWC and linked to an increase in OTU26 (related to *Streptococcus aginosus*). In contrast, the increase in *Veillonellaceae* was more pronounced upon dosing of cRG-I and was attributed to an increase in OTU9 (related to *Dialister succinatiphilus*). Within the *Ruminococcaceae*, two OTUs related to *Faecalibacterium prausnitzii* (i.e., OTU83 and OTU5) increased upon cRG-I, while only OTU5 was stimulated by cRG-I+LMWC and this to a lesser extent.

In the mucosal compartment, both treatments slightly increased *Firmicutes*, while decreasing *Bacteroidetes* levels (Figure 5A). Both cRG-I and cRG-I+LMWC strongly enriched *Lachnospiraceae* (Table 1), due to a marked stimulation of OTU3 (related to *Roseburia hominis*) that increased from 9.8% in the blank control incubations to 64.3% and 74.2%, respectively (Table S1). Although both treatments also significantly increased the proportion of *Streptococcacae* in the mucosal environment, only cRG-I increased mucosal *Actinobacteria* abundances.

To confirm several of the above-mentioned observations obtained through 16S-targeted Illumina sequencing, qPCRs on specific bacterial groups of interest were performed (Supplementary Table S2). This confirmed the key aforementioned conclusions obtained through 16S-targeted Illumina sequencing including that both cRG-I and cRG-I+LMWC stimulated levels of (i) luminal/mucosal *Bifidobacteriaceae* (and not *Lactobacillaceae*); (ii) luminal *Bacteroidetes*; (iii) luminal *Faecalibacterium prausnitzii*; (iv) mucosal *Roseburia* (and *Eubacterium rectale/Clostridium coccoides* group to which it belongs); while not affecting

Akkermansia muciniphila. In addition, both products, but mostly cRG-I+LMWC, increased colonization of *Eubacterium hallii* in the simulated mucus layer.

3.5. Effect of Fermented cRG-I on Intestinal Epithelial Barrier (Test 4)

As cRG-I fermentation enriched several health-associated species and increased production of SCFA, it might exert favorable effects at the host level. To address this question, a Caco-2/PBMC co-culture model was developed. Inflammation-induced barrier disruption was obtained upon 48 h co-culturing of Caco-2 cells with PWM-activated PBMCs and measured as a significant decrease in TEER of the Caco-2 monolayers (Figure S1A). In addition, apical treatment with the positive control sodium butyrate (NaB) prevented this TEER decrease. Likewise, apical treatment with fermented cRG-I showed a significant increase in TEER compared to the blank controls (Figure 6A). Furthermore, effects on T-cell dependent cytokine production were assessed. As shown in Figure S1, NaB significantly decreased the secretion of interferon (IFN)γ, interleukin (IL)-17A, IL-21, IL-4, and IL-9; while increasing the secretion of IL-22; a cytokine involved in maintenance of barrier integrity, wound healing and antimicrobial responses [53]. However, in contrast to its positive effects on IL-10 secretion in the Caco-2/THP1 co-culture assay [29], NaB significantly decreased IL-10 secretion possibly due to toxicity of NaB on IL-10 producing cells at the concentration used [54,55]. Compared to the blank control, fermented cRG-I reduced the secretion of IL-17A, IL-4, and IL-9; reaching statistical significance for IL-17A and IL-4 upon luminal incubations and upon both incubations for IL-9 (Figure 6D,F,G). Furthermore, luminal fermentation of cRG-I tended to increase the secretion of IL-22 and IL-10; of which the latter was already increased upon treatment with the blank controls (Figure 6E,H). In addition, all colonic suspensions completely abolished PWM-induced IL-21 secretion (Figure 6C); while no significant differences were observed on IFNγ secretion (Figure 6B). Hence, metabolites generated from colonic fermentation of cRG-I displayed anti-inflammatory and gut barrier protective properties.

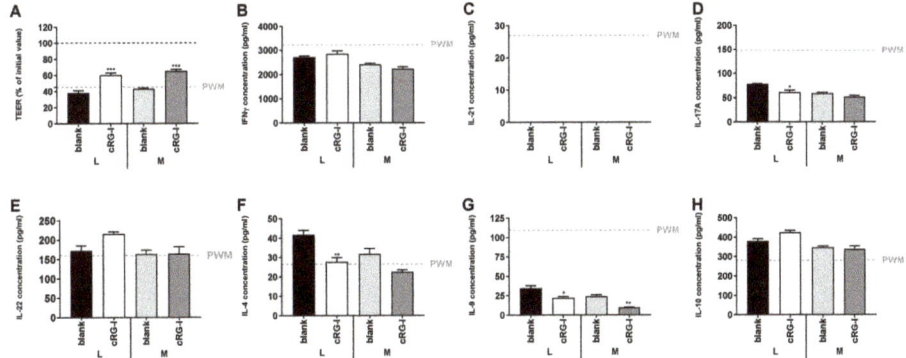

Figure 6. Effect of fermented cRG-I on transepithelial electrical resistance (TEER) and cytokine production in a Caco-2/PBMC co-culture system. Caco-2 cells, cultured 14 days on transwell inserts, were placed on top of pokeweed mitogen (PWM)-activated PBMCs and incubated for 48 h at the apical side with blank or treatment samples collected during the colonic batch incubations containing only a luminal (L) or also a mucosal (M) environment. Average (±SEM) TEER of the Caco-2 monolayers (**A**) and concentration of secreted interferon (IFN)γ (**B**), interleukin (IL)-17A (**C**), IL-21 (**D**), IL-22 (**E**), IL-4 (**F**), IL-9 (**G**) and IL-10 (**H**) in the basolateral medium are shown (n = 3). Statistically significant differences to PWM are represented by (*). (*) = $p < 0.05$, (**) = $p < 0.01$, (***) = $p < 0.001$.

Overall, some minor effects of the incorporation of a mucosal compartment were observed as both blank and treatment colonic suspensions slightly increased TEER; while decreased the secretion of all tested cytokines compared to luminal suspensions (Figure 6).

4. Discussion

In the current study, novel in vitro models and analytical techniques were implemented to investigate whether cRG-I classifies as a potential prebiotic ingredient. First, upon exposure to α-amylase and brush border enzymes (Test 1), unlike the positive controls (cooked starch and maltose, respectively), cRG-I (like the negative control inulin) was not digested to any of the simple sugars measured. This suggests that cRG-I can be considered to be a polysaccharide that likely escapes upper GIT digestion in vivo, thus fulfilling the definition of a prebiotic ingredient that should reach the colon where it could be fermented by the gut microbiota. Secondly, a recently described short-term colonic incubation strategy [29] was upgraded with a simulation of the mucosal microbiota (Test 3). By applying a novel technique to analyze the microbial community composition, i.e., quantitative 16S-targeted Illumina sequencing [33], in-depth quantitative information was obtained at high phylogenetic resolution. Besides elucidating treatment effects of cRG-I, this allowed to validate the implementation of mucin-coated carriers in the short-term incubations by demonstrating a relevant species-specific colonization of the mucosal environment. Indeed, consistent with the well-established long-term M-SHIME® model [12], a wide spectrum of (potential butyrate-producing) *Firmicutes* members specifically colonized the mucosal environment (e.g., OTUs related to *Clostridium butyricum* and *Roseburia hominis*). Furthermore, inclusion of the mucosal environment did not alter the luminal microbiota (except for a minor enrichment in *Akkermansiaceae*), nor did it alter the treatment effects towards luminal microbiota activity and community composition. Overall, including the mucin beads in the current colonic simulations allowed to maintain a higher diversity, thus allowing observation of more complete treatment effects of cRG-I. Finally, application of a model combining gut epithelial and immune cells allowed to point out the gut protective effect of cRG-I fermentation-derived metabolites against an inflammatory stressor (Test 4).

In a first series of short-term colonic incubations (Test 2), cRG-I was found to display prebiotic potential comparable but not identical to that of inulin in modulating microbial activity [19], as followed from increases in health-promoting SCFA (acetate and propionate) and lactate and decreases of bCFA. A side effect of inulin fermentation is the production of high amounts of gas that has been observed in in vitro experiments and clinical studies. Depending on the dose, this can result in mild negative gastro-intestinal symptoms [56–58]. Interestingly, gas production upon dosing of cRG-I was milder compared to inulin, which suggests that in vivo consumption of cRG-I could be less accompanied by adverse side-effects such as bloating and abdominal pain.

Upon fermentation in both short-term colonic incubations (Tests 2/3), cRG-I stimulated acetate, and lactate production which was accompanied with a strong reduction in pH. At community level, this correlated with increases in OTUs related to *Bifidobacterium longum* (OTU7) and *Bifidobacterium adolescentis* (OTU21). *Bifidobacteriaceae* are indeed key acetate and lactate producers [59,60]. Although health effects are to be considered strain-specific, multiple *Bifidobacterium* strains have been associated with beneficial effects on the host health and some strains are widely used as probiotics. A first mechanism by which *Bifidobacteriaceae* contribute to health is by indirectly promoting butyrate production via cross-feeding mechanisms involving for instance *Faecalibacterium prausnitzii* and *Eubacterium hallii* [59,61,62], taxa of which related OTUs were indeed found to be increased upon cRG-I treatment in the current study. In addition, acetate produced by bifidobacteria was also shown to play a key role in their anti-infectious properties against enteropathogens [63]. In terms of host effects, a specific *B. longum* strain has e.g., been shown to exert protective effects in a DSS-induced colitis model in mice by reducing inflammation and enhancing the intestinal epithelial barrier [64]. Moreover, a specific *B. longum* strain reduced chronic mucosal inflammation in ulcerative colitis (UC) patients in a double-blinded, randomized-controlled clinical trial [65]. Likewise, a specific *B. adolescentis* strain protected mice from DSS-induced colitis by increasing IL-10 levels, up-regulation of regulatory T-cells (T_{reg}) and decreasing IL-17A positive T-cells [66]. The strong bifidogenic effect exerted by cRG-I thus supports the prebiotic potential of this novel food ingredient.

Next to acetate and lactate, fermentation of cRG-I increased the production of propionate, which correlated with a stimulation of *Prevotellaceae* and *Bacteroidaceae* due to the stimulation of a wide spectrum of *Bacteroidaceae* OTUs related to e.g., *B. ovatus*, *B. plebeius*, *B. xylanisolvens* and especially *B. dorei*. Indeed, *Bacteriodetes* spp. are known primary fiber degraders that are capable of producing propionate [50]. In the colon, health-related effects of propionate are related to anti-cancer effects [7,8]. Furthermore, propionate was shown to exert anti-lipogenic and cholesterol-lowering effects in the liver [6]. Finally, propionate is a satiety-inducing agent affecting energy intake and feeding behavior [67]. Besides the beneficial effects of propionate, the aforementioned stimulations of specific *Bacteroidaceae* members have also been related to particular health benefits. As an example, in a mouse model of atherosclerosis, *B. dorei* reduced plaque inflammation and decreased intestinal epithelial permeability and systemic endotoxemia [68]. Furthermore, *B. ovatus* reduced mucosal inflammation and stimulated epithelial proliferation and mucin production in a DSS-induced colitis model in mice [69]. Another microbial modulation that could have boosted propionate production upon cRG-I treatment was the increase in *Veillonellaceae* that was solely attributed to an increase in OTU9 (related to *Dialister succinatiphilus*). Interestingly, *D. succinatiphilus* is a succinate-converting, propionate-producing species [70] and as many *Bacteroidetes* spp. are known succinate producers [50], its increase might have contributed to the stronger increase in propionate levels upon dosing of cRG-I. As a final remark, not all *Bacteroidaceae* members increased upon cRG-I treatment, with OTUs relating to *B. caccae* and *B. fragilis* decreasing in abundance upon cRG-I treatment. These species are considered to be opportunistic pathogens carrying virulence factors: enterotoxigenic *B. fragilis* strains secrete the *B. fragilis* toxin (BFT) [71] and *B. caccae* contains the *ompW* gene [72]. Besides its strong bifidogenic effect, cRG-I could further exert health benefits by targeted modulation of specific propionate-producing taxa.

In contrast to propionate, butyrate was not significantly increased upon dosing of cRG-I. However, cRG-I did strongly stimulate *Lachnospiraceae*, containing several butyrate-producing species, in the mucosal compartment. The increase in *Lachnospiraceae* was related to a strong stimulation of an OTU related to *Roseburia hominis*, which has been associated with beneficial effects on barrier function and immune regulation in the gut [73]. Indeed, *R. hominis* showed protective effects in a DSS-model for colitis in mice by reducing pro-inflammatory cytokine expression. Moreover, increased T_{reg} levels were observed in both germ-free and conventional mice fed a supplement containing live *R. hominis*. Also, a significant reduction of *R. hominis* and *F. prausnitzii* was observed in UC and Crohn's disease (CD) patients [74,75]. Interestingly, cRG-I increased the abundance of OTUs related to butyrate-producing species such as *F. prausnitzii* and *Eubacterium hallii*. Like *R. hominis*, *F. prausnitzii* was shown to exert anti-inflammatory potential by increasing IL-10 and promoting T_{reg} differentiation in mice [76]. On the other hand, *E. hallii* improved insulin sensitivity in a mouse model for diabetes [77]. Of note, discrepancy between the stimulation of butyrate producers in the mucosal environment with cRG-I versus the absence of treatment effects on butyrate levels might be explained by the fact that the biofilm which develops on the mucin-coated carriers during short-term colonic incubations (48 h) is still developing during cRG-I treatment. Hence, by the time the biofilm is developed (48 h), all substrate has been consumed (in fact already after 24 h). This may potentially limit the detection of treatment effects resulting from modulation of mucosal microbes on metabolic activity (particularly butyrate production) during short-term incubations. Therefore, testing the impact of cRG-I in a long-term M-SHIME® study could further elucidate the potential impact of cRG-I on butyrate production.

The stimulation of several health-related microbial species and the concomitant increase in health-promoting metabolites suggested that cRG-I may display interesting host beneficial properties in terms of intestinal barrier protection and reduction of inflammation. This hypothesis was confirmed using a Caco-2/PBMC co-culture model in which treatment with fermented cRG-I significantly increased the TEER, indicative for the protective effects of fermentation-derived cRG-I metabolites on inflammation-induced intestinal permeability. To further strengthen this observation, it would be interesting to perform in-depth analysis of the expression and localization of tight junction proteins including occludin, ZO-1, and claudins upon cRG-I treatment in this system. Furthermore, fermented cRG-I metabolites decreased the secretion of the pro-inflammatory cytokines IL-17A, IL-4, and IL-9, while increasing the secretion of IL-22 and of the anti-inflammatory IL-10. This is suggestive of a possible immunoregulatory effect of cRG-I metabolites on the T_{reg}/T_H17 axis; favoring down-regulation of excessive inflammation as IL-10 is necessary for T_{reg} functions [78]. Th17 cells have a dual role in human health as although required for clearance of extracellular pathogens, an elevated frequency of Th17 cells associated with impaired T_{reg} functions has been reported in IBD and other extraintestinal autoimmune disorders [79]. Furthermore, IL-22 plays a role in maintaining the integrity of the mucosal barrier by promoting wound healing and activating antimicrobial responses [53]. Finally, increased levels of IL-4 and IL-9 were associated with UC [80,81]. In addition, IL-9 inhibits wound healing in the intestinal mucosa and impairs intestinal epithelial barrier functions. Also, IL-9 directly regulates tissue recruitment and inflammatory functions of mast cells. Together, these data suggest an interesting immuno-modulatory role of cRG-I metabolites in the gut in terms of increasing barrier tightness and prevention of a "leaky gut".

Finally, a modified formulation of cRG-I was tested which contained small size sugars, i.e., cRG-I+LMWC. Interestingly, the short-term colonic incubation strategy applied in this study was highly sensitive to pick up differences in closely related product compositions. For instance, the presence of these simple sugars resulted in a stronger initial pH decrease upon dosing of cRG-I+LMWC, related to an initial increased production of lactate, which could be linked to a stronger enrichment in a *Streptococcacae* OTU related to *Streptococcus aginosus*. Also, *Enterobacteriaceae* levels were higher upon cRG-I+LMWC treatment. Like *Streptococcaceae*, *Enterobacteriaceae* are expert fermenters of simple sugars [82], specifically present at higher levels in this preparation. Finally, *Coriobacteriaceae* (OTU15 related to *Collinsella aerofaciens*) and *Desulfovibrionaceae* tended to be higher in incubations with cRG-I+LMWC. This suggested a potential co-existence of e.g., *C. aerofaciens* and *Desulfovibrio piger*, based on the fact that the main products of *C. aerofaciens* fermentation (i.e., lactate, H_2, and formate) serve as substrates for *D. piger*, which is the main sulfate-reducing bacterial species in the human gut microbiome [83]. This might also indicate that cRG-I+LMWC might contain small quantities of sulfur (sulfate or sulfur-containing amino acids). These data altogether stress the relevance of testing prebiotic candidates in short-term colonic in vitro incubations to understand their potential impact on the human gut microbiome and to support structure-function studies.

In conclusion, the implementation of novel in vitro models simulating the human colonic environment coupled to cell-based assays mimicking the host gut barrier, allowed to establish the prebiotic potential of cRG-I. This novel fiber is not digested by host enzymes characteristic of the upper gastro-intestinal tract but rapidly fermented by the human colonic microbiota leading to selective stimulation of the growth and activity of intestinal bacterial species associated with human health. cRG-I displays unique properties as it was fermented more rapidly than inulin leading to production of SCFA, especially acetate and propionate, and less gas than inulin. It increases the abundance of several bacterial species reputed for their "anti-inflammatory" profile. In line with this, the metabolites resulting from cRG-I fermentation exhibited a protective effect in an in vitro model of inflamed gut barrier. Overall, the data obtained during this study support future research to further investigate this novel prebiotic candidate in long-term SHIME® models with different fecal sample donors and in clinical trials to confirm the beneficial effect of cRG-I on the microbiota and its impact on human health.

Supplementary Materials: The following are available online at http://www.mdpi.com/2072-6643/12/7/1917/s1, Figure S1: Effect of Sodium butyrate (NaB) on transepithelial electrical resistance (TEER) and cytokine production in a Caco-2/PBMC co-culture system; Table S1: Effect of fermentation of cRG-I and cRG-I+LMWC on microbial community composition at OTU level in short-term colonic batch simulations in absence or presence of a mucosal compartment; Table S2: Effect of fermentation of cRG-I and cRG-I+LMWC on selected bacterial groups in short-term colonic batch simulations in absence or presence of a mucosal compartment as assessed through qPCR.

Author Contributions: Conceptualization, A.M., P.v.d.A., M.M.; Methodology, P.v.d.A.; Formal Analysis, J.G., L.V.; Investigation, J.G., L.V.; Data Curation, P.v.d.A., L.V., J.G.; Writing-Original Draft Preparation, A.M.; P.v.d.A., L.V. Writing-Review and Editing, A.M., R.A., P.v.d.A., L.V.; Supervision, P.v.d.A., M.M.; Project Administration, M.M.; Funding Acquisition, A.M., R.A. All authors have read and agreed to the published version of the manuscript.

Funding: The studies described in this manuscript were performed at the request of and were funded by NutriLeads B.V., Wageningen, The Netherlands. This project has received funding from the European Union's Horizon 2020 research and innovation programme under grant agreements No 811592 and Eurostars E! 10574-NIMF.

Acknowledgments: We thank C. Rösch and H. Schols for their expert advice in the preparation of the cRG-I formulations and sugar analysis. We acknowledge the support of M. Aparicio-Vergara and M. Tzoumaki in performing preliminary work to the experiments.

Conflicts of Interest: A.M. and R.A. are employees of Nutrileads the funder of the study. A.M. participated to the design of the study and the writing of the manuscript. R.A. edited the manuscript.

References

1. Forgie, A.J.; Fouhse, J.M.; Willing, B.P. Diet-Microbe-Host Interactions That Affect Gut Mucosal Integrity and Infection Resistance. *Front. Immunol.* **2019**, *10*, 1802. [CrossRef]
2. Monteagudo-Mera, A.; Rastall, R.A.; Gibson, G.R.; Charalampopoulos, D.; Chatzifragkou, A. Adhesion mechanisms mediated by probiotics and prebiotics and their potential impact on human health. *Appl. Microbiol. Biotechnol.* **2019**, *103*, 6463–6472. [CrossRef]
3. Kachrimanidou, M.; Tsintarakis, E. Insights into the Role of Human Gut Microbiota in Clostridioides difficile Infection. *Microorganisms* **2020**, *8*, 200. [CrossRef]
4. Hooper, L.V.; Midtvedt, T.; Gordon, J.I. How host-microbial interactions shape the nutrient environment of the mammalian intestine. *Annu. Rev. Nutr.* **2002**, *22*, 283–307. [CrossRef]
5. Liu, H.; Wang, J.; He, T.; Becker, S.; Zhang, G.; Li, D.; Ma, X. Butyrate: A Double-Edged Sword for Health? *Adv. Nutr.* **2018**, *9*, 21–29. [CrossRef] [PubMed]
6. Delzenne, N.M.; Williams, C.M. Prebiotics and lipid metabolism. *Curr. Opin. Lipidol.* **2002**, *13*, 61–67. [CrossRef] [PubMed]
7. Li, C.J.; Elsasser, T.H. Butyrate-induced apoptosis and cell cycle arrest in bovine kidney epithelial cells: Involvement of caspase and proteasome pathways. *J Anim. Sci.* **2005**, *83*, 89–97. [CrossRef]
8. Jan, G.; Belzacq, A.S.; Haouzi, D.; Rouault, A.; Métivier, D.; Kroemer, G.; Brenner, C. Propionibacteria induce apoptosis of colorectal carcinoma cells via short-chain fatty acids acting on mitochondria. *Cell Death Differ.* **2002**, *9*, 179–188. [CrossRef]
9. Lin, Y.G.; Vonk, R.J.; Slooff, M.J.H.; Kuipers, F.; Smit, M.J. Differences in propionate-induced inhibition of cholesterol and triacylglycerol synthesis between human and rat hepatocytes in primary culture. *Br. J. Nutr.* **1995**, *74*, 197–207. [CrossRef]
10. Nishina, P.M.; Freedland, R.A. Effects of propionate on lipid biosynthesis in isolated rat hepatocytes. *J. Nutr.* **1990**, *120*, 668–673. [CrossRef]
11. Rinninella, E.; Raoul, P.; Cintoni, M.; Franceschi, F.; Miggiano, G.A.D.; Gasbarrini, A.; Mele, M.C. What is the Healthy Gut Microbiota Composition? A Changing Ecosystem across Age, Environment, Diet, and Diseases. *Microorganisms* **2019**, *7*, 14. [CrossRef] [PubMed]
12. Van den Abbeele, P.; Belzer, C.; Goossens, M.; Kleerebezem, M.; De Vos, W.M.; Thas, O.; De Weirdt, R.; Kerckhof, F.M.; Van de Wiele, T. Butyrate-producing Clostridium cluster XIVa species specifically colonize mucins in an in vitro gut model. *ISME J.* **2013**, *7*, 949–961. [CrossRef] [PubMed]
13. Eckburg, P.B.; Bik, E.M.; Bernstein, C.N.; Purdom, E.; Dethlefsen, L.; Sargent, M.; Gill, S.R.; Nelson, K.E.; Relman, D.A. Diversity of the human intestinal microbial flora. *Science* **2005**, *308*, 1635–1638. [CrossRef] [PubMed]
14. Frank, D.N.; Amand, A.L.S.; Feldman, R.A.; Boedeker, E.C.; Harpaz, N.; Pace, N.R. Molecular-phylogenetic characterization of microbial community imbalances in human inflammatory bowel diseases. *Proc. Natl. Acad. Sci. USA* **2007**, *104*, 13780–13785. [CrossRef]
15. Shen, X.J.; Rawls, J.F.; Randall, T.A.; Burcall, L.; Mpande, C.; Jenkins, N.; Jovov, B.; Abdo, Z.; Sandler, R.S.; Keku, T.O. Molecular characterization of mucosal adherent bacteria and associations with colorectal adenomas. *Gut Microbes* **2010**, *1*, 138–147. [CrossRef]
16. Wang, Y.; Antonopoulos, D.; Zhu, X.; Harrell, L.; Hanan, I.; Alverdy, J.; Meyer, F.; Musch, M.W.; Young, V.B.; Chang, E.B. Laser capture microdissection and metagenomic analysis of intact mucosa-associated microbial communities of human colon. *Appl. Environ. Microbiol.* **2010**, *88*, 1333–1342. [CrossRef] [PubMed]

17. Willing, B.P.; Dicksved, J.; Halfvarson, J.; Andersson, A.F.; Lucio, M.; Zheng, Z.; Järnerot, G.; Tysk, C.; Jansson, J.K.; Engstrand, L. A pyrosequencing study in twins shows that gastrointestinal microbial profiles vary with inflammatory bowel disease phenotypes. *Gastroenterology* **2010**, *139*, 1844–1854. [CrossRef]
18. Hong, P.-Y.; Croix, J.A.; Greenberg, E.; Gaskins, H.R.; Mackie, R.I. Pyrosequencing-based analysis of the mucosal microbiota in healthy individuals reveals ubiquitous bacterial groups and micro-heterogeneity. *PLoS ONE* **2011**, *6*, e25042. [CrossRef]
19. Gibson, G.R.; Hutkins, R.; Sanders, M.E.; Prescott, S.L.; Reimer, R.A.; Salminen, S.J.; Scott, K.; Stanton, C.; Swanson, K.S.; Cani, P.D.; et al. Expert consensus document: The International Scientific Association for Probiotics and Prebiotics (ISAPP) consensus statement on the definition and scope of prebiotics. *Nat. Rev. Gastroenterol. Hepatol.* **2017**, *14*, 491–502. [CrossRef]
20. Minekus, M.; Alminger, M.; Alvito, P.; Balance, S.; Bohn, T.; Bourlieu, C.; Carrière, F.; Boutrou, R.; Corredig, M.; Dupont, D.; et al. A standardised static in vitro digestion method suitable for food—An international consensus. *Food Funct.* **2014**, *5*, 1113–1124. [CrossRef]
21. Hodoniczky, J.; Morris, C.A.; Rae, A.L. Oral and intestinal digestion of oligosaccharides as potential sweeteners: A systematic evaluation. *J. Food Chem.* **2012**, *132*, 1951–1958. [CrossRef]
22. Sonnenburg, E.D.; Zheng, H.; Joglekar, P.; Higginbottom, S.K.; Firbank, S.J.; Bolam, D.N.; Sonnenburg, J.L. Specificity of polysaccharide use in intestinal bacteroides species determines diet-induced microbiota alterations. *Cell* **2010**, *141*, 1241–1252. [CrossRef] [PubMed]
23. Hiippala, K.; Kainulainen, V.; Suutarinen, M.; Heini, T.; Bowers, J.R.; Jasso-Selles, D.; Lemmer, D.; Valentine, M.; Barnes, R.; Engelthaler, D.M.; et al. Isolation of Anti-Inflammatory and Epithelium Reinforcing Bacteroides and Parabacteroides Spp. from A Healthy Fecal Donor. *Nutrients* **2020**, *12*, E935. [CrossRef] [PubMed]
24. Coenen, G.J.; Bakx, E.; Verhoef, R.P.; Schols, H.A.; Voragen, A. Identification of the connecting linkage between homo- or xylogalacturonan and rhamnogalacturonan type I. Carbohydrate. *Polymers* **2007**, *70*, 224–235.
25. Wu, D.; Zheng, J.; Mao, G.; Hu, W.; Ye, X.; Linhardt, R.J.; Chen, S. Rethinking the impact of RG-I mainly from fruits and vegetables on dietary health. *Crit. Rev. Food Sci. Nutr.* **2019**, 1–23. [CrossRef]
26. Chakaroun, R.M.; Massier, L.; Kovacs, P. Gut Microbiome, Intestinal Permeability, and Tissue Bacteria in Metabolic Disease: Perpetrators or Bystanders? *Nutrients* **2020**, *12*, E1082. [CrossRef]
27. Marzorati, M.; Pinheiro, I.; Van den Abbeele, P.; Van de Wiele, T.; Possemiers, S. An in vitro technology platform to assess host microbiota interactions in the gastrointestinal tract. *Agro Food Ind. Hi Tech* **2013**, *23*, 8–11.
28. Satsu, H.; Ishimoto, Y.; Nakano, T.; Mochizuki, T.; Iwanaga, T.; Shimizu, M. Induction by activated macrophage-like THP-1 cells of apoptotic and necrotic cell death in intestinal epithelial Caco-2 monolayers via tumor necrosis factor-alpha. *Exp. Cell Res.* **2006**, *312*, 3909–3919. [CrossRef]
29. Van den Abbeele, P.; Taminiau, B.; Pinheiro, I.; Duysburgh, C.; Jacobs, H.; Pijls, L.; Marzorati, M. Arabinoxylo-Oligosaccharides and Inulin Impact Inter-Individual Variation on Microbial Metabolism and Composition, Which Immunomodulates Human Cells. *J. Agric. Food Chem.* **2018**, *66*, 1121–1130. [CrossRef] [PubMed]
30. Daguet, D.; Pinheiro, I.; Verhelst, A.; Possemiers, S.; Marzorati, M. Arabinogalactan and fructooligosaccharides improve the gut barrier function in distinct areas of the colon in the Simulator of the Human Intestinal Microbial Ecosystem. *J. Funct. Foods* **2016**, *20*, 369–379. [CrossRef]
31. Possemiers, S.; Pinheiro, I.; Verhelst, A.; Van den Abbeele, P.; Maignien, L.; Laukens, D.; Reeves, S.G.; Robinson, L.E.; Raas, T.; Schneider, Y.-J.; et al. A dried yeast fermentate selectively modulates both the luminal and mucosal gut microbiota and protects against inflammation, as studied in an integrated in vitro approach. *J. Agric. Food Chem.* **2013**, *61*, 9380–9392. [CrossRef] [PubMed]
32. Kleiveland, C.R. Peripheral Blood Mononuclear Cells. In *The Impact of Food Bioactives on Health: In vitro and Ex Vivo Models*; Verhoeckx, K., Cotter, P., López-Expósito, I., Kleiveland, C., Lea, T., Mackie, A., Requena, T., Swiatecka, D., Wichers, H., Eds.; Springer Cham (CH): Cham, Switzerland, 2015; Chapter 15.
33. Van den Abbeele, P.; Moens, F.; Pignataro, G.; Schnurr, J.; Ribecco, C.; Gramenzi, A.; Marzorati, M. Yeast-Derived Formulations Are Differentially Fermented by the Canine and Feline Microbiome As Assessed in a Novel In Vitro Colonic Fermentation Model. *J. Agric. Food Chem.* **2020**. [CrossRef] [PubMed]

34. Jonker, D.; Fowler, P.; Albers, R.; Tzoumaki, M.V.; van het Hof, K.H.; Aparicio-Vergara, M. Safety assessment of rhamnogalacturonan-enriched carrot pectin fraction: 90-day oral toxicity study in rats and in vitro genotoxicity studies. *Food Chem. Toxicol.* **2020**, *139*, 111243. [CrossRef]
35. De Weirdt, R.; Possemiers, S.; Vermeulen, G.; Moerdijk-Poortvliet, T.C.W.; Boschker, H.T.S.; Verstraete, W.; Van de Wiele, T. Human faecal microbiota display variable patterns of glycerol metabolism. *FEMS Microbiol. Ecol.* **2010**, *74*, 601–611. [CrossRef] [PubMed]
36. Boon, N.; Top, E.M.; Verstraete, W.; Siciliano, S.D. Bioaugmentation as a tool to protect the structure and function of an activated-sludge microbial community against a 3-chloroaniline shock load. *Appl. Environ. Microbiol.* **2003**, *69*, 1511–1520. [CrossRef]
37. Furet, J.P.; Firmesse, O.; Gourmelon, M.; Bridonneau, C.; Tap, J.; Mondot, S.; Doré, J.; Corthier, G. Comparative assessment of human and farm animal faecal microbiota using real-time quantitative PCR. *FEMS Microbiol. Ecol.* **2009**, *68*, 351–362. [CrossRef]
38. Rinttilä, T.; Kassinen, A.; Malinen, E.; Kroqius, L.; Palva, A. Development of an extensive set of 16S rDNA-targeted primers for quantification of pathogenic and indigenous bacteria in faecal samples by real-time PCR. *J. Appl. Microbiol.* **2004**, *97*, 1166–1177. [CrossRef]
39. Collado, M.C.; Derrien, M.; Isolauri, E.; de Vos, W.M.; Salminen, S. Intestinal integrity and Akkermansia muciniphila, a mucin-degrading member of the intestinal microbiota present in infants, adults, and the elderly. *Appl. Environ. Microbiol.* **2007**, *23*, 7767–7770. [CrossRef]
40. Guo, X.; Xia, X.; Tang, R.; Zhou, J.; Zhao, H.; Wang, K. Development of a real-time PCR method for Firmicutes and Bacteroidetes in faeces and its application to quantify intestinal population of obese and lean pigs. *Lett. Appl. Microbiol.* **2008**, *47*, 367–373. [CrossRef]
41. Nakano, S.; Kobayashi, T.; Funabiki, K.; Matsumura, A.; Nagao, Y.; Yamada, T. Development of a PCR assay for detection of Enterobacteriaceae in foods. *J. Food Prot.* **2003**, *66*, 1798–1804. [CrossRef]
42. Sokol, H.; Seksik, P.; Furet, J.P.; Firmesse, O.; Nion-Larmurier, I.; Beaugerie, L.; Cosnes, J.; Corthier, G.; Marteau, P.; Doré, J. Low counts of Faecalibacterium prausnitzii in colitis microbiota. *Inflamm. Bowel Dis.* **2009**, *15*, 1183–1189. [CrossRef] [PubMed]
43. Ramirez-Farias, C.; Slezak, K.; Fuller, Z.; Duncan, A.; Holtrop, G.; Louis, P. Effect of inulin on the human gut microbiota: Stimulation of Bifidobacterium adolescentis and Faecalibacterium prausnitzii. *Br. J. Nutr.* **2009**, *101*, 541–550. [CrossRef] [PubMed]
44. Props, R.; Kerckhof, F.-M.; Rubbens, P.; De Vrieze, J.; Hernandez Sanabria, E.; Waegeman, W.; Monsieurs, P.; Hammes, F.; Boon, N. Absolute quantification of microbial taxon abundances. *ISME J.* **2017**, *11*, 584–587. [CrossRef] [PubMed]
45. Klindworth, A.; Pruesse, E.; Schweer, T.; Peplies, J.; Quast, C.; Horn, M.; Glöckner, F.O. Evaluation of general 16S ribosomal RNA gene PCR primers for classical and next-generation sequencing-based diversity studies. *Nucleic Acids Res.* **2013**, *41*, e1. [CrossRef] [PubMed]
46. Schloss, P.D.; Westcott, S.L. Assessing and improving methods used in operational taxonomic unit-based approaches for 16S rRNA gene sequence analysis. *Appl. Environ. Microbiol.* **2011**, *77*, 3219–3226. [CrossRef]
47. Kozich, J.J.; Westcott, S.L.; Baxter, N.T.; Highlander, S.K.; Schloss, P.D. Development of a dual-index sequencing strategy and curation pipeline for analyzing amplicon sequence data on MiSeq Illumina sequencing platform. *Appl. Environ. Microbiol.* **2013**, *79*, 5112–5120. [CrossRef]
48. Wang, Q.; Garrity, G.M.; Tiedje, J.M.; Cole, J.R. Naive Bayesian classifier for rapid assignment of rRNA sequences into the new bacterial taxonomy. *Appl. Environ. Microbiol.* **2007**, *73*, 5261–5267. [CrossRef]
49. Cole, J.R.; Wang, Q.; Cardenas, E.; Fish, J.; Chai, B.; Farris, R.J.; Kulam-Syed-Mohideen, A.S.; McGarrell, D.M.; Marsh, T.; Garrity, G.M.; et al. The ribosomal database project: Improved alignments and new tools for rRNA analysis. *Nucleic Acids Res* **2009**, *37*, D141–D145. [CrossRef]
50. Louis, P.; Flint, H.J. Formation of propionate and butyrate by the human colonic microbiota. *Environ. Microbiol.* **2017**, *19*, 29–41. [CrossRef]
51. Hamer, H.M.; De Preter, V.; Windey, K.; Verbeke, K. Functional analysis of colonic bacterial metabolism: Relevant to health. *Am. J. Physiol. Liver Physiol.* **2012**, *302*, G1–G9. [CrossRef]
52. Scott, K.P.; Gratz, S.W.; Sheridan, P.O.; Flint, H.J.; Duncan, S.H. The influence of diet on the gut microbiota. *Pharmacol. Res.* **2013**, *69*, 52–60. [CrossRef] [PubMed]
53. Kempski, J.; Brockmann, L.; Gagliani, N.; Huber, S. TH17 Cell and Epithelial Cell Crosstalk during Inflammatory Bowel Disease and Carcinogenesis. *Front Immunol.* **2017**, *8*, 1373. [CrossRef]

54. Kurita-Ochiai, T.; Fukushima, K.; Ochiai, K. Lipopolysaccharide stimulates butyric acid-induced apoptosis in human peripheral blood mononuclear cells. *Infect. Immun.* **1999**, *67*, 22–29. [CrossRef] [PubMed]
55. Weber, T.E.; Kerr, B.J. Butyrate differentially regulates cytokines and proliferation in porcine peripheral blood mononuclear cells. *Vet. Immunol. Immunopathol.* **2006**, *113*, 139–147. [CrossRef] [PubMed]
56. Bonnema, A.L.; Kolberg, L.W.; Thomas, W.; Slavin, J.L. Gastrointestinal tolerance of chicory inulin products. *J. Am. Diet. Assoc.* **2010**, *110*, 865–868. [CrossRef]
57. Timm, D.A.; Stewart, M.L.; Hospattankar, A.; Slavin, J.L. Wheat Dextrin, Psyllium, and Inulin Produce Distinct FermentationPatterns, GasVolumes, andShort-Chain Fatty AcidProfiles InVitro. *J. Med. Food* **2010**, *13*, 961–996. [CrossRef]
58. Carlson, J.L.; Erickson, J.M.; Hess, J.M.; Gould, T.J.; Slavin, J.L. Prebiotic Dietary Fiber and Gut Health: Comparing the in Vitro Fermentations of Beta-Glucan, Inulin and Xylooligosaccharide. *Nutrients* **2017**, *9*, 1361. [CrossRef]
59. Belenguer, A.; Duncan, S.H.; Calder, A.G.; Holtrop, G.; Louis, P.; Lobley, G.E.; Flint, H.J. Two Routes of Metabolic Cross-Feeding between Bifidobacterium adolescentis and Butyrate-Producing Anaerobes from the Human Gut. *Appl. Environ. Microbiol.* **2006**, *72*, 3593–3599. [CrossRef]
60. De Vuyst, L.; Moens, F.; Selak, M.; Rivière, A.; Leroy, F. Summer Meeting 2013: Growth and physiology of bifidobacteria. *J. Appl. Microbiol.* **2014**, *116*, 477–491. [CrossRef]
61. Milani, C.; Lugli, G.A.; Duranti, S.; Turroni, F.; Mancabelli, L.; Ferrario, C.; Mangifesta, M.; Hevia, A.; Viappiani, A.; Scholz, M.; et al. Bifidobacteria exhibit social behavior through carbohydrate resource sharing in the gut. *Sci. Rep.* **2015**, *5*, 15782. [CrossRef]
62. Moens, F.; Weckx, S.; De Vuyst, L. Bifidobacterial inulin-type fructan degradation capacity determines cross-feeding interactions between bifidobacteria and Faecalibacterium prausnitzii. *Int. J. Food Microbiol.* **2016**, *231*, 76–85. [CrossRef] [PubMed]
63. Fukuda, S.; Toh, H.; Hase, K.; Oshima, K.; Nakanishi, Y.; Yoshimura, K.; Tobe, T.; Clarke, J.M.; Topping, D.L.; Suzuki, T.; et al. Bifidobacteria can protect from enteropathogenic infection through production of acetate. *Nature* **2011**, *469*, 543–547. [CrossRef] [PubMed]
64. Srutkova, D.; Schwarzer, M.; Hudcovic, T.; Zakostelska, Z.; Drab, V.; Spanova, A.; Rittich, B.; Kozakova, H.; Schabussova, I. Bifidobacterium longum CCM 7952 Promotes Epithelial Barrier Function and Prevents Acute DSS-Induced Colitis in Strictly Strain-Specific Manner. *PLoS ONE* **2015**, *10*, e0134050. [CrossRef] [PubMed]
65. Furrie, E.; Macfarlane, S.; Kennedy, A.; Cummings, J.H.; Walsh, S.V.; O'neil, D.A.; Macfarlane, G.T. Synbiotic therapy (Bifidobacterium longum/Synergy 1) initiates resolution of inflammation in patients with active ulcerative colitis: A randomised controlled pilot trial. *Gut* **2005**, *54*, 242–249. [CrossRef]
66. Yu, R.; Zuo, F.; Ma, H.; Chen, S. Exopolysaccharide-Producing Bifidobacterium adolescentis Strains with Similar Adhesion Property Induce Differential Regulation of Inflammatory Immune Response in Treg/Th17 Axis of DSS-Colitis Mice. *Nutrients* **2019**, *11*, E782. [CrossRef] [PubMed]
67. Hosseini, E.; Grootaert, C.; Verstraete, W.; Van de Wiele, T. Propionate as a health-promoting microbial metabolite in the human gut. *Nutr. Rev.* **2011**, *69*, 245–258. [CrossRef] [PubMed]
68. Yoshida, N.; Emoto, T.; Yamashita, T.; Watanabe, H.; Hayashi, T.; Tabata, T.; Hoshi, N.; Hatano, N.; Ozawa, G.; Sasaki, N.; et al. Bacteroides vulgatus and Bacteroides dorei Reduce Gut Microbial Lipopolysaccharide Production and Inhibit Atherosclerosis. *Circulation* **2018**, *138*, 2486–2498. [CrossRef]
69. Ihekweazu, F.D.; Fofanova, T.Y.; Queliza, K.; Nagy-Szakal, D.; Stewart, C.J.; Engevik, M.A.; Hulten, K.G.; Tatevian, N.; Graham, D.Y.; Versalovic, J.; et al. Bacteroides ovatus ATCC 8483 monotherapy is superior to traditional fecal transplant and multi-strain bacteriotherapy in a murine colitis model. *Gut Microbes* **2019**, *10*, 504–520. [CrossRef] [PubMed]
70. Morotomi, M.; Nagai, F.; Sakon, H.; Tanaka, R. Dialister succinatiphilus sp. nov. and Barnesiella intestinihominis sp. nov., isolated from human faeces. *Int. J. Syst. Evol. Microbiol.* **2008**, *58*, 2716–2720. [CrossRef]
71. Sears, C.L. Enterotoxigenic Bacteroides fragilis: A rogue among symbiotes. *Clin. Microbiol. Rev.* **2009**, *22*, 349–366. [CrossRef]
72. Wei, B.; Dalwadi, H.; Gordon, L.K.; Landers, C.; Bruckner, D.; Targan, S.R.; Braun, J. Molecular cloning of a Bacteroides caccae TonB-linked outer membrane protein identified by an inflammatory bowel disease marker antibody. *Infect. Immun.* **2001**, *69*, 6044–6054. [CrossRef] [PubMed]

73. Patterson, A.M.; Mulder, I.E.; Travis, A.J.; Lan, A.; Cerf-Bensussan, N.; Gaboriau-Routhiau, V.; Garden, K.; Logan, E.; Delday, M.I.; Coutts, A.G.P.; et al. Human Gut Symbiont Roseburia hominis Promotes and Regulates Innate Immunity. *Front. Immunol.* **2017**, *8*, 1166. [CrossRef]
74. Machiels, K.; Joossens, M.; Sabino, J.; De Preter, V.; Arijs, I.; Eeckhaut, V.; Ballet, V.; Claes, K.; Van Immerseel, F.; Verbeke, K.; et al. A decrease of the butyrate-producing species Roseburia hominis and Faecalibacterium prausnitzii defines dysbiosis in patients with ulcerative colitis. *Gut* **2014**, *63*, 1275–1283. [CrossRef] [PubMed]
75. Tilg, H.; Danese, S. Roseburia hominis: A novel guilty player in ulcerative colitis pathogenesis? *Gut* **2014**, *63*, 1204–1205. [CrossRef] [PubMed]
76. Qiu, X.; Zhang, M.; Yang, X.; Hong, N.; Yu, C. Faecalibacterium prausnitzii upregulates regulatory T cells and anti-inflammatory cytokines in treating TNBS-induced colitis. *J. Crohns Colitis* **2013**, *7*, e558–e568. [CrossRef] [PubMed]
77. Udayappan, S.; Manneras-Holm, L.; Chaplin-Scott, A.; Belzer, C.; Herrema, H.; Dallinga-Thie, G.M.; Duncan, S.H.; Stroes, E.S.G.; Groen, A.K.; Flint, H.J.; et al. Oral treatment with Eubacterium hallii improves insulin sensitivity in db/db mice. *NPJ Biofilms Microbiomes* **2016**, *2*, 16009. [CrossRef]
78. Murai, M.; Turovskaya, O.; Kim, G.; Madan, R.; Karp, C.L.; Cheroutre, H.; Kronenberg, M. Interleukin 10 acts on regulatory T cells to maintain expression of the transcription factor Foxp3 and suppressive function in mice with colitis. *Nat. Immunol.* **2009**, *10*, 1178–1184. [CrossRef]
79. Kumar, P.; Monin, L.; Castillo, P.; Elsegeiny, W.; Horne, W.; Eddens, T.; Vikram, A.; Good, M.; Schoenborn, A.A.; Bibby, K.; et al. Intestinal Interleukin-17 Receptor Signaling Mediates Reciprocal Control of the Gut Microbiota and Autoimmune Inflammation. *Immunity.* **2016**, *44*, 659–671. [CrossRef] [PubMed]
80. Chen, M.L.; Sundrud, M.S. Cytokine Networks and T-Cell Subsets in Inflammatory Bowel Diseases. *Inflamm. Bowel Dis.* **2016**, *22*, 1157–1167. [CrossRef] [PubMed]
81. Wang, Y.H. Developing food allergy: A potential immunologic pathway linking skin barrier to gut. *F1000Research* **2016**, *5*, F1000. [CrossRef] [PubMed]
82. Clark, D.P. The fermentation pathways of Escherichia coli. *FEMS Microbiol. Rev.* **1989**, *5*, 223–234. [CrossRef]
83. Rey, F.E.; Gonzalez, M.D.; Cheng, J.; Wu, M.; Ahern, P.P.; Gordon, J.I. Metabolic niche of a prominent sulfate-reducing human gut bacterium. *Proc. Natl. Acad. Sci. USA* **2013**, *110*, 13582–13587. [CrossRef] [PubMed]

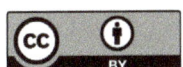

© 2020 by the authors. Licensee MDPI, Basel, Switzerland. This article is an open access article distributed under the terms and conditions of the Creative Commons Attribution (CC BY) license (http://creativecommons.org/licenses/by/4.0/).

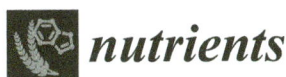

Article

In Vitro Evaluation of Prebiotic Properties of a Commercial Artichoke Inflorescence Extract Revealed Bifidogenic Effects

Pieter Van den Abbeele [1], Jonas Ghyselinck [1], Massimo Marzorati [1,2], Agusti Villar [3], Andrea Zangara [3,4,*], Carsten R. Smidt [5] and Ester Risco [3,6]

1. ProDigest BV, Technologiepark 82, 9052 Ghent, Belgium; Pieter.VandenAbbeele@prodigest.eu (P.V.d.A.); Jonas.Ghyselinck@prodigest.eu (J.G.); massimo.marzorati@prodigest.eu (M.M.)
2. Center of Microbial Ecology and Technology, Ghent University, 9000 Ghent, Belgium
3. Euromed S.A., C/Rec de Dalt, 21-23, Pol. Ind. Can Magarola, Mollet del Valles, 08100 Barcelona, Spain; avillar@euromed.es (A.V.); ERisco@euromed.es (E.R.)
4. Centre for Human Psychopharmacology, Swinburne University, Melbourne, VIC 3122, Australia
5. Smidt Labs, LLC, Sandy, UT 84092, USA; csmidt@smidtlabs.com
6. Unitat de Farmacologia i Farmacognòsia, Facultat de Farmàcia, Universitat de Barcelona, Av. Joan XXIII, s/n. E-08028 Barcelona, Spain
* Correspondence: azangara@euromed.es

Received: 1 May 2020; Accepted: 20 May 2020; Published: 26 May 2020

Abstract: Background: Prebiotics used as a dietary supplement, stimulate health-related gut microbiota (e.g., bifidobacteria, lactobacilli, etc.). This study evaluated potential prebiotic effects of an artichoke aqueous dry extract (AADE) using in vitro gut model based on the Simulator of Human Intestinal Microbial Ecosystem (SHIME®). Methods: Short-term colonic fermentations (48 h) of AADE, fructo-oligosaccharides (FOS), and a blank were performed. Microbial metabolites were assessed at 0, 6, 24, and 48 h of colonic incubation via measuring pH, gas pressure, lactate, ammonium, and short-chain fatty acids (SCFAs) levels. Community composition was assessed via targeted qPCRs. Results: After 24 and 48 h of incubation, bifidobacteria levels increased 25-fold with AADE ($p < 0.05$) and >100-fold with FOS ($p < 0.05$) compared to blank. *Lactobacillus* spp. levels only tended to increase with AADE, whereas they increased 10-fold with FOS. At 6 h, pH decreased with AADE and FOS and remained stable until 48 h; however, gas pressure increased significantly till the end of study. Acetate, propionate, and total SCFA production increased significantly with both at all time-points. Lactate levels initially increased but branched SCFA and ammonium levels remained low till 48 h. Conclusion: AADE displayed prebiotic potential by exerting bifidogenic effects that stimulated production of health-related microbial metabolites, which is potentially due to inulin in AADE.

Keywords: bifidobacteria; colon; fermentation; microbiota; prebiotic; SHIME®; artichoke

1. Introduction

Human gut microbiota consist of over 35,000 bacterial strains, encompassing beneficial and pathogenic species; however, the predominance of positively affecting microbes ensure our well-being [1]. Human gut microbiota are dominated by two main phyla, Firmicutes (including *Lactobacillus* spp.) and Bacteroidetes that are susceptible to alterations. Other phyla are Actinobacteria (including *Bifidobacterium* spp.), Proteobacteria, Fusobacteria, and Verrucomicrobia. Spatial and temporal discrepancies in gut microbial distribution contribute toward specific metabolic, immunological, and gut-protective functions throughout an individual's life span [2,3]. Characterization of such discrepancies can help identify gut-related abnormalities and play an important role in ensuring good health [4].

Prebiotics were first defined as, "Nondigestible food ingredients that beneficially affect a host by selectively stimulating growth and/or activity of one or a limited number of bacteria in the colon that are recognized to improve host health" [5]. Dysbiosis of microbial populations has been postulated as one of the reasons for metabolic disorders such as obesity, type 2 diabetes, and nonalcoholic fatty liver diseases. As prebiotics alter microbiota positively, their use as dietary supplements could effectively improve overall host health [6]. Fructo-oligosaccharides (FOS) are prebiotics that are plant-derived, naturally occurring oligosaccharides, indigestible by human enzymes, and can thus reach the colon unaltered [7]. Daily intake of FOS can increase bifidobacteria counts, a member of the indigenous gut microbiota. However, certain individuals are more sensitive to effects of FOS and suffer side effects such as itching in the throat; puffiness in the eyes, face, and mouth; dizziness; light headedness; fainting; gas; bloating; and itching of the skin [8,9].

There is a constant need for new prebiotics that can target specific bacterial species and most approaches have focused on non-digestible oligosaccharides, such as galacto-oligosaccharides, soya-oligosaccharides, isomaltooligosaccharides, gluco-oligosaccharides, xylo-oligosaccharides, lacto-sucrose, and inulin-type fructans. However, they are known to have varied prebiotic potential. Inulin has been demonstrated to positively alter gut microbiota in a dose range of 4 to 40 g/d [10–16]. Whole food sources, such as artichoke (*Cynara scolymus* L.), chicory (*Cichorium intybus*) roots, and garlic (*Allium sativum*) are rich in inulin and dietary fibers. Inulin from artichoke is recognized to have the highest degree of polymerization known in plants. Degree of polymerization directly contributes to prebiotic effects and persistence in the colon [17]. Inulin promotes host health by positively altering the bacterial metabolites mediated via stimulation of different metabolic pathways within the gut microbial community. Acetate, propionate, and butyrate are the most crucial metabolites. By acidifying the colonic environment, short-chain fatty acids (SCFA) promote growth of beneficial bacteria such as bifidobacteria and lactobacilli, which inhibit the growth of pathogenic bacteria [18]. Additionally, bifidobacteria and lactobacilli exert immunomodulatory activity that contributes to the host defense [19]. Prebiotic potential of artichoke has been demonstrated in several clinical studies and the effect was mainly mediated via increase in *Bifidobacterium* spp. in the gut [20,21]. In addition to inulin, artichoke contains polyphenols, such as dicaffeoylquinic acids and flavonoids, which provide additional nutritional values proposing a novel holistic approach to whole digestive health [22,23].

In the present study, we aimed to evaluate the prebiotic effects of artichoke aqueous dry extract (AADE) through an in vitro approach of highly controlled conditions using short-term colonic incubations based on the Simulator of Human Intestinal Microbial Ecosystem (SHIME®) model [18]. In vitro models offer certain advantages, first they allow dynamic monitoring of gut microbiome at the site of fermentation under a controlled environment and second, in vitro models help avoid large variability that arise during in vivo evaluations owing to host-derived factors such as amount of food intake, immune system, enzyme levels, or transit time. Lastly, using molecular detection methods, microbial changes can be evaluated in detail. Artichoke aqueous dry extract is a standardized herbal powder extract prepared from the edible part of artichoke (*Cynara scolymus* L.); cultivated in Spain, and extracted by the Pure-Hydro Process™ using only water (instead of organic solvents), AADE can be safely used in foods and food supplements.

2. Materials and Methods

2.1. Chemicals and Reagents

All chemicals were obtained from Sigma-Aldrich (Overijse, Belgium), unless stated otherwise. The test product AADE, also known as Cynamed™, was provided by Euromed S.A. (Mollet del Valles, Barcelona, Spain). It is derived from the edible part of the artichoke plant (*Cynara scolymus* L.) cultivated in Mediterranean regions of Spain. The AADE was prepared in accordance with the European Pharmacopoeia monograph extracts (Extracta) (No. 0765) using a proprietary water-based extraction process [24]. This process starts with the milling of dried Artichoke immature edible inflorescences that are extracted with ultrapure water at a temperature between 80 °C and 90 °C. The miscella of extract is filtered until transparency and concentrated under vacuum until a soft paste is obtained that is subsequently dried in a vacuum belt dryer and finally milled to a fine powder. The AADE used in the current study has an exact content of 9.1% caffeoylquinic acids expressed as chlorogenic acid by HPLC and an exact content of 32.2% inulin determined by HPLC. As a nutritional analysis of the AADE, the amount of total carbohydrates is 77% and the amount of protein 8.1% with a negligible content of fat. The FOS preparation used as a positive control in the current study had a purity of 89% FOS with 8% sugar residues. While the degree of polymerization of the ingredient varied between 2 and 10, it was on average 4.

2.2. Short-Term Colonic Fermentation

Short-term colonic fermentations were performed as described recently [18]. Briefly, colonic background medium containing 5.2 g/L K_2HPO_4, 16.3 g/L KH_2PO_4, 2.0 g/L $NaHCO_3$ (Chem-lab NV, Zedelgem, Belgium), 2.0 g/L Yeast Extract, 2.0 g/L pepton (Oxoid, Aalst, Belgium), 1.0 g/L mucin (Carl Roth, Karlsruhe, Germany), 0.5 g/L L-cystein, and 2.0 mL/L Tween80 (Sigma-Aldrich, Bornem, Belgium) was added to incubation reactors (90 vol%), already containing the correct amount of the test products for obtaining a final concentration of 0 g/L (Blank) or 5 g/L (for both AADE and FOS), respectively. The reactors were sealed and anaerobiosis was obtained by flushing with N_2. Subsequently, fresh fecal material of a healthy human donor (no history of antibiotic use in the six months preceding the study) was collected (according to the ethical approval of the University Hospital Ghent with reference number B670201836585; 06/08/2018). After preparation of an anaerobic fecal slurry, this was inoculated at 10 vol% in the aforementioned medium. All incubations were performed in biological triplicate for 48 h at 37 °C under anaerobic conditions with continuous shaking (90 rpm).

2.3. Microbial Metabolic Activity Analysis

Microbial metabolic analyses were performed on samples collected at 0, 6, 24, and 48 h of colonic incubation and levels of pH (Senseline F410; ProSense, Oosterhout, The Netherlands), gas pressure (hand-held pressure indicator CPH6200; Wika, Echt, The Netherlands), lactate, ammonium, and short-chain fatty acids (SCFAs) were measured. Acetate, propionate, butyrate, and branched CFAs (BCFAs) (isobutyrate, isovalerate, and isocaproate) were quantified as described by De Weirdt et al. [25] via GC-FID after performing a diethyl ether extraction. Lactate determination was performed using a commercially available enzymatic assay kit (R-Biopharm, Darmstadt, Germany) as per the manufacturer's instructions. Ammonium analysis was performed using a KjelMaster K-375 device (Büchi, Hendrik-Ido-Ambacht, The Netherlands), wherein ammonium in the sample was liberated as ammonia by addition of 32% NaOH. The released ammonia was then distilled from the sample into a 2% boric acid solution and was titrimetrically determined with a 0.02 M HCl solution.

2.4. Microbial Community Analysis

At the start of colonic incubation and after 24 and 48 h, samples were collected for microbial community analysis. DNA was isolated using the protocol as described by Vilchez-Vargas et al. [26], starting from pelleted cells originating from 1 mL luminal sample. Subsequently, quantitative polymerase chain reaction (qPCR) assays for Bacteroidetes, Firmicutes, *Lactobacillus* spp. (Firmicutes phylum), *Bifidobacterium* spp. (Actinobacteria phylum), and *Akkermansia muciniphila* (Verrucomicrobia phylum) were performed using a StepOnePlus™ real-time PCR system (Applied Biosystems, Foster City, CA, USA). Each sample was analyzed in triplicate. Standard curves for all the different runs had efficiencies between 90–105%. All protocols were initiated for 10 min at 95 °C and terminated with a melting curve from 60 °C to 95 °C. Cycling programs included 40 cycles with a denaturation step of 15 s at 95 °C, an annealing step of 30 s at 60 °C, and an elongation step of 30 s at 72 °C in each cycle. Descriptions of primers used are presented in Table 1.

Table 1. Primers used for quantitative polymerase chain reaction (qPCR) quantification of species-specific 16S rDNA.

Target Species	Primer Sequences 5′-3′ and 3′-5′
Bacteroidetes [27]	GGAACATGTGGTTTAATTCGATGAT AGCTGACGACAACCATGCAG
Firmicutes [27]	GGAGCATGTGGTTTAATTCGAAGCA AGCTGACGACAACCATGCAC
Lactobacillus spp. [20]	AGCAGTAGGGAATCTTCCA CGCCACTGGTGTTCYTCCATATA
Bifidobacterium spp. [28]	TCGCGTCYGGTGTGAAAG CCACATCCAGCYTCCAC
Akkermansia muciniphila [29]	CAGCACGTGAAGGTGGGGAC CCTTGCGGTTGGCTTCAGAT

Besides presenting the absolute levels of the different groups, the ratio between the obtained levels at 24 h and 48 h versus 0 h were calculated for the blank, AADE, and FOS-treated microbiota.

2.5. Statistics

To evaluate differences in microbial metabolites and microbial community composition between blank and treatment incubations at the different time points, a two-way ANOVA with Tukey multiple comparisons test was performed. Differences were found significant if $p < 0.05$. Statistical analysis was performed with the GraphPad Prism software (version 8.3.0, San Diego, USA).

3. Results

3.1. Microbial Composition

While the absolute levels of each of the five targeted microbial groups (*Bifidobacterium* spp., *Lactobacillus* spp., Bacteroidetes, Firmicutes, and *Akkermansia muciniphila*) at each of the three time points (0/6/48 h) are presented in Table 2, the factor increase versus 0 h is presented in Figure 1 for the four microbial groups for which there were significant changes between the treatments (all except *Akkermansia muciniphila*). First, both at 24 h and 48 h, bifidobacteria levels were significantly increased versus the blank for AADE but especially for FOS (Table 2). This was reflected by ~25-fold and ~100-fold increased levels versus 0 h for AADE and FOS, respectively; both after 24 h and 48 h of incubation (Figure 1A). Additionally, *Lactobacillus* spp. were stimulated more profoundly for FOS with ~10-fold increased levels versus 0 h at 24 and 48 h (Figure 1B). AADE exerted more attenuated effects on *Lactobacillus* spp. levels with only statistically significantly increased absolute levels at 48 h. Incubation with FOS increased absolute Firmicutes levels at all time points, while for AADE the increase was only significant at 24 h (Table 2 and Figure 1C). Finally, AADE increased Bacteriodetes levels versus the blank at 48 h (Table 2 and Figure 1D), while FOS decreased *Akkermansia muciniphila* levels versus AADE after 48 h of incubation (Table 2).

Table 2. Mean (±standard deviation) levels of microbial groups as measured via quantitative polymerase chain reaction (qPCR) after 0, 24, and 48 h of treatment of a simulated colonic microbiota with 5 g/L AADE (artichoke aqueous dry extract) or FOS (fructo-oligosaccharides). For each microbial group and within each time point (24 h or 48 h), a value indicated with a different letter (a, b, or c) indicates a statistical difference between AADE, FOS, and/or the blank, as tested with a two-way ANOVA with post-hoc Tukey test ($p < 0.05$). In contrast, when at least one letter is shared between two treatments, there was no significant between these groups.

Incubation Time (h)	Levels of Microbial Groups (log (16S rRNA Copies/mL))						
	0 h	24 h			48 h		
		Blank	AADE	FOS	Blank	AADE	FOS
Firmicutes	9.96 ± 0.36	10.36 ± 0.13 [a]	10.83 ± 0.06 [b]	11.00 ± 0.03 [b]	10.44 ± 0.14 [a]	10.70 ± 0.25 [a]	11.08 ± 0.10 [b]
Bacteroidetes	9.73 ± 0.46	10.64 ± 0.47	11.09 ± 0.05	10.72 ± 0.04	10.44 ± 0.10 [a]	10.99 ± 0.23 [b]	10.87 ± 0.06 [a,b]
Bifidobacteria	8.26 ± 0.25	8.94 ± 0.13 [a]	9.71 ± 0.06 [b]	10.24 ± 0.06 [c]	9.12 ± 0.14 [a]	9.60 ± 0.22 [b]	10.32 ± 0.04 [c]
Lactobacillus spp.	6.58 ± 0.19	6.84 ± 0.10 [a]	7.06 ± 0.03 [a]	7.54 ± 0.03 [b]	6.87 ± 0.06 [a]	7.01 ± 0.15 [b]	7.63 ± 0.06 [c]
Akkermansia muciniphila	7.02 ± 0.51	8.23 ± 0.39	8.30 ± 0.03	7.72 ± 0.08	8.08 ± 0.17 [a,b]	8.19 ± 0.25 [b]	7.85 ± 0.08 [a]

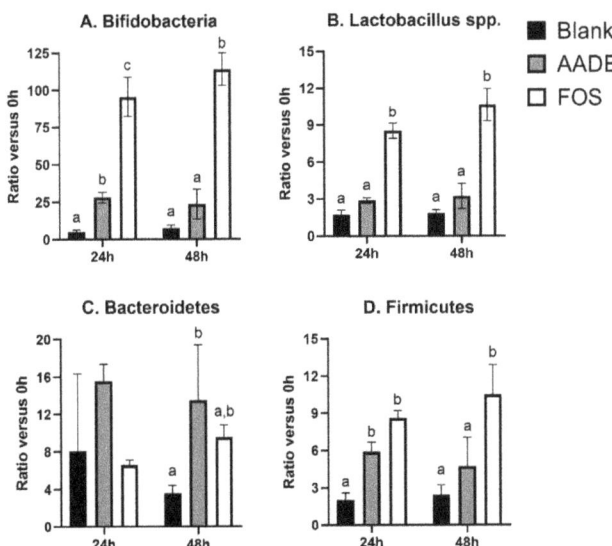

Figure 1. Mean (±standard deviation) ratios of (**A**) *Bifidobacterium* spp., (**B**) *Lactobacillus* spp., (**C**) Firmicutes, and (**D**) Bacteroidetes levels after 24 h or 48 h of treatment of a simulated colonic microbiota with 5 g/L AADE (artichoke aqueous dry extract) or FOS (fructo-oligosaccharides) versus the initial levels (24 h/0 h or 48 h/0 h, respectively) as measured via quantitative polymerase chain reaction (qPCR). For each microbial group and within each time point (24 or 48 h), a bar indicated with a different letter (a, b, or c) indicates a statistical difference between AADE, FOS, and/or the blank at a given time point, as tested with a two-way ANOVA with post-hoc Tukey test ($p < 0.05$). In contrast, when at least one letter is shared between two bars, there was no significant between these treatments.

3.2. pH

A more profound decrease in pH was observed with FOS and to a lesser extent also with AADE compared with blank at 6 h ($p < 0.05$). The pH continued to decrease until 24 h and remained stable thereafter, indicating continued microbial fermentation (Table 3).

Table 3. Mean (±standard deviation) pH and gas pressure after 0, 6, 24, and 48 h of treatment of a simulated colonic microbiota with 5 g/L AADE (artichoke aqueous dry extract) or FOS (fructo-oligosaccharides). For each time point (0, 6, 24, or 48 h), a value indicated with a different letter (a, b, or c) indicates a statistical difference between AADE, FOS, and/or the blank as tested with a two-way ANOVA with post-hoc Tukey test ($p < 0.05$).

Incubation Time (h)	pH		
	Blank	AADE	FOS
0	6.49 ± 0.02	6.51 ± 0.00	6.51 ± 0.00
6	6.39 ± 0.01 [a]	6.22 ± 0.01 [b]	5.64 ± 0.13 [c]
24	6.46 ± 0.02 [a]	6.21 ± 0.01 [b]	5.66 ± 0.02 [c]
48	6.40 ± 0.04 [a]	6.20 ± 0.02 [b]	5.69 ± 0.03 [c]

Incubation Time (h)	Gas Pressure (kPa)		
	Blank	AADE	FOS
6 h	13.2 ± 0.2 [a]	22.8 ± 1.6 [b]	29.9 ± 1.6 [c]
24 h	27.3 ± 0.6 [a]	45.5 ± 0.5 [b]	52.0 ± 2.8 [c]
48 h	31.4 ± 0.6 [a]	48.8 ± 0.6 [b]	54.2 ± 1.1 [c]

3.3. Gas Pressure

As noted in Table 3, as compared with the blank, gas pressure was significant with AADE and FOS on all the time points along the incubation. On all time points, gas production was significantly higher for FOS versus AADE (Table 3).

3.4. Lactate and Carbohydrate (SCFAs, Acetate, Butyrate, and Propionate) and Protein Metabolites (BCFAs and Ammonium)

Compared with the blank, total SCFAs were significantly increased with AADE and FOS at all time-points of incubation ($p < 0.05$), which reflected enhanced microbial metabolic activity upon AADE/FOS administration. However, the overall increase in total SCFAs was higher with FOS compared with AADE (Table 4). Similar patterns of increase in acetate and propionate levels were observed with AADE and FOS as for the total SCFA (Table 4). In contrast, butyrate concentrations were only significantly increased for FOS, and this after 24 h and 48 h.

Table 4. Mean (±standard deviation) carbohydrate- and protein-derived metabolites after 0, 24, and 48 h of treatment of a simulated colonic microbiota with 5 g/L AADE (artichoke aqueous dry extract) or FOS (fructo-oligosaccharides). For each endpoint and within each time point (24 h or 48 h), a value indicated with a different letter (a, b, or c) indicates a statistical difference between AADE, FOS and/or the blank, as tested with a two-way ANOVA with post-hoc Tukey test ($p < 0.05$). In contrast, when at least one letter is shared between two treatments, there was no significant difference between these groups.

Incubation Time (h)	6 h			24 h			48 h		
	Blank	AADE	FOS	Blank	AADE	FOS	Blank	AADE	FOS
	Carbohydrate Metabolite Levels (mean ± SD) (mM)								
Acetate	8.1 ± 0.3 [a]	17.2 ± 1.0 [b]	31.4 ± 3.0 [c]	19.2 ± 0.3 [a]	34.9 ± 0.3 [b]	40.1 ± 0.4 [c]	20.8 ± 0.3 [a]	37.1 ± 0.9 [b]	43.7 ± 0.7 [c]
Butyrate	0.41 ± 0.03	0.26 ± 0.05	0.48 ± 0.01	2.47 ± 0.03 [a]	2.89 ± 0.53 [a]	5.53 ± 0.64 [b]	3.78 ± 0.02 [a]	3.9 ± 0.55 [a]	7.17 ± 0.22 [b]
Propionate	3.5 ± 0.2 [a]	7.6 ± 0.6 [b]	8.7 ± 0.8 [c]	7.1 ± 0.1 [a]	15.6 ± 0.2 [b]	23.6 ± 0.6 [c]	7.8 ± 0.20 [a]	16.3 ± 0.4 [b]	24.1 ± 0.6 [c]
Total SCFAs	12.1 ± 0.5 [a]	25.0 ± 1.6 [b]	40.6 ± 3.9 [c]	31.6 ± 0.4 [a]	56.7 ± 0.5 [b]	69.5 ± 0.9 [c]	38.3 ± 0.7 [a]	65.6 ± 1.2 [b]	75.7 ± 0.8 [c]
Lactate (mean ± SD) (mM)	1.55 ± 0.03 [a]	3.79 ± 0.04 [b]	8.84 ± 1.16 [c]	0.25 ± 0.01	0.33 ± 0.07	0.85 ± 0.78	0.49 ± 0.05	0.47 ± 0.21	0.10 ± 0.07
	Protein Metabolite Levels (mean ± SD) (mg/L)								
BCFAs	0.10 ± 0.00	0.00 ± 0.00	0.00 ± 0.00	1.34 ± 0.24 [a]	1.70 ± 0.37 [a]	0.00 ± 0.00 [b]	4.01 ± 0.13 [a]	3.42 ± 0.02 [b]	0.34 ± 0.26 [c]
Ammonium	0 ± 0	0 ± 0	0 ± 0	328 ± 1 [a]	322 ± 7 [a]	122 ± 5 [b]	414 ± 3 [a]	384 ± 13 [b]	1874 ± 12 [c]

BCFAs, branched short-chain fatty acid; SCFAs, short-chain fatty acids.

As shown in Table 4, no BCFAs were produced during the initial 6 h of incubation in AADE and FOS. After 24 h of incubation, there was a similar production of BCFAs in the blank (1.34 ± 0.24) and upon AADE treatment (1.70 ± 0.37). In contrast, no BCFAs were produced upon FOS administration at the 24 h time point. After 48 h of incubation, BCFAs were produced but were significantly ($p < 0.05$) lower for both AADE (3.42 ± 0.02) and especially FOS (0.34 ± 0.26) when compared with the blank (4.01 ± 0.13). The results for ammonium, another marker for protein fermentation, were similar to those for BCFAs, indicating reduced protein fermentation upon AADE and especially FOS administration. Lactate levels were high ($p < 0.05$) with AADE and even further increased for FOS compared with blank after the initial 6 h of incubation. Thereafter, lactate levels decreased indicating lactate consumption.

4. Discussion

In the present study, although the effects of AADE on microbial activity and composition were milder as compared to the "gold standard" prebiotic FOS, AADE demonstrated marked prebiotic potential. First, AADE significantly decreased pH and increased gas production, which indicated overall increased microbial activity upon administration of the test product. Saccharolytic metabolites such as acetate and propionate, and thus also total SCFAs, increased, while levels of proteolytic metabolites, BCFAs, and ammonium, significantly decreased upon AADE administration at 48 h. A key finding of this study was the growth-promoting action of AADE, mostly on bifidobacteria which are regarded as health-related members of the intestinal microbiome. Further, AADE also affected Bacteroidetes, Firmicutes, and *Lactobacillus* spp. levels.

Based on results of this study, bifidogenic effects of AADE were milder, yet in the same order of magnitude as those of FOS. These findings were similar to those of a previous in vitro study conducted by Barszcz M et al. [28]. Bifidogenic effects were also reported in healthy volunteers [20,21]. The bifidogenic effect of artichoke has been attributed to its inulin content. Inulin exerts most physiological changes through the bacterial metabolites. SCFAs are some of the important metabolites that acidify the colonic environment promoting growth of beneficial bacteria, such as *Lactobacillus* spp. and bifidobacteria, and prevent growth of pathogenic bacteria [30,31].

Moreover, in our study, lactate was produced during the initial 6 h of incubation. Subsequently, lactate was consumed and coincided with an increase in propionate levels for both AADE and FOS, with most marked stimulations being noted for FOS. Butyrate was not stimulated by AADE, suggesting that the majority of lactate (that can be used as a substrate for both propionate and butyrate), was cross-fed to propionate upon AADE supplementation. Some Negativicutes (family Veillonellaceae, phylum Firmicutes) are shown to form propionate [32] and could potentially explain the increase of Firmicutes that was observed for AADE after 24 h in our study. Bacteroidetes also contain potent propionate producers [33,34] and could have further contributed to propionate production upon AADE supplementation since AADE also stimulated this phylum in our study. These alterations in propionate levels correlate with the inulin content of the artichoke [18]. Propionate metabolites have been shown to reduce cholesterol and fatty acid synthesis in liver, improve glucose metabolism, and regulate immune status in adipose tissue, and thus elicit health-promoting activities [18,35]. Finally, another key propionate producer is the mucin-degrading, acetate and propionate producing, *Akkermansia muciniphila*. This taxon was not increased for either AADE or FOS and even decreased upon FOS administration. This was likely due to the fact that FOS more strongly decreased the pH (to 5.66 within 24 h), which is a pH at which *Akkermansia muciniphila* is unable to grow [36]. In vivo, such lower pH could however boost mucin secretion and result in enhanced mucin degradation by *Akkermansia muciniphila* in the distal colon, as shown for inulin in humanized rats [37].

Similarly, acetate and lactate can be cross-fed to butyrate by members of the Ruminococcaceae, Lachnospiraceae, Clostridiaceae, Eubacteriaceae, all members of the Firmicutes phylum [18,38]. Butyrate is a major energy source for the gut microbiota and may also reduce oxidative stress, improve gut function, and restrict inflammatory response. In this study, butyrate levels were increased majorly with FOS and were usually produced during the later stage of incubation period. As our study duration was limited to 48 h, additional studies with longer incubation periods are warranted to make accurate conclusions. Moreover, cross-feeding between microbial communities should be taken into account when drawing definite conclusions [39].

Furthermore, propionate and acetate have been shown to stimulate release of peptide hormones leading to short-term signaling of satiation and satiety to appetite centers in the brain, resulting in reduced food intake by the host [35,40,41]. Several metabolic disorders such as obesity, insulin resistance, and metabolic syndrome are associated with impaired carbohydrate and lipid metabolism by the host, and are accompanied by changes in the gut microbiota [32]. Inulin could stimulate different metabolic pathways within the gut microbial community and could potentially elicit varied health-promoting activities [18].

Ammonia and BCFAs are toxic metabolites produced from protein fermentation [39]. In this investigation, the reduction in BCFAs and ammonia production in part explains the increase in carbohydrate metabolism. In vivo studies have also demonstrated that generation and accumulation of ammonia can be reduced by lowering protein supply and by colonic fermentation of suitable non-digestible carbohydrates from food [39,42].

Short-term colonic incubations have often been used to gather information on the prebiotic potential of novel ingredients. Results of the present study using an incubation strategy based on the SHIME® model indicate the prebiotic potential of AADE. These findings could be further validated using different models, such as M-SHIME® (Mucosal Simulator of the Human Intestinal Microbial Ecosystem) which focuses not only on luminal but also mucosal gut-colonizing microbes [43]. Moreover, studies with repeated administration are required in order to simulate gradual changes that occur in vivo with long-term use and to assess any beneficial microbial shift.

5. Conclusions

The present preliminary evaluation, conducted using the SHIME® model, demonstrated that AADE has promising prebiotic potential. Incubation with AADE resulted in an increase of beneficial microbes, which was correlated with their metabolite profile. The promising results of this study justify future investigations using multiple doses in upgraded models to further validate these findings.

Author Contributions: Conceptualization, M.M.; study method, investigation, and data analysis, P.V.d.A. and J.G.; funding acquisition, A.V. and A.Z.; and writing—original draft, reviewing, and editing manuscript, all authors. All authors have read and agreed to the published version of the manuscript.

Funding: The study was funded by Euromed S.A.

Acknowledgments: Authors acknowledge CBCC Global Research for providing statistical analysis and medical writing assistance in the development of this manuscript, which was funded by Euromed S.A.

Conflicts of Interest: A.V., A.Z., and E.R. are employed by Euromed S.A. The study funders (Euromed S.A.) had no role in the design, collection, or analysis of the data.

References

1. Frank, D.N.; Amand, A.L.S.; Feldman, R.A.; Boedeker, E.C.; Harpaz, N.; Pace, N.R. Molecular-phylogenetic characterization of microbial community imbalances in human inflammatory bowel diseases. *Proc. Natl. Acad. Sci.* **2007**, *104*, 13780–13785. [CrossRef] [PubMed]
2. Jandhyala, S.M.; Talukdar, R.; Subramanyam, C.; Vuyyuru, H.; Sasikala, M.; Reddy, D.N. Role of the normal gut microbiota. *World J. Gastroenterol.* **2015**, *21*, 8787. [CrossRef] [PubMed]
3. Jandhyala, S.M.; Madhulika, A.; Deepika, G.; Rao, G.V.; Reddy, D.N.; Subramanyam, C.; Sasikala, M.; Talukdar, R. Altered intestinal microbiota in patients with chronic pancreatitis: Implications in diabetes and metabolic abnormalities. *Sci. Rep.* **2017**, *7*, 43640. [CrossRef]
4. Blaser, M.J. The microbiome revolution. *J. Clin. Investig.* **2014**, *124*, 4162–4165. [CrossRef] [PubMed]

5. Gibson, G.R.; Roberfroid, M.B. Dietary modulation of the human colonic microbiota: Introducing the concept of prebiotics. *J. Nutr.* **1995**, *125*, 1401–1412. [CrossRef] [PubMed]
6. A. Parnell, J.; A. Reimer, R. Prebiotic fiber modulation of the gut microbiota improves risk factors for obesity and the metabolic syndrome. *Gut Microbes* **2012**, *3*, 29–34. [CrossRef] [PubMed]
7. Oku, T.; Tokunaga, T.; Hosoya, N. Nondigestibility of a new sweetener, "Neosugar", in the rat. *J. Nutr.* **1984**, *114*, 1574–1581. [CrossRef]
8. Spiegel, J.E.; Rose, R.; Karabell, P.; Frankos, V.H.; Schmitt, D.F. Safety and benefits of fructooligosaccharides as food ingredients. *Food Technol. (Chic.)* **1994**, *48*, 85–89.
9. Johnson, J. Are Fructooligosaccharides Safe? In *Medical News Today*. Available online: https://www.medicalnewstoday.com/articles/319299.php (accessed on 15 October 2018).
10. Williams, C.; Witherly, S.; Buddington, R. Influence of dietary neosugar on selected bacterial groups of the human faecal microbiota. *Microb. Ecol. Health Dis.* **1994**, *7*, 91–97. [CrossRef]
11. Gibson, G.R.; Beatty, E.R.; Wang, X.; Cummings, J.H. Selective stimulation of bifidobacteria in the human colon by oligofructose and inulin. *Gastroenterology* **1995**, *108*, 975–982. [CrossRef]
12. Buddington, R.K.; Williams, C.H.; Chen, S.-C.; Witherly, S.A. Dietary supplement of neosugar alters the fecal flora and decreases activities of some reductive enzymes in human subjects. *Am. J. Clin. Nutr.* **1996**, *63*, 709–716. [CrossRef] [PubMed]
13. Kleessen, B.; Sykura, B.; Zunft, H.-J.; Blaut, M. Effects of inulin and lactose on fecal microflora, microbial activity, and bowel habit in elderly constipated persons. *Am. J. Clin. Nutr.* **1997**, *65*, 1397–1402. [CrossRef] [PubMed]
14. Bouhnik, Y.; Vahedi, K.; Achour, L.; Attar, A.; Salfati, J.; Pochart, P.; Marteau, P.; Flourie, B.; Bornet, F.; Rambaud, J.-C. Short-chain fructo-oligosaccharide administration dose-dependently increases fecal bifidobacteria in healthy humans. *J. Nutr.* **1999**, *129*, 113–116. [CrossRef]
15. Kruse, H.-P.; Kleessen, B.; Blaut, M. Effects of inulin on faecal bifidobacteria in human subjects. *Br. J. Nutr.* **1999**, *82*, 375–382. [CrossRef] [PubMed]
16. Den Hond, E.; Geypens, B.; Ghoos, Y. Effect of high performance chicory inulin on constipation. *Nutr. Res.* **2000**, *20*, 731–736. [CrossRef]
17. Van De Wiele, T.; Boon, N.; Possemiers, S.; Jacobs, H.; Verstraete, W. Inulin-type fructans of longer degree of polymerization exert more pronounced in vitro prebiotic effects. *J. Appl. Microbiol.* **2007**, *102*, 452–460. [CrossRef]
18. Van den Abbeele, P.; Taminiau, B.; Pinheiro, I.; Duysburgh, C.; Jacobs, H.; Pijls, L.; Marzorati, M. Arabinoxylo-Oligosaccharides and Inulin Impact Inter-Individual Variation on Microbial Metabolism and Composition, Which Immunomodulates Human Cells. *J. Agric. Food Chem.* **2018**, *66*, 1121–1130. [CrossRef]
19. Hardy, H.; Harris, J.; Lyon, E.; Beal, J.; Foey, A.D. Probiotics, prebiotics and immunomodulation of gut mucosal defences: Homeostasis and immunopathology. *Nutrients* **2013**, *5*, 1869–1912. [CrossRef]
20. Kleessen, B.; Schwarz, S.; Boehm, A.; Fuhrmann, H.; Richter, A.; Henle, T.; Krueger, M. Jerusalem artichoke and chicory inulin in bakery products affect faecal microbiota of healthy volunteers. *Br. J. Nutr.* **2007**, *98*, 540–549. [CrossRef]
21. Costabile, A.; Kolida, S.; Klinder, A.; Gietl, E.; Bäuerlein, M.; Frohberg, C.; Landschütze, V.; Gibson, G.R. A double-blind, placebo-controlled, cross-over study to establish the bifidogenic effect of a very-long-chain inulin extracted from globe artichoke (*Cynara scolymus*) in healthy human subjects. *Br. J. Nutr.* **2010**, *104*, 1007–1017. [CrossRef]
22. D'Antuono, I.; Garbetta, A.; Linsalata, V.; Minervini, F.; Cardinali, A. Polyphenols from artichoke heads (*Cynara cardunculus* (L.) subsp. scolymus Hayek): In vitro bio-accessibility, intestinal uptake and bioavailability. *Food Funct.* **2015**, *6*, 1268–1277. [PubMed]
23. Rocchetti, G.; Giuberti, G.; Lucchini, F.; Lucini, L. Polyphenols and sesquiterpene lactones from artichoke heads: Modulation of starch digestion, gut bioaccessibility, and bioavailability following in vitro digestion and large intestine fermentation. *Antioxidants* **2020**, *9*, 306. [CrossRef] [PubMed]
24. Council of Europe. *European Pharmacopoeia*; Council of Europe: Strasbourg, France, Ph. Eur. 10.1 04/2019:0765.

25. De Weirdt, R.; Possemiers, S.; Vermeulen, G.; Moerdijk-Poortvliet, T.C.; Boschker, H.T.; Verstraete, W.; Van de Wiele, T. Human faecal microbiota display variable patterns of glycerol metabolism. *FEMS Microbiol. Ecol.* **2010**, *74*, 601–611. [CrossRef] [PubMed]
26. Vilchez-Vargas, R.; Geffers, R.; Suarez-Diez, M.; Conte, I.; Waliczek, A.; Kaser, V.S.; Kralova, M.; Junca, H.; Pieper, D.H. Analysis of the microbial gene landscape and transcriptome for aromatic pollutants and alkane degradation using a novel internally calibrated microarray system. *Environ. Microbiol.* **2013**, *15*, 1016–1039. [CrossRef] [PubMed]
27. Freire, F.C.; Adorno, M.A.T.; Sakamoto, I.K.; Antoniassi, R.; Chaves, A.C.S.D.; Dos Santos, K.M.O.; Sivieri, K. Impact of multi-functional fermented goat milk beverage on gut microbiota in a dynamic colon model. *Food Res. Int.* **2017**, *99*, 315–327. [CrossRef]
28. Barszcz, M.; Taciak, M.; Skomiał, J. The effects of inulin, dried Jerusalem artichoke tuber and a multispecies probiotic preparation on microbiota ecology and immune status of the large intestine in young pigs. *Arch. Anim. Nutr.* **2016**, *70*, 278–292. [CrossRef]
29. Van Hoek, M.J.; Merks, R.M. Emergence of microbial diversity due to cross-feeding interactions in a spatial model of gut microbial metabolism. *BMC Syst. Biol.* **2017**, *11*, 56.
30. Cummings, J.H.; Macfarlane, G.T.; Englyst, H.N. Prebiotic digestion and fermentation. *Am. J. Clin. Nutr.* **2001**, *73*, 415s–420s. [CrossRef]
31. Blaut, M. Relationship of prebiotics and food to intestinal microflora. *Eur. J. Nutr.* **2002**, *41*, i11–i16. [CrossRef]
32. Rios-Covian, D.; Salazar, N.; Gueimonde, M.; de Los Reyes-Gavilan, C.G. Shaping the Metabolism of Intestinal Bacteroides Population through Diet to Improve Human Health. *Front. Microbiol.* **2017**, *8*, 376. [CrossRef]
33. Aguirre, M.; Eck, A.; Koenen, M.E.; Savelkoul, P.H.; Budding, A.E.; Venema, K. Diet drives quick changes in the metabolic activity and composition of human gut microbiota in a validated in vitro gut model. *Res. Microbiol.* **2016**, *167*, 114–125. [CrossRef]
34. Salonen, A.; Lahti, L.; Salojärvi, J.; Holtrop, G.; Korpela, K.; Duncan, S.H.; Date, P.; Farquharson, F.; Johnstone, A.M.; Lobley, G.E.; et al. Impact of diet and individual variation on intestinal microbiota composition and fermentation products in obese men. *ISME J.* **2014**, *8*, 2218–2230. [CrossRef] [PubMed]
35. Chambers, E.S.; Viardot, A.; Psichas, A.; Morrison, D.J.; Murphy, K.G.; Zac-Varghese, S.E.; MacDougall, K.; Preston, T.; Tedford, C.; Finlayson, G.S. Effects of targeted delivery of propionate to the human colon on appetite regulation, body weight maintenance and adiposity in overweight adults. *Gut* **2015**, *64*, 1744–1754. [CrossRef] [PubMed]
36. Herreweghen, F.; Van den Abbeele, P.; De Mulder, T.; De Weirdt, R.; Geirnaert, A.; Hernandez-Sanabria, E.; Vilchez-Vargas, R.; Jauregui, R.; Pieper, D.H.; Belzer, C.; et al. In vitro colonisation of the distal colon by *Akkermansia muciniphila* is largely mucin and pH dependent. *Benef. Microbes* **2017**, *8*, 81–96. [CrossRef] [PubMed]
37. Van den Abbeele, P.; Gérard, P.; Rabot, S.; Bruneau, A.; El Aidy, S.; Derrien, M.; Kleerebezem, M.; Zoetendal, E.G.; Smidt, H.; Verstraete, W.; et al. Arabinoxylans and inulin differentially modulate the mucosal and luminal gut microbiota and mucin-degradation in humanized rats. *Environ. Microbiol.* **2011**, *13*, 2667–2680. [CrossRef] [PubMed]
38. Baxter, N.T.; Schmidt, A.W.; Venkataraman, A.; Kim, K.S.; Waldron, C.; Schmidt, T.M. Dynamics of Human Gut Microbiota and Short-Chain Fatty Acids in Response to Dietary Interventions with Three Fermentable Fibers. *mBio* **2019**, *10*, e02566-18. [CrossRef]
39. Maathuis, A.J.; van den Heuvel, E.G.; Schoterman, M.H.; Venema, K. Galacto-oligosaccharides have prebiotic activity in a dynamic in vitro colon model using a 13C-labeling technique. *J. Nutr.* **2012**, *142*, 1205–1212. [CrossRef]
40. Tolhurst, G.; Heffron, H.; Lam, Y.S.; Parker, H.E.; Habib, A.M.; Diakogiannaki, E.; Cameron, J.; Grosse, J.; Reimann, F.; Gribble, F.M. Short-chain fatty acids stimulate glucagon-like peptide-1 secretion via the G-protein–coupled receptor FFAR2. *Diabetes* **2012**, *61*, 364–371. [CrossRef]
41. Freeland, K.R.; Wolever, T.M. Acute effects of intravenous and rectal acetate on glucagon-like peptide-1, peptide YY, ghrelin, adiponectin and tumour necrosis factor-α. *Br. J. Nutr.* **2010**, *103*, 460–466. [CrossRef]

42. Geboes, K.P.; De Hertogh, G.; De Preter, V.; Luypaerts, A.; Bammens, B.; Evenepoel, P.; Ghoos, Y.; Geboes, K.; Rutgeerts, P.; Verbeke, K. The influence of inulin on the absorption of nitrogen and the production of metabolites of protein fermentation in the colon. *Br. J. Nutr.* **2006**, *96*, 1078–1086. [CrossRef]
43. Van den Abbeele, P.; Roos, S.; Eeckhaut, V.; MacKenzie, D.A.; Derde, M.; Verstraete, W.; Marzorati, M.; Possemiers, S.; Vanhoecke, B.; Van Immerseel, F. Incorporating a mucosal environment in a dynamic gut model results in a more representative colonization by lactobacilli. *Microb. Biotechnol.* **2012**, *5*, 106–115. [CrossRef] [PubMed]

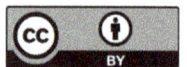

© 2020 by the authors. Licensee MDPI, Basel, Switzerland. This article is an open access article distributed under the terms and conditions of the Creative Commons Attribution (CC BY) license (http://creativecommons.org/licenses/by/4.0/).

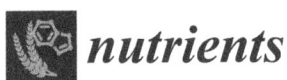

Article

Possible Protective Effects of TA on the Cancerous Effect of Mesotrione

Agata Jabłońska-Trypuć [1,*], Urszula Wydro [1], Elżbieta Wołejko [1], Joanna Rodziewicz [2] and Andrzej Butarewicz [1]

[1] Division of Chemistry, Biology and Biotechnology, Faculty of Civil Engineering and Environmental Sciences, Bialystok University of Technology, 15-351 Białystok, Poland; u.wydro@pb.edu.pl (U.W.); e.wolejko@pb.edu.pl (E.W.); a.butarewicz@pb.edu.pl (A.B.)
[2] Faculty of Geoengineering, Department of Environmental Engineering, University of Warmia and Mazury in Olsztyn, 10-719 Olsztyn, Poland; joanna.rodziewicz@uwm.edu.pl
* Correspondence: a.jablonska@pb.edu.pl; Tel.: +48-797-995-971

Received: 25 March 2020; Accepted: 6 May 2020; Published: 8 May 2020

Abstract: The interaction of different food ingredients is now a very important and often emerging topic of research. Pesticides and their breakdown products, which may be carcinogenic, are one of the frequently occurring food contaminants. Compounds like traumatic acid (TA), which originates from plants, are beneficial, antioxidant, and anticancer food ingredients. Previously obtained results from our research group indicated antioxidative in normal human fibroblasts and prooxidative in cancer cells activity of TA. Since the literature data show an undoubted connection between the presence of pesticides in food and the increased incidence of different types of cancers, we attempted to clarify whether TA can abolish the effect of mesotrione stimulating the growth of cancer cells. In order to study the influence of mesotrione on breast cancer cells, we decided to carry out cytotoxicity studies of environmentally significant herbicide concentrations. We also analyzed the cytotoxicity of TA and mixtures of these two compounds. After selecting the most effective concentrations of both components tested, we conducted analyses of oxidative stress parameters and apoptosis in ZR-75-1 cells. The obtained results allow us to conclude that traumatic acid by stimulating oxidative stress and apoptosis contributes to inhibiting the growth and development of cells of the ZR-75-1 line strengthened by mesotrione. This may mean that TA is a compound with pro-oxidative and proapoptotic effects in cancer cells whose development and proliferation are stimulated by the presence of mesotrione. The presented results may be helpful in answering the question of whether herbicides and their residues in edibles may constitute potential threat for people diagnosed with cancer and whether compounds with proven pro-oxidative effects on cancer cells can have potential cytoprotective functions.

Keywords: mesotrione; traumatic acid; breast cancer; herbicide; antioxidant; oxidative stress

1. Introduction

Different chemical substances from the group of pesticides are used in the food production process to ensure seasonal availability and good quality of products. However, it should be mentioned that the frequent and widespread use of pesticides carries the risk of their penetration into the human body. Pesticides are a group of chemical compounds, both natural and synthetic, that are used in order to destroy plant and animal parasites, reduce the risk of plant diseases, and control weeds. The massive use of pesticides results from the growing number of consumers, and thus from an increased demand for food. Pesticide residues may remain in food after their application to crops. The maximum permissible levels of pesticides residues in food are determined by the regulatory authorities in the European Union, mostly at the level of the European Commission. Exposure of a given population to pesticides and their residues most often occurs as a result of the consumption of processed food or close contact with pesticide treated areas, such as farms [1,2].

Mesotrione (Mes) is an herbicide which controls most broadleaf weeds and weed grasses in crops cultivation. Due to its frequent use in agriculture, the detectable level of this compound in countries such as North America and Canada fluctuates around 4.1µg/L [3,4]. According to its chemical structure, Mes is 2-[4-methylsulfonyl-2-nitrobenzoyl]-1,3-cyclohexanedione and it belongs to the family of triketone. Its main role is an inhibition of the enzyme 4-hydroxy-phenyl-pyruvate-dioxygenase, which converts tyrosine to plastoquinone (PQ) and alpha-tocopherol [5]. Mes is a quite water soluble compound, which, in combination with its widespread application and soil retention capacity, contributes to the fact that this herbicide easily contaminates surface and groundwater [6]. According to Bonnet et al., Mes decomposition products appear to be more dangerous and harmful than the parent compound [7].

The endocrine-disrupting influence of selected pesticides has caused great concerns due to the hormonal activity of many well-documented risk factors for breast cancer. Literature data suggest that selected pesticides could be related to an increase in breast cancer risk and urge researchers to examine environmental risk factors and possible compounds, preferably of natural origin, that could reduce side effects of pesticide use and thus the incidence of this disease [8–10]. Many pesticides are considered as analogues of human hormones. They may exert influence through estrogen receptors. Therefore, we chose to examine the ZR-75-1 breast cancer cell line, which is commonly used for endocrine-based research, rather than choosing on the other breast cancer cell line or nonhuman cell line. Discordances in scientific data regarding possible herbicides cancerogenic properties may result from the different test models. Therefore, for the experiment, we decided to choose the human estrogen-dependent breast cancer cell line, which is characterized by the presence of the estrogen receptor (ER+). The aim of this paper was to study the mutual interaction mechanisms of two opposite compounds, one of which is highly undesirable food contaminant (Mes), and traumatic acid (TA), which is a promising food ingredient. In already published papers, we indicated that TA is characterized by antioxidative activity in normal human fibroblasts and pro-oxidative properties in malignant cells [11,12]. In our preliminary studies on the toxicological effects of Mes and TA in various breast cancer lines, we showed that TA, depending on the concentration used, has an effect on the selected herbicides including Mes [13]. The literature, which has documented relationship between the consumption of food contaminated with pesticides and the increased incidence of different types of cancers, led us to investigate whether TA can counteract the stimulating influence of mesotrione on the proliferation and growth of malignant cells.

2. Materials and Methods

2.1. Reagents

Phosphate buffered saline (PBS), without Ca and Mg, was provided PAN Biotech (Aidenbach, Germany). SDS (Sodium dodecyl sulphate), TCA (trichloroacetic acid), TBA (thiobarbituric acid), Folin-Ciocalteu reagent, and Mesotrione were provided by Sigma-Aldrich and DTNB (dithiobis-2-nitrobenzoic acid, Ellman's reagent) by Serva. Dichlorodihydrofluorescein diacetate assay (DCFH-DA) and cell stain double staining kit containing propionium iodide and calcein AM was provided by Sigma-Aldrich, St. Louis, MO, USA. The fluorescein isothiocyanate (FITC) Annexin V Apoptosis Detection Kit I was purchased from BD Pharmingen (San Diego, CA, USA). The Cayman's Catalase Assay Kit, Cayman's Superoxide Dismutase Assay Kit, and Cayman GPx Assay were obtained from Cayman Chemical (Ann Arbor, MI, USA).

2.2. Cell Culture

The effect of herbicide, TA (Cayman Chemical Company (1180 East Ellsworth Road, Ann Arbor, MI, USA), purity ≥ 98%; formal name: 2E-dodecenedioic acid; CAS number: 6402-36-4; formulation: A crystalline solid) and the mix of herbicide with TA was studied in the ZR-75-1 cell line, which was obtained from American Type Culture Collection (ATCC, Manassas, VA, USA). The ZR-75-1 cells were cultured in RPMI-1640 Medium containing glucose at 4.5 mg/mL (25 mM) supplemented with 10% fetal bovine serum (FBS) (PAN Biotech), penicillin (100 U/mL) (PAN Biotech), and streptomycin (100 µg/mL) (PAN Biotech) at 37 °C in a humidified atmosphere of 5% CO_2 in air.

2.3. Cytotoxicity Assay

Cytotoxicity were studied according to the method of Carmichael using 3-(4,5-dimethylthiazol-2-yl)-2,5-diphenyltetrazolium bromide (MTT) (Sigma-Aldrich, St. Louis, MO, USA) [14].

TA cytotoxicity was studied at selected concentrations of 0.5 µM, 0.75 µM, 1 µM, 10 µM, 20 µM, 50 µM, 100 µM, 200 µM, 500 µM, 750 µM, and 1000 µM. Mes cytotoxicity was estimated at concentrations of 0.01 µM, 0.025 µM, 0.05 µM, 0.1 µM, 0.5 µM, 1 µM, 5 µM, 10 µM, 25 µM, and 50 µM. The concentrations of both compounds selected for the analysis of the effect of the tested chemicals mixture on the cells have been chosen on the basis of MTT cytotoxicity tests performed. The concentration of Mes with the highest stimulating effect on the ZR-75-1 cells was selected. The control cells were cultured without test compounds.

Breast cancer cells were seeded in a 96-well plate at a density of 2×10^4 cells/well. Cells cultured for 24 h and 48 h were first treated with TA in the concentration range from 0.5 µM to 1000 µM, then Mes in the concentration range from 0.01 µM to 50 µM, and finally TA mixed with Mes: TA in the concentration range from 0.5 µM to 1000 µM mixed with 0.05 µM Mes. The analysis was conducted according to Jabłońska-Trypuć et al. using a microplate reader GloMax®-Multi Microplate Multimode Reader (Promega Corporation, Madison, WI, USA) [13]. The viability of breast cancer cells was presented as a percentage of control cells. All the experiments were done in triplicate.

2.4. Caspase 3/7 Activity Assay

The activity of caspases 3/7 was examined at TA concentrations of 100µM and 200 µM, Mes concentration of 0.05 µM, and the combination of two compounds (TA + Mes, concentrations: 100 µM + 0.05 µM and 200 µM + 0.05 µM, respectively) after 24 h and 48 h of incubation. Breast cancer cells were seeded in 96-well white plate at a density of 2×10^4 cells/well. Luminescent assay was applied according to manufacturer's instructions (Promega Corporation, Madison, WI, USA) as described previously [15]. A microplate reader GloMax®-Multi Microplate Multimode Reader was used and the experiments were done in triplicate.

2.5. Fluorescent Microscopy Analysis

For the analysis of apoptotic and necrotic cells nuclear morphology, two fluorescent dyes, propionium iodide and calcein-AM, were applied. Cells were seeded on cell imaging dishes with coverglass bottoms at a density of 2×10^5 cells/well with 200 µM TA, 0.05 µM Mes, the mix of two compounds, and without the tested compound for 24 h. Subsequently, cells were washed twice with PBS and then stained with dyes solution in the dark in 37 °C for 15 min. The mixture of dyes was removed and the cells were washed with phosphate buffer and analyzed with the use of Olympus IX83 fluorescent microscope with SC180 camera with Cell Sens Dimension 1.17 program (200 × magnification). Calcein-AM stains viable cells and PI pass only through damaged membrane in dead cells. The following criteria were used: Living cells were characterized by regularly distributed green chromatin nucleus and are stained with green color. Dead cells, probably apoptotic cells, were characterized by red nuclei with chromatin condensation or fragmentation. Necrotic cells showed red-stained cell nuclei.

2.6. Analysis of Apoptosis Using Flow Cytometry

Breast cancer cells were seeded in six-well plates at a density of 2×10^5 cells/well. Cells were exposed to 100 µM TA, 200 µM TA, 0.05 µM Mes, and the mix of two compounds (TA + Mes, concentrations: 100 µM + 0.05 µM, 200 µM + 0.05 µM, respectively) and incubated for 24 h and

48 h. Apoptosis was studied by flow cytometry on FACSCalibura II cytometer (Becton-Dickinson). After trypsinization, cells were resuspended in RPMI-1640. Then, cells were suspended in binding buffer for staining with FITC (Annexin V) and propidium iodide (PI) for 15 min at room temperature in the dark following the manufacturer's instructions (FITC Annexin V apoptosis detection Kit I). The signal obtained from cells stained with Annexin V or PI alone was used for fluorescence compensation. Data were analyzed with FACStationTM software (BD PharmingenTM, San Diego, CA, USA).

2.7. Total Protein Content

ZR-75-1 cells were exposed to 100 μM TA, 200 μM TA, 0.05 μM Mes, and the mix of two compounds (TA + Mes, concentrations: 100 μM + 0.05 μM, 200 μM + 0.05 μM, respectively) and incubated for 24 h and 48 h. ZR-75-1 cells (2.5×10^5 cells/mL) were cultured with tested compounds. The protein concentration was determined as described previously [15]. All the experiments were done in triplicate.

2.8. Determination of SH Groups

SH groups content was analyzed using Rice-Evans method (1991) as described previously [15]. ZR-75-1 cells were exposed to 100 μM TA, 200 μM TA, 0.05 μM Mes, and the mix of two compounds (TA + Mes, concentrations: 100 μM + 0.05 μM, 200 μM + 0.05 μM, respectively) and incubated for 24 h and 48 h. ZR-75-1 cells (2.5×10^5 cells/mL) were cultured with tested compounds. All the experiments were done in triplicate.

2.9. Determination of TBA Reactive Species (TBARS) Level

The Rice-Evans method (1991) was used for measuring membrane lipid-peroxidation products level (TBARS), as described previously [15]. ZR-75-1 cells were exposed to 100 μM TA, 200 μM TA, 0.05 μM Mes, and the mix of two compounds (TA + Mes, concentrations: 100 μM + 0.05 μM, 200 μM + 0.05 μM, respectively) and incubated for 24 h and 48 h. ZR-75-1 cells (2.5×10^5 cells/mL) were cultured with test compounds. All the experiments were done in triplicate.

2.10. Determination of GSH/GSSG

GSH/GSSG (GSH–reduced form of glutathione, GSSG–oxidized form of glutathione) ratio was examined at TA concentrations of 100 μM and 200 μM, Mes concentration of 0.05 μM, and the mixture of these two compounds (TA + Mes, concentrations: 100 μM + 0.05 μM and 200 μM + 0.05 μM, respectively) after 24 h and 48 h of incubation. Breast cancer cells were seeded in 96-well white plates at a density of 2×10^4 cells/well. GSH/GSSG ratio was assayed in triplicate via GSH/GSSG-Glo™ kit (Promega Madison, WI, USA) following manufacturer's instructions as described [15].

2.11. Intracellular ROS Detection

Intracellular ROS level was examined at TA concentrations of 100 μM and 200 μM, Mes concentration of 0.05 μM, and the mixture of these two compounds (TA + Mes, concentrations: 100 μM + 0.05 μM and 200 μM + 0.05 μM, respectively) after 24 h and 48 h of incubation. Breast cancer cells were seeded in 96-well white plates at a density of 2×10^4 cells/well. Dichlorodihydrofluorescein diacetate (DCFH-DA), (Sigma, St. Louis, MO, USA) and GloMax®-Multi Detection System (Promega Corporation, Madison, WI, USA) were used in order to measure the level of intracellular reactive oxygen species (ROS) [16]. The method was described previously [12]. All the experiments were done in triplicate.

2.12. Catalase Activity

Catalase is an enzyme which is involved in the detoxification processes, mainly the metabolism of hydrogen peroxide, which originates during normal aerobic metabolism and pathogenic reactive oxygen species (ROS) generation. Cells were cultured in six-well plates at 1×10^5 cells/well (Sarstedt), treated with 100 μM and 200 μM TA, 0.05 μM Mes, and the mix of two compounds (TA + Mes, concentrations: 100 µM + 0.05 µM, 200 µM + 0.05 µM, respectively) for 24 h and 48 h. For the determination of catalase activity, the Catalase Assay Kit (Cayman Chemical Company Ann Arbor, MI, USA) was used following manufacturer's instructions. The absorbance of final product was read at 540 nm using the GloMax®-Multi Microplate Multimode Reader. All the experiments were done in triplicate.

2.13. Glutathione Peroxidase Activity

Glutathione peroxidase is involved in cells protection against oxidative stress by catalyzing the reduction of hydroperoxides by reduced GSH. Cells were cultured in six-well plates at 1×10^5 cells/well (Sarstedt), and treated with 100 µM and 200 µM TA, 0.05 µM Mes, and the mix of two compounds (TA + Mes, concentrations: 100 µM + 0.05 µM, 200 µM + 0.05 µM, respectively) for 24 h and 48 h. Prior to the analysis, cells were washed with phosphate buffer. Cells were collected using rubber policeman and homogenized in a cold buffer, then centrifuged at $10,000\times g$ for 15 min at 4 °C. Supernatant was used for the assay. For the determination of glutathione peroxidase activity GPx Assay kit (Cayman Chemical Company Ann Arbor, MI, USA) was used following manufacturer's instructions. The absorbance at 340 nm was read using the GloMax®-Multi Microplate Multimode Reader. All the experiments were done in triplicate.

2.14. Superoxide Dismutase Activity

Superoxide dismutases belong to the group of metalloenzymes. They catalyze the superoxide anion dismutation to molecular oxygen and hydrogen peroxide and therefore play an important role in the cellular antioxidant defense system. Cells were seeded in six-well plates at 1×10^5 cells/well (Sarstedt), and treated with 100 µM and 200 µM TA, 0.05 µM Mes, and the mix of two compounds (TA + Mes, concentrations: 100 µM + 0.05 µM, 200 µM + 0.05 µM, respectively) for 24 h and 48 h. Prior to the analysis, cells were washed with phosphate buffer. Cells were collected using rubber policeman and homogenized in a cold buffer, then centrifuged at $10,000\times g$ for 15 min at 4 °C. Supernatant was used for the assay. For the determination of SOD activity, the Superoxide Dismutase Assay Kit (Cayman Chemical Company Ann Arbor, MI, USA) was applied following manufacturer's instructions. The absorbance (440–460 nm) was read using the GloMax®-Multi Microplate Multimode Reader. All the experiments were done in triplicate.

2.15. Statistical Analysis

Statistical analysis for the obtained results was performed. The effect of TA, Mes, and the combination of TA and Mes on apoptosis and oxidative stress parameters in ZR-75-1 cells was calculated as a means and compared in analysis of variance using the post-hoc test of ANOVA. The significant differences were estimated by Tukey test at $p < 0.05$. A biplot graph was used in order to present correlation between parameters. Staistica 13 (StatSoft, Kraków, Poland) was used to present data analysis.

3. Results

3.1. Cytotoxicity

An MTT assay was applied in order to estimate potential TA cytotoxicity (Figure 1A). The analyzed compound caused significant decreases in relative ZR-75-1 cell viability, which was observed right after 24 h treatment. It was effective even in lower concentrations. At 1 µM TA concentration, a 37% decrease was noticed after 24 h treatment. Concentrations of 100 µM and 200 µM decreased the viability of cells by about 40% and more than 50%, respectively, after 24 h treatment. None of the tested TA concentrations stimulated studied cells viability. On the other hand, Mes significantly increased relative cell viability. The most significant increase in the relatively shorter time of incubation was observed under the influence of 0.05 µM of Mes, which is presented in Figure 1B. Therefore, one of Mes concentrations, 0.05 µM, was selected for further analysis, and was applied together with all of the studied concentrations of TA. We noticed significant decline in relative cell viability in both incubation times, especially in combination of Mes with TA in 0.05 µM + 100 µM and 0.05 µM + 200 µM, respectively (Figure 1C). Taking into account the results of the above-mentioned experiments, we decided to choose two combinations of analyzed compounds for further analysis of the mechanisms by which they affect breast cancer cells. TA concentrations of 100 µM and 200 µM are close to IC50 value, and more importantly, TA concentrations higher than 400 µM could be potentially cytotoxic for the human organism. For studying oxidative stress parameters and apoptosis, we analyzed the influence of 0. 05 µM Mes + 100 µM TA and 0.05 µM Mes + 200 µM TA.

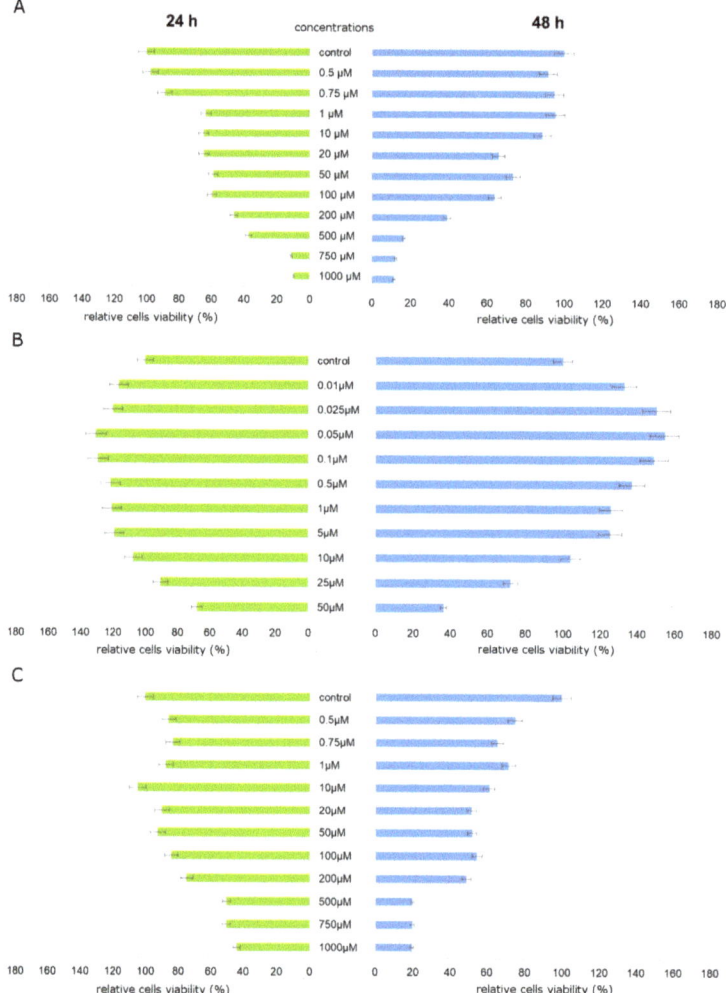

Figure 1. Relative cell viability. The ZR-75-1 cell line was exposed to (**A**) graded concentrations of TA (traumatic acid), (**B**) graded concentrations of Mes (mesotrione), and (**C**) graded concentrations of TA mixed with 0.05 µM of Mes. Mean values from three independent experiments ± standard deviation (SD) are shown.

3.2. Apoptosis

Before conducting the Caspase-Glo® 3/7 Assay, cells were subjected to 0.05 μM Mes, 100 μM TA, 200 μM TA, and the combination of 0.05 μM of Mes with 100 μM TA and 0.05 μM of Mes with 200 μM of TA (Figure 2A). Mes treatment did not induce apoptosis in studied cell line. TA slightly enhanced the activity of analyzed caspases, especially after 48 h of treatment. However, the most significant changes in caspases 3/7 activity caused by two mixed compounds were observed when TA concentration was about 200 μM.

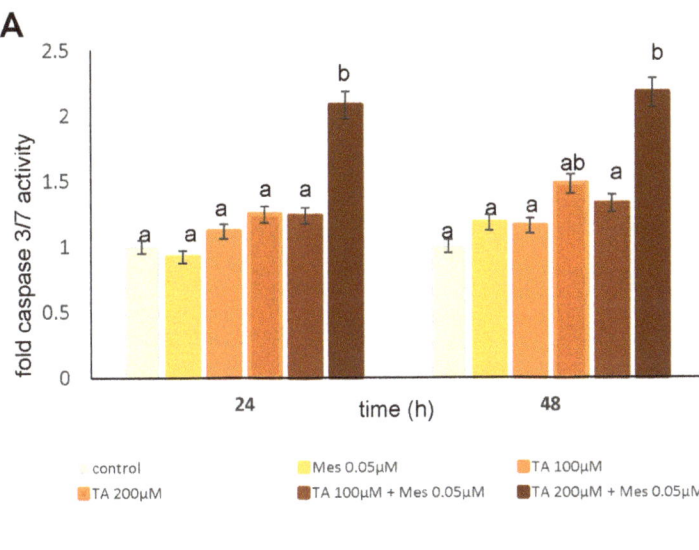

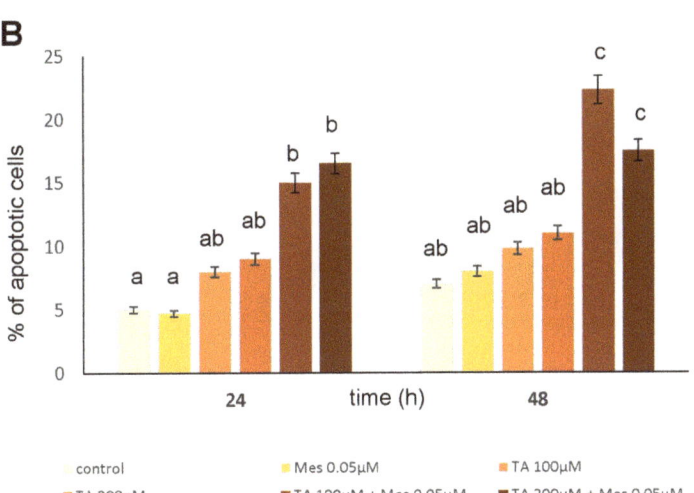

Figure 2. The effect of TA, Mes, and the combination of TA+Mes on apoptosis in ZR-75-1 cells, which were incubated with 100 μM of TA, 200 μM of TA, 0.05 μM of Mes, and a mix of 100 μTA + 0.05 μM Mes, 200 μM TA + 0.05 μM Mes. (**A**) Caspase 3/7 activity in ZR-75-1 cells under the influence of TA, Mes and TA + Mes on, (**B**) Bar graphs presenting the percentage of apoptotic cells. Mean values from three independent experiments ± SD are shown. Different letters indicate statistical differences ($p \leq 0.05$) between treatments estimated by Tukey's test.

Apoptosis was also estimated using flow cytometry, and the results are presented in Figure 2B. In Figure 2B, the percent of apoptotic cells cultured for 24 h and 48 h with TA, Mes, and the mixture of TA and Mes is depicted. The values obtained for herbicide treatment indicate that tested compound did not enhance apoptosis. However, TA treatment, both alone and in combination with Mes, enhanced apoptosis. The results obtained in the flow cytometry experiment confirmed the studied caspases activity.

A fluorescent microscopy assay was used in order to confirm the occurrence of apoptosis (Figure 3). We evaluated apoptotic and necrotic cells morphology using fluorescent staining. Similar to luminescence and flow cytometry analysis, we observed differences between control, TA, and TA + Mes treatments. We did not observe differences between control and pesticide-treated cells. Calcein—AM stained only viable cells, while propidium iodide stained viable and death cells.

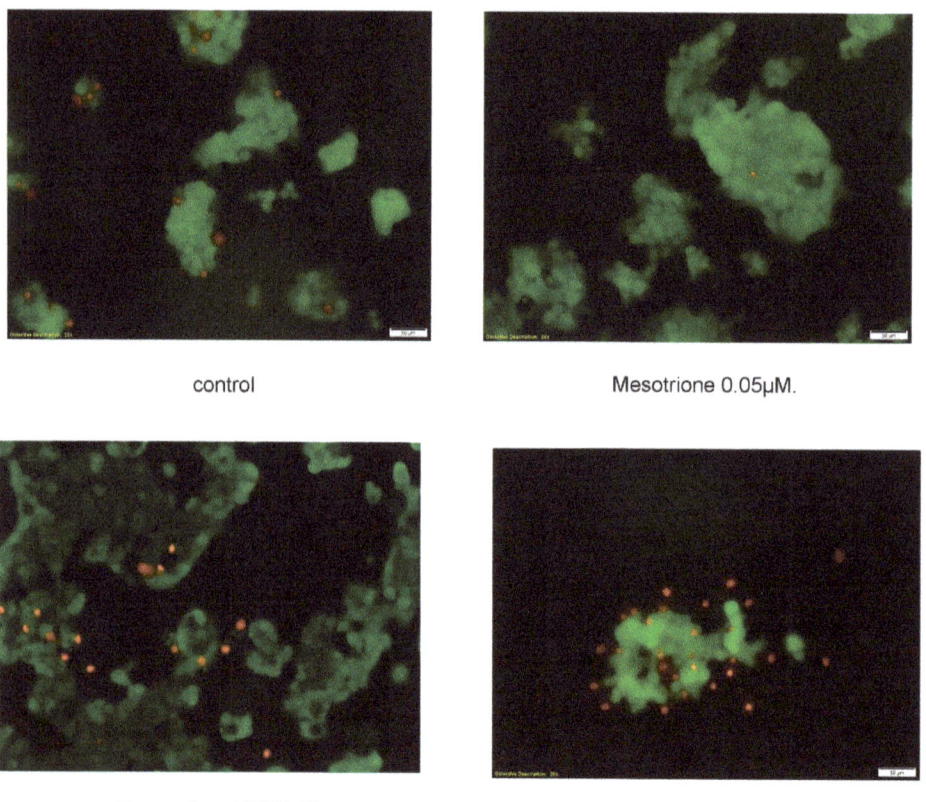

Figure 3. The influence of TA (200 µM), Mes (0.05 µM), and the mix of TA + Mes (200 µM + 0.05 µM) on apoptosis and necrosis in the ZR-75-1 cell line estimated using fluorescence microscope assay (200 × magnification). The cells were cultured with TA and Mes for 24 h and stained with Calcein-AM and propidium iodide. Three independent experiments were conducted and representative images are depicted.

3.3. Oxidative Stress

In the combination of Mes and TA, unsaturated dicarboxylic fatty acid demonstrates anticancer properties against Mes-induced breast cancer development by enhancing the stimulatory effect on oxidative stress parameters.

The influence of TA and Mes on the amount of SH groups is presented in Figure 4A. A statistically significant increase in thiol group content by approximately 68% was noticed under the influence of Mes after 24 h. Exposure to TA after 24 h incubation also caused an increase in analyzed parameter. However, 48 h incubation with tested compounds caused a significant decrease in thiol group content. Notably, the decrease was observed in case of the TA pretreatment of cells. The obtained results indicate that 100 µM of TA delayed the antioxidative effect of Mes on breast cancer cells, because we noticed a decrease in thiol group content caused by 0.05 µM Mes in the culture pretreated with 100 µM TA. The presented data may indicate that TA could be a compound, which intensifies oxidative stress in cancer cells, even in the presence of herbicide.

Lipid peroxidation in cancer cells is a very important process, which consists a source of free radicals inevitable for fast cancer cell proliferation (Figure 4B). Incubation with all of the analyzed compounds after 24 h caused an increase in TBARS content, which was analyzed as an index of lipid peroxidation. However, statistically significant changes in tested parameter were observed after 48 h treatment. Both TA alone and 100 µM TA in combination with Mes caused a very high increase in TBARS level. However, 200 µM TA mixed with Mes caused a decrease of about 75% as compared to the first analyzed mix, which could be explained by the presence of the other lipid peroxidation products, for example HNE. The obtained results suggest that TA may demonstrate protective properties by increasing membrane phospholipid peroxidation to such a high level, which is toxic to cancer cells.

Figure 5B shows the influence of TA and Mes on the production of ROS in the ZR-75-1 breast cancer cells. The intensity of fluorescence of 2′7′-dichlorodihydrofluorescein (DCF) for the ZR-75-1 cells cultured with TA and Mes for 24 h and 48 h is shown as a relative ROS amount. An incubation of cells with tested compounds caused an increase in ROS content in both analyzed times. At a concentration of 200 µM, TA caused an increase, which was very high, at about 95% after 24 h. Treatment with 100 µM and 200 µM of TA significantly reduced the ROS amount in the Mes-treated cell culture as compared to TA-treated cells. The presented data show an enhancing effect of TA on ROS formation.

The influence of Mes, TA, and the mixture of Mes with TA on GSH/GSSG ratio is depicted in Figure 5A. Reduced glutathione belongs to the group of very important antioxidants, which maintain oxidative balance within the cell. At a concentration of 200 µM, TA significantly decreased GSH/GSSG ratio after 24 h of incubation, while 100 µM of TA combined with 0.05 µM Mes significantly increased the tested parameter after 48 h incubation time compared to the control. Treatment with 200 µM of TA caused a reduced ratio of GSH/GSSG after 24 h and 48 h of culturing, even after addition of Mes. Treatment with the Mes and TA mixture for 24 h reduced the level of GSH compared to untreated cells. Based on the results obtained, we conclude that TA had a rather inhibitory effect and Mes had a stimulatory effect on the GSH/GSSG ratio in the ZR-75-1 cell line.

The first line of antioxidant defense that plays a key role in maintaining redox homeostasis in the cell are enzymes such as GPx, catalase and SOD. A significant increase in catalase activity under the influence of TA combined with 0.05 µM Mes was observed after 48 h incubation only (Figure 6A). At concentrations of 100 µM and 200 µM, TA, applied as a pretreatment before adding Mes, increased catalase activity by about 40% and 23%, respectively, as compared to the control untreated cells. At a concentration of 0.05 µM, Mes decreased catalase activity in both treatment times, however statistically insignificantly. The opposite results were observed in case of glutathione peroxidase (Figure 6B). The GPx activity was the highest under the influence of 100 µM TA + 0.05 µM Mes after 24 h incubation. Longer treatment with all of the tested compounds caused declines in GPx activity, but statistically insignificant. Our results showed that SOD activity was enhanced not only by the action of Mes, but also TA. The combination of these two compounds revealed decreases in SOD activity as compared to free Mes or free TA (Figure 6C).

In Figure 7, PCA analysis is depicted. It presents the correlation between the studied variables concerning the oxidative stress and apoptosis resulting from the activity of tested compounds and their mixture in the ZR-75-1 cell line. Figure 7 shows that 24 h treatment with TA was positively correlated with TBARS content, ROS content, and SOD activity, and was also correlated with the first component, which explains the 48.82% variability. However, Mes treatment was correlated with GSH/GSSG ratio, which is represented by the second component, explaining the 36.49% variability. After 48 h treatment, the previously observed correlation between TA and ROS content and TA + M and caspase 3/7 activity was maintained.

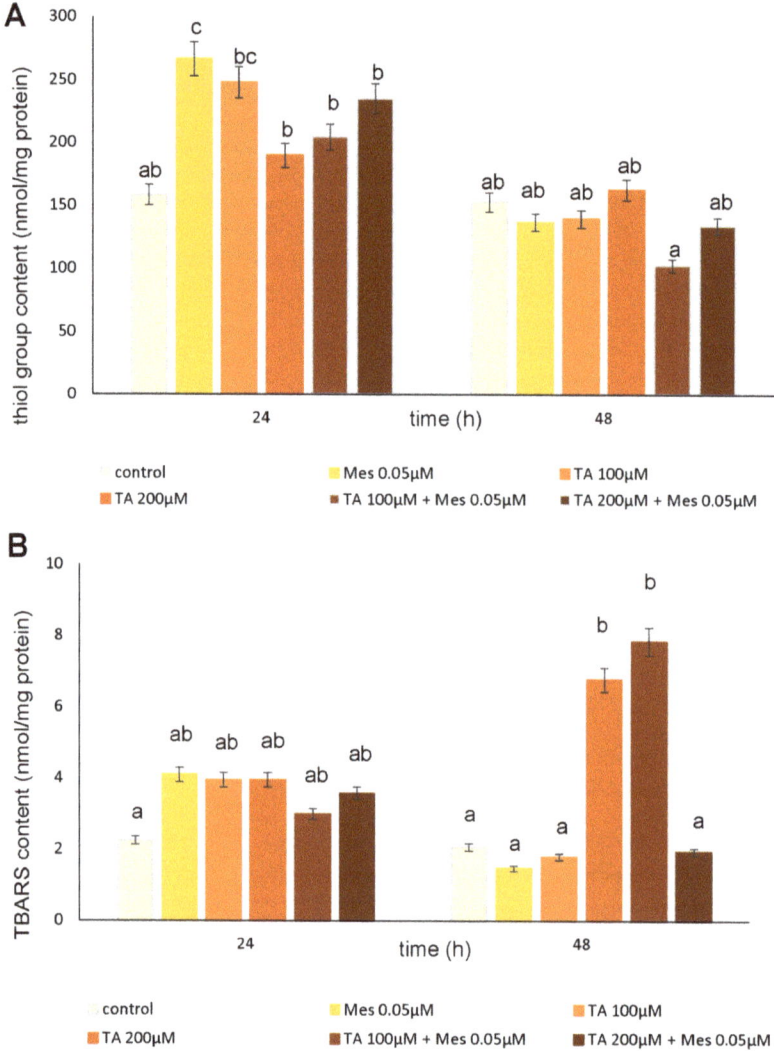

Figure 4. The influence of TA, Mes, and the mix of TA and Mes on SH group content (**A**) and TBARS content (**B**) in ZR-75-1 cells. The cells were cultured with 100 µM of TA, 200 µM of TA, 0.05 µM of Mes, mix of 100 µM TA + 0.05 µM Mes, and 200 µM TA + 0.05 µM Mes for 24 h and 48 h. Mean values from three independent experiments ± SD are shown. Different letters indicate statistical differences ($p \leq 0.05$) between each treatment estimated by Tukey's test.

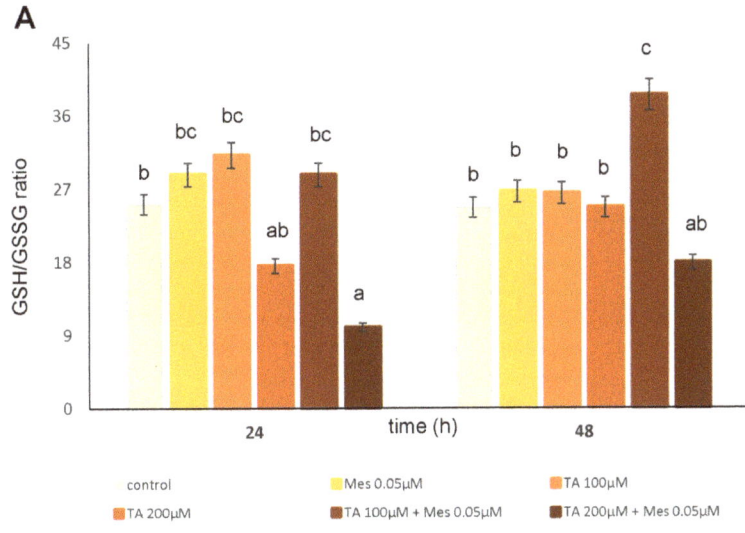

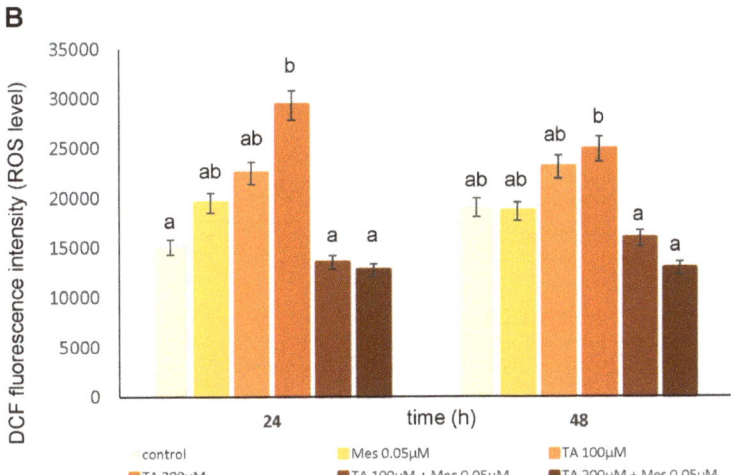

Figure 5. The influence of TA, Mes and the mix of TA and Mes on GSH/GSS (GSH–reduced form of glutathione, GSSG–oxidized form of glutathione) ratio (**A**) and reactive oxygen species (ROS) content (**B**) in ZR-75-1 cells. The cells were cultured with 100 μM TA, 200 μM TA, 0.05 μM Mes, and a mix of 100 μTA + 0.05 μM Mes, 200 μM TA + 0.05 μM Mes for 24 h and 48 h. Mean values from three independent experiments ± SD are shown. Different letters indicate statistical differences ($p \leq 0.05$) between each treatment estimated by Tukey's test.

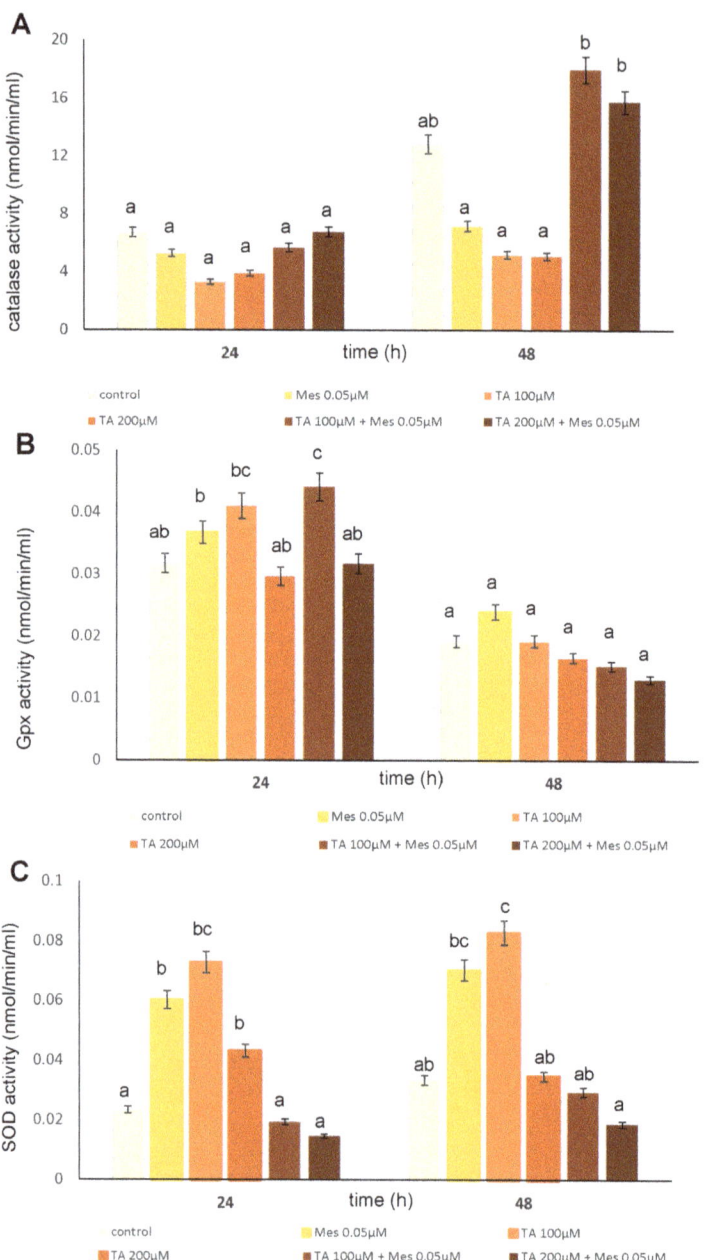

Figure 6. The influence of TA, Mes, and the mix of TA and Mes on catalase activity (**A**) GPx (glutathione peroxidase) activity (**B**) and SOD (superoxide dismutase) activity (**C**) in ZR-75-1 cells. The cells were cultured with 100 μM of TA, 200 μM of TA, 0.05 μM of Mes, and a mix of 100 μM TA + 0.05 μM Mes, 200 μM TA + 0.05 μM Mes for 24 h and 48 h. Mean values from three independent experiments ± SD are shown. Different letters indicate statistical differences ($p \leq 0.05$) between each treatment estimated by Tukey's test.

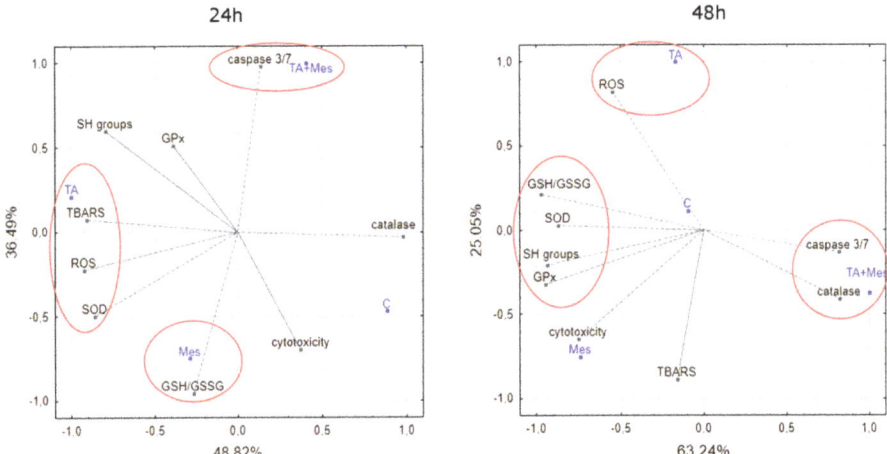

Figure 7. Biplot showing variables (SH groups (thiol groups), TBARS (thiobarbituric acid reactive species) content, GSH/GSSG ratio, ROS content, SOD, catalase, GPX activity, caspase 3/7 activity, cytotoxicity) and cases (tested compounds: Mes, TA, and TA+Mes—mix of two analyzed compounds) in two dimensions.

4. Discussion

Due to the increasing popularity of diets based mainly on products of plant origin, we should be aware of the presence in everyday meals of both ingredients having a beneficial effect on the human body, but also compounds that are residues from the method of growing and preserving food of plant origin. The first group of compounds mentioned above includes TA, which is a plant hormone with beneficial antioxidant and probably anticancer effects. While the second group of compounds present in the crop plants are undoubtedly pesticides, an example of which is analyzed Mes. Taking into account its chemical structure TA belongs to the group of unsaturated fatty acids, whose positive effect on the human body has been quite well documented in the scientific literature. Although unsaturated fatty acids are fairly well known and their anti-cancer properties are investigated and described, there is literally scarce of literature data on TA. Our previous papers have shown that TA has a positive effect on healthy human fibroblasts by reducing oxidative stress level and that TA exhibits toxicity towards breast cancer cells by stimulating apoptosis through an increased level of oxidative stress [11,12]. In our preliminary study we also did an experiment regarding the mixtures of TA with selected herbicides frequently used in Poland and in EU on three breast cancer cell lines and one normal healthy cell line obtained from mammary gland [13]. Based on conducted experiments we concluded that TA in a dose–dependent manner may exert some toxicological effects in analyzed cells subjected also to herbicides. Therefore, as a next step, in this study we want to start investigating the mechanisms by which these two compounds may interact with each other and therefore influence growth and development of breast cancer cells.

First, the influence of analyzed compounds on the ZR-75-1 cell line proliferation was investigated. The MTT test was the basic experiment on the basis of which the concentrations were selected for further determinations. Cells under analysis were subjected to wide range of TA and Mes concentrations for 24 h and 48 h. The relative cell viability was monitored, and subsequently, one of Mes concentrations (0.05 µM) was selected for the experiment with the combination of two tested compounds. In the third part of the experiment, cells were pretreated with TA in the wide range of concentrations, and then Mes in the concentration of 0.05 µM was added. The most significant declines in Mes-treated cells viability were noticed as a result of 100 µM and 200 µM of TA treatment. The presented results are in agreement with our previously published data regarding TA influence on MCF-7 cells, where we indicated a decline in cancer cell proliferation and viability caused by TA [12]. Literature data has indicated that pesticides may stimulate cancer cells proliferation through different mechanisms, e.g., glyphosate stimulates human breast cancer cells growth through estrogen receptors pathways, diuron acts in a tissue-specific manner and ROS play a role in its toxicity, and bifenox and dichlobenil exhibit enhancing effects on oxidative stress, simultaneously stimulating cancer cell proliferation and inhibiting apoptosis [17–19]. There is a large amount of literature data indicating a link between elevated levels of oxidative stress and a simultaneous increase in tumor cell proliferation [20–22]. Therefore, in our work, we focused primarily on the analysis of various parameters of oxidative stress. Cancer cells of different types are characterized by high level of ROS as compared to normal cells. This is primarily due to genetic disorders which appear in cancer cells, resulting in uncontrolled proliferation. In order to analyze the possible inhibiting effect of TA on the proliferation of Mes-treated cells, we conducted an MTT assay. The results indicate that TA exhibits antiproliferative properties.

In our studies, we noticed a decline in the amount of ROS in Mes-treated cells preincubated with TA, which may be associated with the cytotoxic effect of TA in cancer cells. Cancer cells usually use elevated level of oxidative stress caused, among others, by ROS generation in order to reduce the body's antioxidant protection. This allows the initial defeat of the first defense line against metastasis and angiogenesis, which are key stages in the development and progression of cancer [23,24]. This is in agreement with our research results indicating the relationship between an observed increase in ROS content and an increase in proliferation in Mes-treated cells and the decrease in ROS content in TA preincubated cells with a decrease in their proliferation level.

Many compounds of natural origin from the cytokinin group have antioxidant activity in healthy cells and pro-oxidative in cancer cells, which we also showed in our previous papers [12,25]. TA, as an unsaturated fatty acid, shows an increased susceptibility to oxidative processes. According to the literature, breast cancer cells are also definitely predisposed to oxidation of the macromolecules, which build them as compared to healthy cells. Unsaturated fatty acids have been shown to induce increased synthesis in *inter alia* lipid hydroperoxides in lipids that are part of cell membranes [26,27]. According to O'Shea M. et al., conjugated linoleic acid causes an increase in lipid peroxidation in breast cancer cells with a simultaneous decrease in cell proliferation [28]. We observed similar results in our research. We noticed increases in TBARS levels, which are correlated with changes in the content of SH groups. Incubation with TA for 48 h caused a decrease in thiol groups, even in Mes-treated cells. Mes stimulates the growth of cancer cells and causes an increase in the level of SH groups, which can probably also increase their resistance to oxidative stress and possible damage and enhance proliferation. Changes in the level of TBARS content and SH groups were also accompanied by changes in the GSH/GSSG ratio, particularly decreases under the influence of preincubation with 200 µM TA in cells treated with Mes. The correspondingly high level of GSH, which is one of the most important low molecular weight antioxidants in breast cancer cells, is usually correlated with the resistance of these cells to the induction of apoptosis and with their increased proliferation [29]. Our results indicate statistically significant decreases in GSH level under the influence of 200 µM TA in cells treated with Mes, with simultaneous statistically significant increases in the level of effector caspases 3/7 activity. The analysis of the activity of caspases 3/7, confirmed by the results obtained from flow cytometry and fluorescence microscopy, demonstrates that, at a concentration of 0.05 µM, Mes induces a decrease in the percentage of apoptotic cells as compared to control and to TA-treated cells. After both 24 h and after 48 h, we observed that TA at 200 µM significantly induced apoptosis even in combination with Mes, which may mean that TA is capable of overcome activity of pesticide and stimulate apoptosis in breast cancer cells.

Due to the application of TA, especially at a concentration of 200 µM, we noticed a significant increase in the activity of caspase 3/7, a decrease in ROS content, and a decrease in GSH content. However, it should be noted that the cells antioxidant defense system are divided into two parts: Enzymatic and nonenzymatic. Primary endogenous antioxidants are superoxide dismutase (SOD), catalase and glutathione peroxidase [30]. Our results clearly show that TA caused an increase in oxidative toxicity in Mes-treated ZR-75-1 cells. It was manifested by a decrease in GPx activity and GSH/GSSG ratio and increase in TBARS content. Lipid hydroperoxides and other ROS are a major cause of oxidative damage within the cell membrane lipids, leading to increase in TBARS content. The GSH pool in the cells decreases due to an excessive generation of lipid peroxidation products and other oxygen species [31]. In turn, an excess in TA-induced ROS generation causes a significant decline in GSH synthesis and inhibition of antioxidant enzymes [32]. The reduced form of glutathione is an antioxidant low in molecular mass for appropriate cell integrity and redox balance, although GPx is an antioxidant enzyme, which contains selenium and its main role is scavenging of ROS. Catalase in breast cancer cells is characterized by high activity and expression level [33]. In our research, a decrease in catalase activity was observed under the influence of Mes and both analyzed concentrations of TA. However, under the influence of TA mixed with Mes, significant increases were noticed in both analyzed TA concentrations, especially after 48 h incubation. The presented results are consistent with literature data, indicating that catalase activity is induced in MCF-7 breast cancer cell line exposed to conjugated linoleic acid [34]. However, SOD activity, similar to GPx activity under the influence of Mes in TA-preincubated cells, was significantly lower as compared to the control or to the TA-treated and Mes-treated cells. Mes enhanced the activity of both SOD and GPx, but TA was effective enough to withstand the stimulating effect of the Mes and reduce the activity of the enzymes studied. Ding WQ et al. also observed that cancer cell treatment with docosahexaenoic acid reduced significantly SOD1 expression [35]. Literature data describing in vivo studies have shown divergent results of analyses regarding the effect of fatty acids on antioxidant enzyme activity. Some studies have indicated higher activity of antioxidant enzymes analyzed in animals consuming PUFA-enriched feed, while others have indicated that PUFAs caused a decline in the activity of these enzymes in the tissues of noncancerous rats [36,37]. In the present study, we found that TA inhibits SOD activity in Mes-treated ZR-75-1 cells, which has not been reported previously. Selected unsaturated fatty acids are known to modulate genes expression in malignant cells [38]. After being transported into cell nucleus, fatty acids such as TA are bounded to peroxisome proliferator-activated receptor [39]. This receptor response element is in the SOD1 gene promoter in rats [40]. Therefore, the transcription of the SOD1 gene could be influenced by TA in ZR-75-1 cells. On the other hand, SOD1 mRNA destabilization could be influenced by DHA, which subsequently causes its lower expression. The target reduction of SOD activity was a way to increase intracellular peroxide amount, hence causing an increase in mitochondrial damage and stimulating apoptosis in cancer cells [41].

In our experiments, we observed a 45% decrease of SOD activity in the ZR-75-1 cells treated with 200 µM TA and incubated with Mes. According to our biplot analysis results, this was not correlated the growth rate of cells but was significantly correlated with the effect on TA-induced lipid peroxidation and ROS content after 24 h and with GPx activity, GSH/GSSG ratio, and SH group content. Our results support the idea that compounds, which influence antioxidant enzymes activity and oxidative balance in cancer cells, could be applied in the elimination of tumor cells through the induction of apoptosis.

5. Conclusions

The presented results allow us to conclude that TA may act as pro-oxidative and pro-apoptotic agent against Mes-stimulated breast cancer growth and development. TA could be considered as a plant, alternative source of unsaturated fatty acids that can eliminate the positive effect of pesticides on the growth and development of breast cancer cells. By stimulating oxidative stress and inhibiting the enzymatic antioxidative defense system in cancer cells, this compound can inhibit the growth and development of breast cancer. It should be also mentioned that TA acts as a pro-oxidative and pro-apoptotic agent in other breast cancer cell lines, simultaneously acting as antioxidant in normal human cells. Due to its unique properties, it could be considered as an important food ingredient. Exposure to herbicides present in food is dangerous for both healthy people and certainly for women diagnosed with breast cancer. This is also evidenced by the results of our research showing the positive and stimulating effect of Mes on the development and growth of cancer cells. However, TA seems to be a compound with high anti-cancer potential, which may endure the negative impact of herbicides on the human body.

Author Contributions: A.J.-T.—corresponding author, wrote the paper, planned experiments; performed experiments; analysed data; U.W.—performed statistical analysis; analysed data; E.W.—analysed data; J.R.—analysed data; A.B.—analyzed the data; funding acquisition. All authors have read and agreed to the published version of the manuscript.

Funding: This work was financially supported by Ministry of Science and Higher Education, Poland, under the research project number WZ/WBiIŚ/3/2019.

Acknowledgments: This work was financially supported by Ministry of Science and Higher Education, Poland, under the research project number WZ/WBiIŚ/3/2019.

Conflicts of Interest: The authors declare no conflict of interest.

Compliance with Ethical Standards: The manuscript does not contain clinical studies or patient data.

References

1. Jabłońska-Trypuć, A.; Wołejko, E.; Wydro, U.; Butarewicz, A. The impact of pesticides on oxidative stress level in human organism and their activity as an endocrine disruptor. *J. Environ. Sci. Health B* **2017**, *52*, 483–494. [CrossRef] [PubMed]
2. Hamilton, D.; Crossley, S. *Pesticide Residues in Food and Drinking Water: Human Exposure and Risks*; John Wiley & Sons, Ltd.: Chichester, UK, 2004.
3. Mitchell, G.; Bartlett, D.W.; Fraser, T.E.M.; Hawkes, T.R.; Holt, D.C.; Townson, J.K.; Wichert, R.A. Mesotrione: A new selective herbicide for use in maize. *Pest Manag. Sci.* **2001**, *57*, 120–128. [CrossRef]
4. Chrétien, F.; Giroux, I.; Thériault, G.; Patrick, G.; Corriveau, J. Surface Runoff and Subsurface Tile Drain Losses of Neonicotinoids and Companion Herbicides at Edge-Of-Field. *Environ. Pollut.* **2017**, *224*, 255–264. [CrossRef] [PubMed]
5. Norris, S.R.; Barrette, T.R.; Della Penna, D. Genetic dissection of carotenoid synthesis in arabidopsis defines plastoquinone as an essential component of phytoene desaturation. *Plant Cell* **1995**, *7*, 2139–2149. [PubMed]
6. Zhang, F.; Yao, X.; Sun, S.; Wang, L.; Liu, W.; Jiang, X.; Wang, J. Effects of mesotrione on oxidative stress, subcellular structure, and membrane integrity in Chlorella vulgaris. *Chemosphere* **2019**, *247*, 125668. [CrossRef] [PubMed]
7. Bonnet, J.L.; Bonnemoy, F.; Dusser, M.; Bohatier, J. Toxicity assessment of the herbicides sulcotrione and mesotrione toward two reference environmental microorganisms: Tetrahymena pyriformis and Vibrio fischeri. *Arch. Environ. Contam. Toxicol.* **2008**, *55*, 576–583. [CrossRef]
8. Bonefeld-Jørgensen, E.C.; Andersen, H.R.; Rasmussen, T.H.; Vinggaard, A.M. Effect of highly bioaccumulated polychlorinated biphenyl congeners on estrogen and androgen receptor activity. *Toxicology* **2001**, *158*, 141–153. [CrossRef]
9. Ellsworth, R.E.; Mamula, K.A.; Costantino, N.S.; Deyarmin, B.; Kostyniak, P.J.; Chi, L.H.; Shriver, C.D.; Ellsworth, D.L. Abundance and distribution of polychlorinated biphenyls (PCBs) in breast tissue. *Environ. Res.* **2015**, *138*, 291–297. [CrossRef]
10. Engel, L.S.; Werder, E.; Satagopan, J.; Blair, A.; Hoppin, J.A.; Koutros, S.; Lerro, C.C.; Sandler, D.P.; Alavanja, M.C.; Beane Freeman, L.E. Insecticide Use and Breast Cancer Risk among Farmers' Wives in the Agricultural Health Study. *Environ. Health Perspect.* **2017**, *125*, 097002. [CrossRef]
11. Jabłońska-Trypuć, A.; Pankiewicz, W.; Czerpak, R. Traumatic Acid Reduces Oxidative Stress and Enhances Collagen Biosynthesis in Cultured Human Skin Fibroblasts. *Lipids* **2016**, *51*, 1021–1035. [CrossRef]
12. Jabłońska-Trypuć, A.; Krętowski, R.; Wołejko, E.; Wydro, U.; Butarewicz, A. Traumatic acid toxicity mechanisms in human breast cancer MCF-7 cells. *Regul. Toxicol. Pharmacol.* **2019**, *106*, 137–146. [CrossRef] [PubMed]
13. Jabłońska-Trypuć, A.; Wydro, U.; Wołejko, E.; Butarewicz, A. Toxicological Effects of Traumatic Acid and Selected Herbicides on Human Breast Cancer Cells: In Vitro Cytotoxicity Assessment of Analyzed Compounds. *Molecules* **2019**, *24*, 1710. [CrossRef] [PubMed]

14. Carmichael, J.; DeGraff, W.G.; Gazdar, A.F.; Minna, J.D.; Mitchell, J.B. Evaluation of a tetrazolium-based semiautomated colorimetric assay: Assessment of chemosensitivity testing. *Cancer Res.* **1987**, *47*, 936–942. [PubMed]
15. Jabłońska-Trypuć, A.; Krętowski, R.; Kalinowska, M.; Świderski, G.; Cechowska-Pasko, M.; Lewandowski, W. Possible Mechanisms of the Prevention of Doxorubicin Toxicity by Cichoric Acid—Antioxidant Nutrient. *Nutrients* **2018**, *10*, 44. [CrossRef] [PubMed]
16. Krętowski, R.; Kusaczuk, M.; Naumowicz, M.; Kotyńska, J.; Szynaka, B.; Cechowska-Pasko, M. The Effects of Silica Nanoparticles on Apoptosis and Autophagy of Glioblastoma Cell Lines. *Nanomaterials* **2017**, *7*, 230. [CrossRef] [PubMed]
17. Thongprakaisang, S.; Thiantanawat, A.; Rangkadilok, N.; Suriyo, T.; Satayavivad, J. Glyphosate induces human breast cancer cells growth via estrogen receptors. *Food Chem. Toxicol.* **2013**, *59*, 129–136. [CrossRef] [PubMed]
18. Huovinen, M.; Loikkanen, J.; Naarala, J.; Vähäkangas, K. Toxicity of diuron in human cancer cells. *Toxicol. Vitro* **2015**, *29*, 1577–1586. [CrossRef] [PubMed]
19. Jabłońska-Trypuć, A.; Wydro, U.; Serra-Majem, L.; Wołejko, E.; Butarewicz, A. The Analysis of Bifenox and Dichlobenil Toxicity in Selected Microorganisms and Human Cancer Cells. *Int. J. Environ. Res. Public Health* **2019**, *16*, 4137. [CrossRef] [PubMed]
20. Kumari, S.; Badana, A.K.; Malla, R. Reactive Oxygen Species: A Key Constituent in Cancer Survival. *Biomark. Insights* **2018**, *13*, 1177271918755391. [CrossRef]
21. Coughlin, S.S. Oxidative Stress, Antioxidants, Physical Activity, and the Prevention of Breast Cancer Initiation and Progression. *J. Environ. Health Sci.* **2018**, *4*, 55–57.
22. Jezierska-Drutel, A.; Rosenzweig, S.A.; Neumann, C.A. Role of oxidative stress and the microenvironment in breast cancer development and progression. *Adv. Cancer Res.* **2013**, *119*, 107–125. [PubMed]
23. Hecht, F.; Pessoa, C.F.; Gentile, L.B.; Rosenthal, D.; Carvalho, D.P.; Fortunato, R.S. The role of oxidative stress on breast cancer development and therapy. *Tumor Biol.* **2016**, *37*, 4281–4291. [CrossRef] [PubMed]
24. Gorrini, C.; Harris, I.S.; Mak, T.W. Modulation of oxidative stress as an anticancer strategy. *Nat. Rev. Drug Discov.* **2013**, *12*, 931–947. [CrossRef] [PubMed]
25. Jabłońska-Trypuć, A.; Matejczyk, M.; Czerpak, R. N6-benzyladenine and kinetin influence antioxidative stress parameters in human skin fibroblasts. *Mol. Cell. Biochem.* **2016**, *413*, 97–107. [CrossRef] [PubMed]
26. Takeda, S.; Horrobin, D.F.; Manku, M.; Sim, P.G.; Ells, G.; Simmons, V. Lipid peroxidation in human breast cancer cells in response to gamma-linolenic acid and iron. *Anticancer Res.* **1992**, *12*, 329–333. [PubMed]
27. Menendez, J.A.; Ropero, S.; Mehmi, I.; Atlas, E.; Colomer, R.; Lupu, R. Overexpression and hyperactivity of breast cancer-associated fatty acid synthase (oncogenic antigen-519) is insensitive to normal arachidonic fatty acid-induced suppression in lipogenic tissues but it is selectively inhibited by tumoricidal alpha-linolenic and gamma-linolenic fatty acids: A novel mechanism by which dietary fat can alter mammary tumorigenesis. *Int. J. Oncol.* **2004**, *24*, 1369–1383.
28. O'Shea, M.; Devery, R.; Lawless, F.; Murphy, J.; Stanton, C. Milk fat conjugated linoleic acid (CLA) inhibits growth of human mammary MCF-7 cancer cells. *Anticancer Res.* **2000**, *20*, 3591–3601.
29. Malla, J.A.; Umesh, R.M.; Yousf, S.; Mane, S.; Sharma, S.; Lahiri, M.; Talukdar, P. A Glutathione Activatable Ion Channel Induces Apoptosis in Cancer Cells by Depleting Intracellular Glutathione Levels. *Angew. Chem. Int. Ed. Engl.* **2020**. [CrossRef]
30. Chio, I.I.C.; Tuveson, D.A. ROS in cancer: The burning question. *Trends Mol. Med.* **2017**, *23*, 411–429. [CrossRef]
31. Nazıroglu, M. New molecular mechanisms on the activation of TRPM2 channels by oxidative stress and ADP-ribose. *Neurochem. Res.* **2007**, *32*, 1990–2001. [CrossRef]
32. Nazıroglu, M.; Tokat, S.; Demirci, S. Role of melatonin on electro-magnetic radiation-induced oxidative stress and Ca2þ signaling molecular pathways in breast cancer. *J. Recept. Signal Transduct. Res.* **2012**, *32*, 290–297. [CrossRef] [PubMed]
33. Kattan, Z.; Minig, V.; Leroy, P.; Dauça, M.; Becuwe, P. Role of manganese superoxide dismutase on growth and invasive properties of human estrogen-independent breast cancer cells. *Breast Cancer Res. Treat.* **2008**, *108*, 203–215. [CrossRef] [PubMed]
34. O'Shea, M.; Stanton, C.; Devery, R. Antioxidant enzyme defence responses of human MCF-7 and SW480 cancer cells to conjugated linoleic acid. *Anticancer Res.* **1999**, *19*, 1953–1959.

35. Ding, W.Q.; Vaught, J.L.; Yamauchi, H.; Lind, S.E. Differential sensitivity of cancer cells to docosahexaenoic acid-induced cytotoxicity: The potential importance of down-regulation of superoxide dismutase 1 expression. *Mol. Cancer Ther.* **2004**, *3*, 1109–1117.
36. Venkatraman, J.T.; Chandrasekar, B.; Kim, J.D.; Fernandes, G. Effects of n-3 and n-6 fatty acids on the activities and expression of hepatic antioxidant enzymes in autoimmune-prone NZB × NZW F1 mice. *Lipids* **1994**, *29*, 561–568. [CrossRef] [PubMed]
37. Venkatraman, J.T.; Angkeow, P.; Satsangi, N.; Fernandes, G. Effects of dietary n-6 and n-3 lipids on antioxidant defense system in livers of exercised rats. *J. Am. Coll. Nutr.* **1998**, *17*, 586–594. [CrossRef]
38. Hughes-Fulford, M.; Chen, Y.; Tjandrawinata, R.R. Fatty acid regulates gene expression and growth of human prostate cancer PC-3 cells. *Carcinogenesis* **2001**, *22*, 701–707. [CrossRef]
39. Huang, H.; Starodub, O.; McIntosh, A.; Kier, A.B.; Schroeder, F. Liver fatty acid-binding protein targets fatty acids to the nucleus. Real time confocal and multiphoton fluorescence imaging in living cells. *J. Biol. Chem.* **2002**, *277*, 29139–29151. [CrossRef]
40. Chang, M.S.; Yoo, H.Y.; Rho, H.M. Positive and negative regulatory elements in the upstream region of the rat Cu/Zn-superoxide dismutase gene. *Biochem. J.* **1999**, *339*, 335–341. [CrossRef]
41. Huang, P.; Feng, L.; Oldham, E.A.; Keating, M.J.; Plunkett, W. Superoxide dismutase as a target for the selective killing of cancer cells. *Nature* **2000**, *407*, 390–395. [CrossRef]

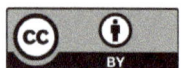

© 2020 by the authors. Licensee MDPI, Basel, Switzerland. This article is an open access article distributed under the terms and conditions of the Creative Commons Attribution (CC BY) license (http://creativecommons.org/licenses/by/4.0/).

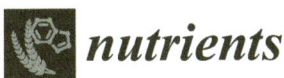

Article

Is Acrylamide as Harmful as We Think? A New Look at the Impact of Acrylamide on the Viability of Beneficial Intestinal Bacteria of the Genus *Lactobacillus*

Katarzyna Petka [1], Tomasz Tarko [2] and Aleksandra Duda-Chodak [2,*]

[1] Department of Plant Products Technology and Nutrition Hygiene, Faculty of Food Technology, University of Agriculture in Krakow, 30-149 Krakow, Poland; katarzyna.petka@urk.krakow.pl
[2] Department of Fermentation Technology and Microbiology, Faculty of Food Technology, University of Agriculture in Krakow, 30-149 Krakow, Poland; tomasz.tarko@urk.edu.pl
* Correspondence: aleksandra.duda-chodak@urk.krakow.pl; Tel.: +48-12-662-47-92

Received: 20 March 2020; Accepted: 18 April 2020; Published: 21 April 2020

Abstract: The impact of acrylamide (AA) on microorganisms is still not clearly understood as AA has not induced mutations in bacteria, but its epoxide analog has been reported to be mutagenic in *Salmonella* strains. The aim of the study was to evaluate whether AA could influence the growth and viability of beneficial intestinal bacteria. The impact of AA at concentrations of 0–100 μg/mL on lactic acid bacteria (LAB) was examined. Bacterial growth was evaluated by the culture method, while the percentage of alive, injured, and dead bacteria was assessed by flow cytometry after 24 h and 48 h of incubation. We demonstrated that acrylamide could influence the viability of the LAB, but its impact depended on both the AA concentration and the bacterial species. The viability of probiotic strain *Lactobacillus acidophilus* LA-5 increased while that of *Lactobacillus plantarum* decreased; *Lactobacillus brevis* was less sensitive. Moreover, AA influenced the morphology of *L. plantarum*, probably by blocking cell separation during division. We concluded that acrylamide present in food could modulate the viability of LAB and, therefore, could influence their activity in food products or, after colonization, in the human intestine.

Keywords: lactic acid bacteria; probiotic; acrylamide; viability; flow cytometry

1. Introduction

Acrylamide (AA) is a chemical compound used in many industries. It is produced as a substrate for the synthesis of polymers widely used in the paper, chemical, and cosmetics industries. In 1994, the International Agency for Research on Cancer (IARC) included acrylamide in a group of compounds "probably carcinogenic to humans" after laboratory tests in mice and rats [1].

Acrylamide in foods is formed mainly by the reaction of free asparagine with reducing sugars (especially fructose and glucose) during the Maillard reaction, but it can also be formed by other pathways, e.g., the acrolein pathway [2]. The most important factors for AA formation are time and the temperature of the thermal processing of food products, and it is thought that a prerequisite for AA formation is temperature exceeding 120 °C.

Acrylamide has been shown to be a reproductive toxicant in animal models [3,4]. It exerts neurotoxic activity [5–7], and many studies have proved that AA also has genotoxic, cytotoxic, and carcinogenic impacts on the human organism [6,8–10]. However, due to the fact that acrylamide does not exert a mutagenic effect in bacterial cells [3,11], it has been agreed that its carcinogenic activity is related to glycidamide (GA)—an acrylamide metabolite formed in mammalian cells. The mutagenic and genotoxic effects of GA have already been confirmed in various in vitro and in vivo studies, showing that this AA metabolite can induce the formation of DNA adducts, resulting in mutagenesis and the development of cancers [6,8,9,12].

The impact of AA on microorganisms is still unclear. The results of many assays made by various laboratories are consistent in showing that AA is not a mutagen in *Salmonella* Typhimurium tested strains at concentrations up to 5 mg/plate, with or without metabolic activation [3]. However, three epoxide analogs of acrylamide, e.g., glycidamide, have been reported to be mutagenic in *Salmonella* strains ± S9 activation [11,13]. Tsuda et al. [14] reported that AA did not induce any gene mutations in *Salmonella*/microsome test systems (TA98, TA100, TA1535, TA1537) and in *Escherichia coli*/microsome assays (WP2 uvrA$^-$) up to a dose of 50 mg AA/plate, but acrylamide did show a strong positive response in a *Bacillus subtilis* spore-rec assay (induced DNA damage) at 10–50 mg/disc. According to the authors, the results suggested that AA had the potential to induce gross DNA damage rather than point mutations detected by the Ames test. There are also studies demonstrating that after introducing 1%–3% acrylamide into the growth medium, *Escherichia coli* cells undergo various changes, such as blockage of cell division, elongation of cells, inhibition of DNA synthesis, decreased osmotic stability, and ultrastructural alterations of the outer membrane [15].

Taking into account eukaryotic cells, it is worth citing the research of Kwolek-Mirek et al. [16]. They demonstrated that acrylamide caused impairment of growth of *Saccharomyces cerevisiae* yeast deficient in Cu, Zn-superoxide dismutase (Δsod1) in a concentration-dependent manner. This inhibitory effect was not due to cell death but to decreased cell vitality and proliferative capacity. Exposing Δsod1 yeast to acrylamide caused the increased generation of reactive oxygen species and decreased glutathione levels.

It has also been proven that some microorganisms have the ability to use acrylamide as a carbon and nitrogen source for their growth and that amidases are the main factor involved in AA degradation. Amidases are enzymes (EC. 3.5.1.4) that occur ubiquitously in nature and are characterized by a broad spectrum of catalyzed reactions [17]. Classification on the basis of catalytic activity takes into account the substrate specificity profile of the particular amidase and divides known amidases into six classes. During the amidase-catalyzed deamination reaction of acrylamide, acrylic acid and ammonia are formed. Then, acrylic acid can be reduced to propionate or transformed into β-hydroxypropionate, lactate, or CO_2, in a pathway involving coenzyme-A [2,5,8].

To date, laboratory tests have shown the ability to degrade AA by many environmental microorganisms, mainly bacteria, such as *Ralstonia eutropha* [18], *Pseudomonas chlororaphis* [19], *Enterobacter aerogenes* [20], *Pseudomonas aeruginosa* [21,22], *Bacillus cereus* [23], *Rhodococcus* sp., *Klebsiella pneumoniae* [24,25], and *Burkholderia* sp. [26]. It is worth highlighting that among the amidase producers are certain species that naturally occur in human organisms or are delivered with food, such as *Escherichia coli* [27], *Bacillus clausii* [28], *Enterococcus faecalis* [29], and *Helicobacter pylori* [30,31]. However, the substrate specificity of their amidases and the potential for reaction with acrylamide have not yet been confirmed. In some cases, it has even been proved that those bacteria produce only cell wall amidases, such as N-acetylmuramoyl-L-alanine amidase [32], with no affinity to acrylamide. Either way, there is a possibility that members of microbiota could degrade acrylamide directly in the human intestine.

Lactic acid bacteria (LAB) constitute very important members of intestinal microbiota and play an important role in proper organism functioning and maintenance of our health [33–36]. Representatives of LAB are also important in the food industry, both as starter culture added during production and as native microbiota of raw materials used for food production [37–39]. The positive role of LAB could also be related to their ability to reduce AA levels in organisms or foodstuffs. To date, the possibility of degrading AA by amidase production has not been confirmed, although synthesis of N-acetylmuramoyl-L-alanine amidase, involved in the degradation of peptidoglycan and hydrolysis of the amide bond between N-acetylmuramic acid and L-amino acids of the bacterial cell wall, has been reported in LAB [40,41]. Other studies [42,43] have shown that *Lactobacillus reuteri* NRRL 14171 and *Lactobacillus casei* Shirota are able to remove acrylamide in aqueous solution by physically binding the toxin to the bacterial cell wall, probably with a significant role of the teichoic acid structure. Later, Rivas-Jimenez [44] demonstrated that both mentioned bacterial strains were able to remove dietary AA (commercial potato chips with an average AA content of ~34,000 µg/kg) under different simulated gastrointestinal conditions. The percentage of AA removed by each bacterium exposed to different concentrations of the toxin (10–350 µg/mL) had a similar tendency; the lower the concentration of AA, the higher the percentage of toxin removed. The results showed that *L. casei* Shirota showed a higher percentage (68%) of AA removed than *L. reuteri* (53%) when bacteria were exposed to the lowest concentration of toxin (10 µg/mL), but no significant differences ($p < 0.05$) were observed in the percentage of toxin removed by both strains (~2%) when ≥100 mg/mL of AA was used. These findings proved that strains of the genus *Lactobacillus* could be employed to reduce the bioavailability of dietary AA. However, the strong dependence on AA concentration suggests that the mechanism of AA reduction is still the physical binding of AA by bacteria.

To the best of our knowledge, no one has investigated how acrylamide affects the viability of lactic acid bacteria so far, and this is an important issue considering their important role in the human body. First of all, lactic acid bacteria can be exposed to acrylamide just in food products. There are many fermented milk products that contain various "additives" rich in AA, such as biscuits, muesli, roasted almonds, nuts and seeds, dried fruit, breakfast cereals, and bran flake cereals. Also, so-called pro-health foods, such as probiotic bars and cereals, contain live strains of LAB, as well as crispy cereals, roasted nuts, almonds and seeds, almond and peanut butter, dried fruits, flakes, etc. Moreover, intestinal LAB can also be exposed to dietary acrylamide after intake of various fried, grilled, toasted, roasted, or baked foods. Although acrylamide is rapidly absorbed from the intestine, there are studies suggesting that some food matrices (or components) can reduce the intestinal absorption of AA. For example, a high protein concentration in the human diet may reduce acrylamide uptake [45], causing unmetabolized acrylamide to reach the colon. Therefore, the aim of this study was to evaluate whether acrylamide could influence the growth and viability of lactic acid bacteria belonging to the *Lactobacillus* genus.

2. Materials and Methods

2.1. Bacteria

Pure cultures of lactic acid bacteria belonging to the *Lactobacillus* genus were used in the study. For the experiments, 4 strains constituting a typical microbiota of fermented milk products and 2 probiotic strains were chosen: *Lactobacillus plantarum* DSMZ 20205, *Lactobacillus brevis* DSMZ 20054, *Lactobacillus lactis* subsp. *lactis* DSMZ 20481, and *Lactobacillus casei* DSMZ 20011. All were purchased from Leibniz Institut DSMZ (Deutsche Sammlung von Mikroorganismen und Zelkulturen GmbH, Braunschweig, Germany). Two probiotic strains—*Lactobacillus acidophilus* LA-5 and *L. casei* LC01—were obtained from Christian Hansen (Hørsolm, Denmark).

Bacteria were delivered as freeze-dried cultures and were handled according to supplier protocol. Briefly, after opening the ampoule, bacteria were rehydrated and then transferred to a tube with sterile liquid De Man, Rogosa, and Sharpe (MRS) agar medium (BioMaxima, Lublin, Poland) and incubated at a temperature optimal for strain. For *L. acidophilus* LA-5 and both *L. casei* strains, the optimal temperature was 37 °C, while, for other *Lactobacillus* species, it was 30 °C.

2.2. Measurement of Optical Density of Bacterial Suspension: Calibration

To tubes containing 5 mL of sterile MRS medium, a volume of 0.1 mL of 24-h liquid bacterial culture was added, the contents were mixed, and the tubes were incubated for 24 h at the optimum temperature for the tested strain. After incubation, bacterial cultures were centrifuged at 194× *g* for 15 min (MPW-35JR centrifuge, MPW MED Instruments, Warsaw, Poland), and the supernatant was discarded. The pellets were rinsed by mixing with 5 mL of sterile distilled water followed by centrifugation (using previous parameters). The resulting pellets were resuspended in sterile water so as to obtain an optical density of the bacterial suspensions equal to McFarland standard 1.0 (using a Den-1B densitometer, Biosan, Latvia). Then, serial 10-fold dilutions were made in sterile water, and 1 mL of subsequent dilution was spread over the surface of the MRS medium (in triplicate). After 72 h of incubation at an optimal temperature, bacterial colonies were counted, mean bacterial cell density in cfu/mL from 3 replicates was calculated for each tested strain, and the relationship between the optical density of McFarland = 1 and bacterial cell density was determined. The relationships obtained for individual strains were as follows (1 McFarland unit equivalent): *L. plantarum*, 1.55×10^8 cfu/mL; *L. brevis*, 4.5×10^7 cfu/mL; *L. lactis* subsp. *lactis*, 1.6×10^8 cfu/mL: *L. casei*, 4.9×10^7 cfu/mL; *L. acidophilus* LA-5, 4.45×10^7 cfu/mL; *L. casei* LC01, 4.8×10^7 cfu/mL. Before each experiment, a 24 h culture of adequate *Lactobacillus* strain was centrifuged, washed in sterile water, and resuspended (as described above). The optical density of the bacterial suspension was adjusted to a value corresponding to 2×10^7 cfu/mL.

2.3. Model Medium for Experiments

All experiments were carried out in carbon- and nitrogen-limiting conditions because model medium composed of 0.45% NaCl (POCh, Gliwice, Poland), and 0.45% bacteriological peptone (BioMaxima, Lublin, Poland) was used. If a solid medium was required, bacteriological agar was added in a final concentration of 2% (BioMaxima, Lublin, Poland). All media were sterilized using a Microjet Microwave Autoclave (process parameters: 135 °C, 80 s, 3.6 bar; Enbio Technology Sp. z o.o., Gdynia, Poland).

2.4. Preparation of Acrylamide "Stock" Solution

Concentrated (20 g/L) aqueous solution of acrylamide (purum, ≥98% (GC) provided by Sigma-Aldrich Sp. z o.o, Poznan, Poland) was sterilized by filtering through a sterile membrane filter (pore $\varphi = 0.22$ μm; PES Millex-GP, Bionovo, Poland) and diluted (if needed) with sterile distilled water to obtain "stock" solutions of acrylamide (concentrations: 0.5, 1.0, 2.0, 5.0, 10.0, and 20.0 g/L).

2.5. Preliminary Assessment of Acrylamide Impact on Lactobacillus Growth

The impact of acrylamide on *Lactobacillus* was assessed by evaluating visible bacterial growth on the solid model medium containing acrylamide at various concentrations: 10, 50, 100, 250, 500, and 1000 μg/mL. Serial 10-fold dilutions of the suspension of tested bacteria (2×10^7 cfu/mL) were made in sterile water. Then, a volume of 1 mL of acrylamide "stock" solution of adequate concentration was added to 18 mL of sterile, cooled, but still, liquid, model medium and poured into a sterile Petri plate containing 1 mL of the diluted bacterial suspension. Positive controls were Petri plates with 19 mL of the model medium (without acrylamide) mixed with 1 mL of a diluted suspension of tested bacteria. After media solidification, all plates were incubated for 72 h at a proper temperature optimal for the tested strain, and then the bacterial growth was assessed according to the following scale:

++++   very intense growth (colonies cover the whole surface, creating lawn plates)
+++   intense growth (too many colonies to count, but they are distinguishable)
++   good growth (30–300 colonies/plate)
+   only a few colonies (<30 colonies/plate)
−   no growth

First, the growth of bacteria on plates with positive control was evaluated, and the dilution of bacterial suspension with good growth (30–300 colonies/plate) was chosen. For the same dilution, growth in the presence of AA was assessed. The experiment was performed in 5 replicates.

2.6. Determination of Cell Concentration and Viability by Flow Cytometry

The *Lactobacillus* strains whose growth was influenced by acrylamide in the preliminary analysis were chosen for this stage of the experiment. A volume of 1 mL of bacterial suspension (containing

2×10^7 cfu/mL) was inoculated into 19 mL of liquid model medium, with the addition of acrylamide to a final concentration of 7.5, 15, 30, or 100 µg/mL, and incubated for 48 h. The final bacterial cell density was 10^6 cells/mL, which corresponded to the average number of LAB cells found in fermented milk drinks (FAO/WHO Food Standards). The proposed AA concentrations were selected based on the literature [42,46], and the 100 µg/mL concentration is higher than the possible level reached in the human gastrointestinal tract or in food products. The positive control was medium with 1 mL of sterile distilled water added instead of an acrylamide "stock" solution (marked as 0 µg/mL). Immediately after adding bacteria to the medium (marked as 0 h, but taking into account staining times and cytometric measurement, the analysis was actually done about 2 h after adding the bacteria), after 24 h and 48 h of incubation at an optimal temperature, the cell concentration (cell/mL) was evaluated by flow cytometry (BD Accuri™ C6 Flow cytometer, BD Biosciences, Bio-Rad, Poland) equipped with fluorescence detectors FL1 533/30, FL2 585/40, FL3 670LP. For this purpose, the commercially available BD™ Cell Viability Kit with BD Liquid Counting Beads (cat. # 349480, Becton, Dickinson and Company, BD Biosciences, San Jose, CA, USA) was used. According to the protocol, cells were stained with provided dyes, and cytometric analysis was conducted using the following parameters: fluidic flow rate 14 µL/min, the threshold set at 10,000 on (Forward Scatter-Height), sample volume set at 10 µL. The bacterial cells and counting beads were gated based on (Side Scatter) parameters and FL2, while the populations of alive, injured, and dead bacteria were discriminated based on an FL1 (thiazole orange) vs. FL3 (propidium iodide) plot. In live cells, the membrane is intact and impermeable to dyes, such as propidium iodide (PI), while when cells are injured or dead, the propidium iodide can leak into the cells because of their compromised membranes. PI is a nucleic acid intercalator, so it stains nucleic acids. On the other side, thiazole orange is a permeant dye that also reacts with nucleic acids but enters all cells—alive, injured, and dead, to varying degrees. Therefore, it will stain all cells containing nucleic acids. Thus a combination of these two dyes provides a rapid and reliable method for discriminating live, injured, and dead bacteria. To determine the concentrations of cell populations (expressed as cell/mL), Equation (1) was used:

$$\frac{\text{\# of events in cell region}}{\text{\# of events in bead region}} \times \frac{\text{\# of beads per test}^*}{\text{test volume}} \times \text{dilution factor} = \text{concentration of cell population} \quad (1)$$

* This value was found on the vial of BD Liquid Counting Beads and could vary from lot to lot.

In the case of *Lactobacillus plantarum*, changes in cell morphology under the influence of acrylamide were noted, which manifested in the form of cells with twice or several times stronger FL1 signal. Analysis of microscopic preparations stained by the Gram method confirmed that they were *Lactobacillus plantarum* cells appearing individually (bacillus), in pairs (diplobacillus), or in the form of chains (streptobacillus).

2.7. Statistical Analysis

All experiments were carried out in 5 replicates, and results are expressed as mean ± standard deviation (SD). When the impact of acrylamide on bacterial cell number was assessed, one-way analysis of variance (ANOVA) with Tukey's honest significant difference (HSD) posthoc test was used to compare mean values and determine the significance of differences. The Brown–Forsythe test was used to verify the hypothesis of homogeneity of variances, while Shapiro–Wilk test was used to test the normality of distribution. A p-value < 0.05 was considered statistically significant. This part of statistical analysis was carried out in Dell Statistica (Data Analysis Software System, version 13, 2016, software.dell.com). Two-way ANOVA in a mixed model was used to assess data from flow cytometry, which means the interrelationship of two independent variables (incubation times and acrylamide concentrations) with a dependent variable (% of particular cell types), using IBM SPSS Statistics for Windows (2017, Version 25.0; IBM Corp., Armonk, NY, USA). Bonferroni posthoc test was used, and the differences were considered significant when p-value < 0.05.

3. Results

3.1. Impact of Acrylamide on LAB Growth on Solid Medium

The model medium used for experiments was low nitrogen and low carbon; therefore, the growth of *Lactobacillus* was significantly limited compared to the MRS medium. Acrylamide added to such medium did not show bactericidal or bacteriostatic activity against tested bacteria from the *Lactobacillus* genus even in very big concentrations, not reported in food (Table 1).

Table 1. Impact of acrylamide on the growth of *Lactobacillus* strains on solid medium.

Bacteria Strain	AA Concentration (µg/mL)	Growth Evaluation (Mean of 5 Replicates)
Lactobacillus plantarum	Control	++
	10	++
	50	++
	100	++
	250	++
	500	++
	1000	+++
Lactobacillus brevis	Control	++
	10	++
	50	++
	100	++
	250	++
	500	+++
	1000	+++
Lactobacillus lactis sp. *lactis*	Control	++
	10	++
	50	++
	100	++
	250	++
	500	+++
	1000	+++
Lactobacillus casei	Control	++
	10	++
	50	++
	100	++
	250	++
	500	++
	1000	++

Table 1. *Cont.*

Bacteria Strain	AA Concentration (µg/mL)	Growth Evaluation (Mean of 5 Replicates)
Lactobacillus acidophilus LA-5	Control	++
	10	++
	50	++
	100	++
	250	++
	500	++
	1000	+++
Lactobacillus casei LC-01	Control	++
	10	++
	50	++
	100	++
	250	++
	500	++
	1000	++

Scale: ++++ very intense growth (colonies cover whole surface creating lawn plates); +++ intense growth (too many colonies to count, but they are distinguishable); ++ good growth (30–300 colonies/plate); + only a few colonies (<30 colonies/plate); − no growth. AA, acrylamide.

Moreover, it was surprising that AA could stimulate the growth of *L. plantarum* and probiotic strain *L. acidophilus* LA-5 at a concentration of 1000 µg/mL, while *L. brevis* and *L. lactis* sp. *lactis* growth was more intense compared to control in the presence of 500 µg and 1000 µg of acrylamide per mL. The acrylamide concentration used in that part of the study was much higher than that detected in food. The concentrations of acrylamide reported in the literature vary from <10 to even 80,920 µg/kg, with the highest levels in potato chips, French fries, roasted coffee, and coffee extract [44,47–50]. Considering the quantities of particular foodstuffs we consume each day, it has been estimated that total AA uptake varies from 0.3 to 1.4 µg per kg body weight per day [48], depending on the age group (high consumption of coffee in adults) and eating habits. In particular cases, it can reach up to 5 µg/kg/day [5].

The obtained results suggested that some lactic acid bacteria probably could utilize acrylamide as a source of carbon and nitrogen if they lack in the environment (medium). The possibility of acrylamide degradation (not binding) by LAB has been suggested by the results of a study conducted on rats fed with acrylamide 3 h after consumption of four species of *Bifidobacterium*. A significant reduction in the degree of liver damage [51] has been observed. Other studies have demonstrated that in portions of potatoes prepared for French fries subjected to 15 min of fermentation before frying, the AA level is reduced by 90% [52]. However, these results only confirm that lactic acid bacteria can utilize substances that are precursors of acrylamide for their own use; the possibility of AA degradation by LAB has not been studied.

Another strategy to reduce acrylamide formation in bread was proposed by Nachi et al. [53] by using selected lactic acid bacteria strains for dough fermentation. When the LAB was used to inoculate sourdough, the acrylamide concentration in the bread was reduced. This was due to the lower pH of the LAB-inoculated sourdough after fermentation for 16 h compared to the spontaneous sourdough (using only baker's yeast). The acidification was accompanied by a significant increase in the concentration of reducing sugars, which were then used as electron acceptors by LAB and reduced to mannitol. The lack of sugar and low pH prevented the Maillard reaction. The most pronounced reduction of acrylamide formation (by 84.7%) was obtained in bread made with *Pediococcus acidilactici* strain S16.

3.2. Impact of AA on Lactic Acid Bacteria Concentration in Medium

Three LAB strains were chosen for further experiments: *L. brevis*, *L. plantarum*, and probiotic strain *L. acidophilus* LA-5. The bacteria concentration was measured by flow cytometry immediately and after 24 h and 48 h of acrylamide addition at various concentrations (Figure 1). The number of bacteria cells in the medium was determined according to Equation (1) using the number of events in the bacteria and bead regions and expressed as cell number per 1 mL.

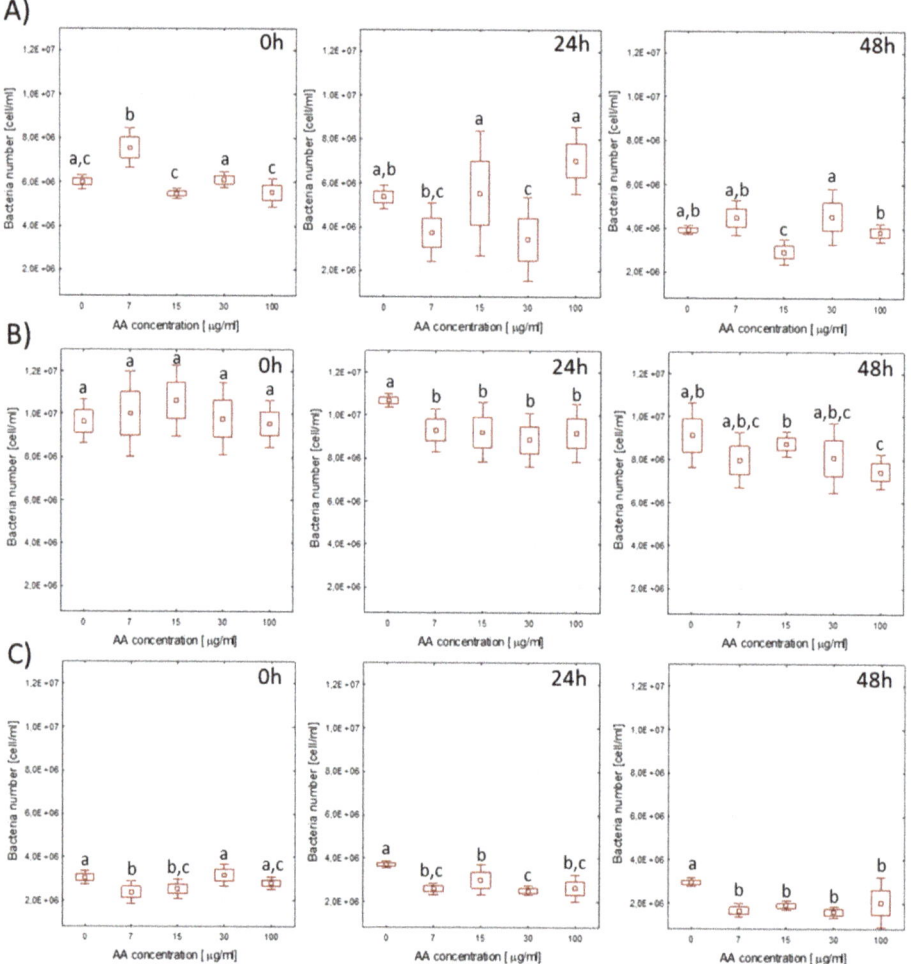

Figure 1. Impact of acrylamide (AA) concentration in medium (0, 7.5, 15, 30, and 100 µg/mL) on bacterial cell number in culture (cells/mL) determined by cytometric method immediately after AA addition and after 24 h and 48 h incubation. (**A**) *L. acidophilus* LA-5, (**B**) *L. brevis*, (**C**) *L. plantarum*. Values in graphs with different letters differ from each other at the level of $p < 0.05$ (Tukey's HSD test).

Already at 0 h, some influence of AA on the number of bacteria in the limiting medium could be seen. It should be recalled that preparing cells for cytometric analysis takes about 2 h from the addition of AA to the medium, so the bacteria have time to change their metabolism and can already start using AA as a source of carbon or nitrogen. The presence of AA in the medium resulted in a decrease in *L. brevis* number after 24 h and 48 h incubation, but not significantly correlated with the AA concentration used (Figure 1B). For *L. acidophilus* LA-5, differences in population size compared to controls and between AA doses were not statistically significant (Figure 1A). The initial increase in cell number in the sample with 7.5 μg AA might have resulted from the use of small amounts of AA, but the concentration was too low to guarantee adequate conditions for bacterial growth and multiplication over a longer period of time. After 24 h, very large fluctuations in culture were reported, but after 48 h, the observed differences were not statistically significant, except for incubation in the presence of 15 μg/mL AA, when LA-5 was lower than in other samples.

These results suggested that *L. acidophilus* LA-5 was sensitive to AA because of decreased cell numbers, which would be consistent with the results of studies on other bacteria. However, these studies have used a medium-low in nitrogen and carbon, and not, as in most other studies, an optimal medium for LAB growth. Therefore, the LAB number also decreased in the medium without the addition of AA. This environment is, therefore, ideal for assessing the impact of AA in the absence of other, more absorbable sources of carbon and nitrogen. In milk, lactic acid bacteria use casein as a source of amino acids, thanks to having appropriate proteolytic enzymes [54]. Gene encoding the cell-wall bound proteinase (PrtP) is only found on the chromosome of *L. acidophilus*; neither *L. plantarum* nor *L. brevis* [55] has it. Also, some peptidases are unique to individual species. The presence of these enzymes, however, is important primarily in the environment typical for these microorganisms (milk) and affects the rate of multiplication of individual bacteria due to various assimilation possibilities of proteins available in the environment, as well as the final effect of the fermentation process, including the resulting secondary metabolites.

In the medium used in this experiment, the only source of carbon and nitrogen was 0.45% of peptone obtained as enzymatic meat tissue hydrolysate, while, in MRS, usually about 2.5% of nitrogen compounds and 2% glucose are present. Furthermore, *L. acidophilus* and *L. brevis* possess all three known LAB peptide transport systems: the di/tripeptide Dpp and DtpT systems and the oligopeptide Opp system [55]. LAB are auxotrophs relative to amino acids, and, depending on the species, they can synthesize only a few amino acids, while the others must be provided with the medium. This means that a medium-low in protein and amino acids will quickly become a factor that limits bacterial growth because bacterial growth and multiplication require the assimilation of substrates to supply the cell with the necessary energy, carbon, and nitrogen to build new structures. That is why the ability to degrade acrylamide to be used as a source of nitrogen (released by NH_4^+ amidase) and carbon was so important in this experiment.

It should be recalled that in this part of the study, all cells were counted: those that were alive and able to function properly and further divide, those that were damaged and whose metabolism was temporarily switched to repair the damage, and dead cells that had not yet broken down.

The situation differed in the case of *L. plantarum* (Figure 1C). After 24 h in the control medium without AA, an increase in the number of bacteria was observed; however, by analyzing their morphology, it was clear that this correlated with the grouping type in which these cells occurred. In the initial population (0 h), 92.55 ± 0.08% of cells appeared as single bacilli and 7.41 ± 0.08% as diplobacilli, while no streptobacilli were observed. After 24 h, the number of cells in culture without AA increased slightly; however, this was mainly due to the fact that the diplobacilli split into single cells. A lack of division meant that after another 24 h, 99% of the population were single rods, and their numbers significantly decreased compared to the initial value.

3.3. Acrylamide Impact on LAB Viability

Cell concentration and viability were measured by flow cytometry immediately and 24 h and 48 h after acrylamide addition at various concentrations. Populations of dead, injured, and alive bacteria were discriminated based on fluorescence signal after staining with thiazole orange (FL1) and propidium iodide (FL2) provided in the assay. The concentrations of various cell populations were determined using counting beads.

First, it was checked whether incubation time, regardless of acrylamide concentration, had a significant impact on the percentages of specific cell types (main effect of incubation time). All tested main effects of incubation time were statistically significant, except for dead cells of *Lactobacillus brevis* (Table 2). The viability of *L. brevis* increased after AA addition, while the percentage of injured cells was significantly diminished. Contrary to that was the viability of *Lactobacillus acidophilus* LA-5. The highest percentage of live cells was at the beginning of the experiment, while the lowest was after 24 h. Tracking changes in the percentage of injured cells, it appeared that some were repaired, and after 48 h, they were considered to be fully viable. Moreover, some dead cells underwent autolysis, and the cell content released in the medium was utilized by survivors. Lactic acid bacteria are characterized by differentiated autolytic activity, but the process allows them to eliminate weak or impaired cells from the population [56]. In the mentioned study, *L. plantarum* strains were autolyzed more than other LAB strains; however, the authors did not test the autolytic activity of *L. brevis* or *L. acidophilus* [56]. It is well known that some lactic acid bacteria can undergo enzymatic cleavage of cell wall peptidoglycans by peptidoglycan hydrolases present in the bacterial cells and that the autolysis depends on factors, such as carbon source, temperature, osmotic concentration, and pH [56]. It has also been demonstrated that N-acetylmuramidase has a critical function in *Lactobacillus bulgaricus* autolysis [57] as one of the major degraders of the cell wall.

Table 2. The main effect of incubation time: impact of time on percentage of specific cell types, regardless of AA concentration.

Bacteria Strain	% of Cells	Time			F	p
		0 h	24 h	48 h		
Lactobacillus acidophilus LA-5	alive	99.6 ± 0.35 [a]	91.92 ± 2.08 [b]	93.04 ± 3.43 [c]	761.35	<0.001
	injured	0.39 ± 0.35 [a]	6.60 ± 1.85 [b]	5.34 ± 2.57 [c]	937.62	<0.001
	dead	0.02 ± 0.02 [a]	1.48 ± 0.48 [b]	1.63 ± 0.93 [b]	183.83	<0.001
Lactobacillus brevis	alive	98.76 ± 0.27 [a]	99.51 ± 0.25 [b]	99.54 ± 0.10 [b]	107.44	<0.001
	injured	0.89 ± 0.26 [a]	0.16 ± 0.06 [b]	0.14 ± 0.03 [b]	227.62	<0.001
	dead	0.35 ± 0.03	0.33 ± 0.20	0.32 ± 0.08	0.47	0.630
Lactobacillus plantarum	alive	97.42 ± 0.51 [a]	97.62 ± 0.89 [a]	95.09 ± 1.23 [b]	143.33	<0.001
	injured	1.00 ± 0.17 [a]	1.20 ± 0.36 [a]	3.70 ± 1.33 [c]	851.52	<0.001
	dead	1.58 ± 0.43 [a]	1.18 ± 0.62 [b]	1.21 ± 0.61 [b]	7.59	0.002
Morphology Lactobacillus plantarum	bacillus	95.09 ± 2.35 [a]	98.15 ± 0.50 [b]	73.46 ± 15.96 [c]	3358.82	<0.001
	diplobacillus	4.91 ± 2.35 [a]	1.77 ± 0.50 [b]	24.03 ± 13.47 [c]	2909.62	<0.001
	streptobacillus	0 ± 0.01 [a]	0.08 ± 0.02 [b]	2.52 ± 3.18 [c]	1078.97	<0.001

a, b, c—Means indicated with different letters differ from each other at the level of $p < 0.05$ (Bonferroni test). Values given are mean ± SD of the percentage of cells of a certain type.

In our experiment, the percentage of live *L. plantarum* cells was significantly lower after 48 h than at the beginning or after 24 h. Moreover, significant differences in *L. plantarum* morphology were observed. After 48 h of incubation in the presence of acrylamide, fewer cells were present in the form of single bacilli, while the amounts of diplobacilli and streptobacilli were significantly increased (Table 2 and Figure 2). Such an effect was not observed in other LAB strains.

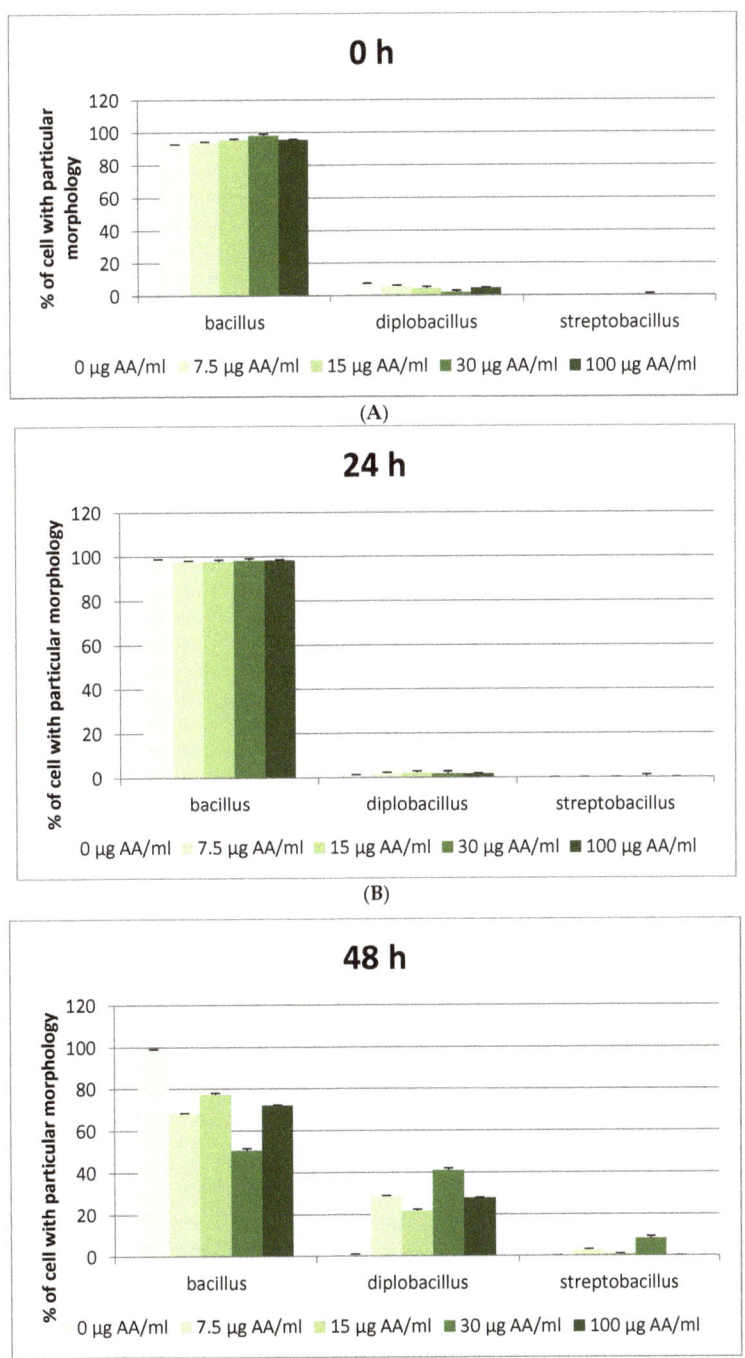

Figure 2. Impact of acrylamide concentration on the morphology of *Lactobacillus plantarum*. (**A**) 0 h, (**B**) 24 h, (**C**) 48 h.

Then, it was tested whether the acrylamide concentration, regardless of the time of incubation, had a significant effect on the percentage of specific cell types (alive, injured, dead) or *L. plantarum* morphology (main effect of acrylamide concentration). The ANOVA results are presented in Table 3 and posthoc tests in Table 4.

Table 3. The main effect of acrylamide concentration: influence of acrylamide concentration on the percentage of occurrence of certain cell types (expressed as arithmetic mean (SD)), regardless of the incubation time.

Bacteria Strain	% of Cells	Acrylamide Concentration (µg/mL)					F	p
		0	7.5	15	30	100		
Lactobacillus acidophilus LA-5	alive	93.86 (0.34) [a]	94.79 (0.68) [a]	93.48 (0.93) [a]	97.18 (0.10) [b]	94.95 (0.43) [a]	31.67	<0.001
	injured	5.02 (0.27) [a]	4.34 (0.54) [a]	4.99 (0.57) [a]	2.11 (0.03) [b]	4.07 (0.44) [b]	39.50	<0.001
	dead	1.12 (0.07) [a]	0.86 (0.23) [a]	1.54 (0.44) [a]	0.71 (0.09) [a]	0.97 (0.06) [a]	9.62	<0.001
Lactobacillus brevis	alive	99.15 (0.02)	99.33 (0.04)	99.30 (0.16)	99.23 (0.19)	99.33 (0.04)	2.43	0.081
	injured	0.47 (0.01)	0.34 (0.03)	0.34 (0.03)	0.46 (0.18)	0.38 (0.01)	2.79	0.054
	dead	0.39 (0.01)	0.32 (0.03)	0.36 (0.13)	0.31 (0.02)	0.28 (0.04)	2.12	0.115
Lactobacillus plantarum	alive	97.81 (0.08) [a]	96.76 (0.18) [b]	95.84 (0.57) [c]	96.51 (0.28) [b]	96.64 (0.42) [b]	19.95	<0.001
	injured	1.14 (0.04) [a]	1.92 (0.09) [b]	2.71 (0.17) [c]	2.33 (0.13) [d]	1.72 (0.19) [b]	98.90	<0.001
	dead	1.05 (0.06) [a]	1.32 (0.15) [a]	1.45 (0.42) [a]	1.16 (0.18) [a]	1.64 (0.26) [b]	4.50	0.009
Morphology *Lactobacillus plantarum*	bacillus	96.77 (1.03) [a]	86.73 (0.51) [b]	90.17 (0.29) [c]	82.25 (0.38) [d]	88.57 (0.71) [b]	341.41	<0.001
	diplobacillus	3.17 (1.03) [a]	12.21 (0.39)	9.51 (0.28)	14.95 (0.25)	11.36 (0.7) [a]	263.77	<0.001
	streptobacillus	0.06 (0.01) [a]	1.06 (0.13) [b]	0.33 (0.04) [c]	2.80 (0.24) [d]	0.08 (0.01) [a]	420.58	<0.001

a, b, c—Means with different letters differ from each other at the level of $p < 0.05$ (Bonferroni test).

The analysis showed that the main effect of acrylamide concentration did not occur in the *L. brevis* strain, which meant that in this case, acrylamide (regardless of the incubation time) had no effect on their viability. The AA impact was observed in other tested strains and when the morphology of *L. plantarum* was taken into account. Posthoc analysis showed that acrylamide significantly increased the percentage of alive cells of *L. acidophilus* LA-5 strain, but this was only observed at a concentration of 30 µg/mL and was accompanied by a significant decrease in the number (percentage) of injured cells. In the *L. plantarum* strain, acrylamide at each concentration significantly reduced viability while also significantly increasing the number of injured cells. In addition, morphological examination of *L. plantarum* showed a decrease in the proportion of single cells (bacilli), mainly in favor of increasing their frequency in pairs (diplobacilli). The number of cells in the form of chains (streptobacillus) also increased, but to a lesser extent.

Finally, the interaction effects (simultaneous impact) of incubation time and acrylamide concentration were tested. Acrylamide significantly increased the viability of *L. acidophilus* LA-5 cells at a concentration of 30 µg/mL after 24 h incubation and at 0, 30, and 100 µg/mL after 48 h, when compared to the model medium without acrylamide (Table 5). The increase in alive cells was mainly accompanied by a reduction in injured cells, rather than dead ones. In turn, the viability of *L. acidophilus* LA-5 decreased at an acrylamide concentration of 15 µg/mL after 48 h.

Table 4. The main effect of acrylamide concentration: posthoc Bonferroni test.

Bacteria Strain	AA Concentration (µg/mL)	% of Cells *					
		Alive/Bacillus		Injured/Diplobacillus		Dead/Streptobacillus	
		Difference between Means	p	Difference between Means	p	Difference between Means	p
Lactobacillus acidophilus LA-5	0 vs. 7.5	−0.93	0.182	0.68	0.197	0.26	0.898
	0 vs. 15	0.38	1.000	0.03	1.000	−0.42	0.093
	0 vs. 30	−3.32	<0.001	2.91	<0.001	0.42	0.093
	0 vs. 100	−1.10	0.067	0.95	0.020	0.15	1.000
Lactobacillus brevis	0 vs. 7.5	−0.19	0.187	0.12	0.332	0.06	1.000
	0 vs. 15	−0.16	0.460	0.13	0.223	0.02	1.000
	0 vs. 30	−0.09	1.000	0.01	1.000	0.08	0.724
	0 vs. 100	−0.19	0.180	0.08	1.000	0.10	0.197
Lactobacillus plantarum	0 vs. 7.5	1.05	0.002	−0.78	<0.001	−0.27	1.000
	0 vs. 15	1.97	<0.001	−1.57	<0.001	−0.40	0.186
	0 vs. 30	1.30	<0.001	−1.19	<0.001	−0.11	1.000
	0 vs. 100	1.17	<0.001	−0.58	<0.001	−0.59	0.012
morphology *Lactobacillus plantarum*	0 vs. 7.5	10.04	<0.001	−9.05	<0.001	−1.00	<0.001
	0 vs. 15	6.60	<0.001	−6.34	<0.001	−0.27	0.034
	0 vs. 30	14.52	<0.001	−11.78	<0.001	−2.74	<0.001
	0 vs. 100	8.20	<0.001	−8.19	<0.001	−0.01	1.000

* In a morphological study, percentages of bacillus, diplobacillus, and streptobacillus cells were compared.

Table 5. The interaction effect of incubation time and concentration of acrylamide on the viability of *Lactobacillus acidophilus* LA-5 (Bonferroni test).

Incubation Time (h)	AA Concentration (µg/mL)	% of Cells					
		Alive		Injured		Dead	
		Difference between Means	p	Difference between Means	p	Difference between Means	p
0	0 vs. 7.5	−0.10	<0.001	0.08	0.001	0.02	1.000
	0 vs. 15	0.01	1.000	−0.02	1.000	0.01	1.000
	0 vs. 30	−0.02	0.334	0.01	1.000	0.01	1.000
	0 vs. 100	0.83	<0.001	−0.83	<0.001	0	1.000
24	0 vs. 7.5	0.58	1.000	−0.38	1.000	−0.20	1.000
	0 vs. 15	−2.15	0.149	2.23	0.015	−0.08	1.000
	0 vs. 30	−3.89	0.001	3.83	<0.001	0.06	1.000
	0 vs. 100	0.02	1.000	0.27	1.000	−0.29	1.000
48	0 vs. 7.5	−3.28	<0.001	2.33	<0.001	0.96	0.003
	0 vs. 15	3.29	<0.001	−2.12	<0.001	−1.17	<0.001
	0 vs. 30	−6.06	<0.001	4.88	<0.001	1.18	<0.001
	0 vs. 100	−4.13	<0.001	3.40	<0.001	0.73	0.029

In the case of *Lactobacillus brevis*, acrylamide at each concentration decreased the percentage of injured cells after 24 h and 48 h incubation (compared to control), although a statistically significant reduction in the percentage of alive bacteria was observed only after 48 h at 100 µg/mL (Table 6). All other changes were not statistically significant.

Table 6. The interaction effect of incubation time and concentration of acrylamide on the viability of *Lactobacillus brevis* (Bonferroni test).

Incubation Time (h)	AA Concentration (µg/mL)	% of Cells					
		Alive		Injured		Dead	
		Difference between Means	p	Difference between Means	p	Difference between Means	p
0	0 vs. 7.5	−0.11	1.000	0.15	1.000	−0.04	0.365
	0 vs. 15	−0.20	1.000	0.21	1.000	−0.01	1.000
	0 vs. 30	0.19	1.000	−0.15	1.000	−0.04	0.561
	0 vs. 100	−0.06	1.000	0.06	1.000	0.00	1.000
24	0 vs. 7.5	−0.32	0.435	0.15	<0.001	0.16	1.000
	0 vs. 15	−0.17	1.000	0.12	0.001	0.05	1.000
	0 vs. 30	−0.29	0.633	0.12	0.001	0.17	1.000
	0 vs. 100	−0.33	0.401	0.13	<0.001	0.20	1.000
48	0 vs. 7.5	−0.13	0.352	0.06	0.004	0.06	1.000
	0 vs. 15	−0.10	1.000	0.06	0.001	0.03	1.000
	0 vs. 30	−0.15	0.121	0.05	0.015	0.10	0.540
	0 vs. 100	−0.18	0.046	0.06	0.004	0.12	0.277

After 24 h and 48 h of incubation in the presence of acrylamide at concentrations higher than 7.5 µg/mL, reduced viability of *L. plantarum* cells was observed, while the number of injured cells increased compared with medium without acrylamide (Table 7).

Table 7. The interaction effect of incubation time and concentration of acrylamide on the viability of *Lactobacillus plantarum* (Bonferroni test).

Incubation Time (h)	AA Concentration (µg/mL)	% of Cells					
		Alive		Injured		Dead	
		Difference between Means	p	Difference between Means	p	Difference between Means	p
0	0 vs. 7.5	1.01	0.009	−0.09	1.000	−0.92	0.002
	0 vs. 15	0.75	0.098	−0.21	0.373	−0.53	0.149
	0 vs. 30	0.44	1.000	−0.04	1.000	−0.39	0.648
	0 vs. 100	0.48	0.789	−0.26	0.115	−0.22	1.000
24	0 vs. 7.5	1.00	0.153	−0.55	0.001	−0.45	1.000
	0 vs. 15	2.08	<0.001	−0.88	<0.001	−1.20	0.007
	0 vs. 30	1.46	0.010	−0.77	<0.001	−0.69	0.311
	0 vs. 100	1.44	0.011	−0.37	0.049	−1.07	0.019
48	0 vs. 7.5	1.12	0.260	−1.70	<0.001	0.57	0.481
	0 vs. 15	3.07	<0.001	−3.61	<0.001	0.53	0.652
	0 vs. 30	2.00	0.004	−2.76	<0.001	0.76	0.115
	0 vs. 100	1.58	0.028	−1.10	0.001	−0.48	0.911

We observed that the morphology of one of the tested bacteria, *Lactobacillus plantarum*, was significantly influenced by acrylamide. Based on the fact that cells with both twofold and several times stronger FL1 fluorescence signal (thiazole orange) appeared in the population, we concluded that acrylamide did not inhibit or even stimulate the division of *L. plantarum* but blocked cell separation; hence bacteria in the form of diplobacilli and streptobacilli were present in the population. This conclusion was confirmed by microscopic preparations. A statistically significant reduction in the number of single rods (bacilli) in the presence of AA in amounts of 7.5 and 15 µg/mL after 24 h incubation and in all AA concentrations after 48 h was demonstrated compared to the medium without acrylamide. This was mainly accompanied by a significant increase in the number of cells found in pairs (diplobacilli) and to a much lower extent in chains (streptobacilli). For each analyzed concentration of AA, this increase was especially significant after 48 h, reaching even ~50% at 30 µg/mL (Table 8).

Table 8. The interaction effect of incubation time and concentration of acrylamide on the morphology of *Lactobacillus plantarum* (Bonferroni test).

Incubation Time (h)	AA Concentration (µg/mL)	% of Cells					
		Bacillus		Diplobacillus		Streptobacillus	
		Difference between Means	p	Difference between Means	p	Difference between Means	p
0	0 vs. 7.5	−1.51	1.000	1.52	1.000	0	1.000
	0 vs. 15	−2.77	0.140	2.77	0.140	0	1.000
	0 vs. 30	−5.42	<0.001	5.42	<0.001	0	1.000
	0 vs. 100	−2.82	0.127	2.81	0.127	0	1.000
24	0 vs. 7.5	0.87	0.024	−0.86	0.023	−0.01	1.000
	0 vs. 15	0.98	0.008	−0.98	0.007	0	1.000
	0 vs. 30	0.59	0.280	−0.57	0.313	−0.02	0.417
	0 vs. 100	0.48	0.692	−0.45	0.791	−0.02	0.598
48	0 vs. 7.5	30.77	<0.001	−27.80	<0.001	−2.98	<0.001
	0 vs. 15	21.60	<0.001	−20.81	<0.001	−0.80	0.033
	0 vs. 30	48.37	<0.001	−40.18	<0.001	−8.19	<0.001
	0 vs. 100	26.95	<0.001	−26.93	<0.001	−0.01	1.000

4. Discussion

In this study, we demonstrated that the tested lactic acid bacteria strains were tolerant of acrylamide even at high concentrations (up to 1 g/mL). Moreover, the growth of *Lactobacillus plantarum*, *L. lactis* sp. *Lactis*, and *L. brevis*, as well as probiotic strain *L. acidophilus* LA-5, was more intense in the presence of acrylamide at high concentration than in medium with limited accessibility of carbon and nitrogen compounds. The obtained results suggested that: (1) acrylamide had no toxic impact on LAB; (2) some lactic acid bacteria probably could utilize acrylamide as a source of carbon and nitrogen if they lack in the environment/medium. Of course, fermented milk beverages and the human gut cannot be considered nutrient-poor environments, as the availability of easily digestible food for bacteria is large, but the possibility of using acrylamide by lactic acid bacteria might be beneficial for both bacteria and the human intestine where the LAB reside.

Our results proved that acrylamide not only influenced the number of lactic acid bacteria but also their viability. The impact of acrylamide on LAB viability depended on both the AA concentration and the bacteria species. First of all, when the impact of incubation time on bacterial viability was analyzed, all the main effects were statistically significant, except the percentage of dead cells of *Lactobacillus brevis*. Secondly, the main effect of acrylamide concentration on the percentage of alive, injured, and dead cells was not observed only in *L. brevis*. This suggested that *L. brevis* was less sensitive to acrylamide among the tested bacteria strains, and it was confirmed in the further analysis as almost all observed differences were not statistically significant.

The posthoc tests showed that acrylamide caused a significant increase in the percentage of alive cells of probiotic strain *L. acidophilus* LA-5 at an AA concentration of 30 µg/mL compared to the cultures without AA. This increase was mainly accompanied by a reduction in the number of injured cells rather than dead ones. On the other side, acrylamide reduced the viability of *L. plantarum* cells after 24 h and 48 h incubation at each AA concentration except 7.5 µg/mL, simultaneously increasing the amount of injured cells. Moreover, we observed a strong influence of acrylamide (especially at a concentration of 30 µg/mL) on the morphology of bacteria only in *L. plantarum*. Based on the fact that cells with both twofold and several times stronger FL1 fluorescence signal (thiazole orange) appeared in the population, we concluded that acrylamide had no impact on the division of *L. plantarum*, but at the same time, it inhibited cell separation, as cells in the form of diplobacilli and streptobacilli were present in the population (confirmed in microscopic preparations). This suggested that in this case, acrylamide could have a harmful or even mutagenic impact on *L. plantarum*.

It is known that many proteins and hydrolytic enzymes are involved in the proper growth and division of bacteria. Various enzymes participate in turnover (remodeling) of peptidoglycan, and their proper activity and specificity are critical, as bacterial division requires both localized hydrolysis and de novo biosynthesis of the peptidoglycan layer. For example, amidase and glucosaminidase displaying murein hydrolase activity are necessary for the generation of the equatorial ring on the staphylococcal cell surface and complete cell division and separation [58]. *Escherichia coli* division requires the activity of amidases—AmiA, AmiB, and AmiC [59]. It is important that muralytic enzymes distinguish elements of peptidoglycan of specific species. Generally, these enzymes are secreted into the surrounding medium, so they need to distinguish between the cell walls of other species and their own. It seems likely that the targeting mechanisms of murein hydrolases employ species-specific receptors for either physiological cell-wall turnover or the bacteriolytic killing of competing microorganisms [58,60,61]. Most Gram-positive bacteria contain a structurally similar peptidoglycan layer [62]. Thus, targeting of muralytic enzymes cannot be achieved by simple enzyme-substrate interactions but requires specific surface receptors [63]. For example, choline within teichoic acid moieties serves as a receptor for the LytA enzyme of *Streptococcus pneumoniae* [64]. A mutant of *S. pneumoniae* showing complete deletion in the lytA gene coding for N-acetylmuramyl-L-alanine amidase has been isolated. It shows a normal growth rate, and the most remarkable biological consequences of the absence of amidase are the formation of short chains (six to eight cells) and the absence of lysis in the stationary phase of growth. In our study, *L. plantarum* morphology changed in the presence of acrylamide, and bacteria started to form diplobacilli and streptobacilli. It is possible that acrylamide reacted with the active site of muralytic amidases and, therefore, blocked cell separation during division.

Different influence of AA on *Lactobacillus* species tested in the study could also be caused by the diversity of their teichoic acid (TA) structure. Teichoic acids in lactic acid bacteria consist of poly(ribitol phosphate) polymers with attached glucose, D-alanine, and/or glycerol molecules, among others [43]. Their structure is highly variable; thus, even closely related strains can differ in their ability to bind toxins. This is coincident with our results, showing that *L. brevis* was less and *L. plantarum* most sensitive to acrylamide among tested LAB strains. Serrano-Nino et al. [43] proved a significant correlation between the binding percentage of acrylamide and the content of some constituents of cell wall TAs. They proposed that H-bonds could occur between the carbonyl oxygen and the amino group (NH ⋯ OC) between adjacent acrylamide and D-alanine attached to the ribitol. Moreover, the amine group of D-alanine might react with acrylamide units by means of a Michael addition, while hydrogen bonds might also occur between carbonyl (C=O) oxygens of acrylamide and the hydroxyl groups of glucose residue or glycerol phosphate substituents attached to the poly (ribitol phosphate) chain. Moreover, they demonstrated that acrylamide binding to teichoic acids in *Lactobacillus* was irreversible.

The role of teichoic acids in cell division and morphogenesis has been investigated in some bacteria species, and it appears that wall teichoic acids (WTAs) are involved in elongation of bacteria, while lipoteichoic acids (LTAs) participate in the cellular division [65]. By obtaining the mutants of *L. plantarum*, it has been revealed that WTAs are not essential for survival, but they are required for proper cell elongation and cell division [66]. Therefore, the reaction of acrylamide with teichoic acids could impede division and cause that *L. plantarum* remains in the form of chains and diplobacillus.

Studies of Zhang [67] showed that the ability of acrylamide binding also depended on the peptidoglycan structure. The peptidoglycan of *L. plantarum* (strain 1.0065) had the highest affinity for AA binding (87.14%), whereas peptidoglycans of *L. casei* ATCC393 and *L. acidophilus* KLDS1.0307 showed lower affinity (75.50% and 56.75%, respectively). This binding ability of *L. plantarum* positively correlated with the carbohydrate content in peptidoglycan and the contents of four amino acids (alanine, aspartic acid, glutamic acid, and lysine). Additionally, it was demonstrated that C–O (carboxyl, polysaccharides, and arene), C=O amide, and N–H amines groups were involved in the AA binding.

Analyzing the interaction of acrylamide with peptidoglycan, one should take into account the differences in the structure of cell wall stem peptides. The amino acid sequence of stem peptide involved in linking glycan chains in LAB peptidoglycan is L-Ala–D-Glu–X–D-Ala. The third amino acid (X) is a diamino acid, which in LAB usually is L-Lys (e.g., *L. lactis* and most lactobacilli), but can also be meso-diaminopimelic acid (mDAP) (e.g., in *L. plantarum*) or L-ornithine (e.g., in *L. fermentum*) [62]. Peptidoglycan with mDAP is typical for Gram-negative bacteria, and in such cell walls, a direct cross-connection between neighboring stem peptides takes place (the mDAP in position 3 of one peptide chain binds to D-Ala in position 4 of another chain). In lactic acid bacteria with Lys-type peptidoglycan, an additional interpeptide bridge made of one D-amino acid (e.g., D-Asp or D-Asn in *L. lactis, L. casei*, and most lactobacilli) is included [62]. It means that the structure of *L. plantarum* is unusual among LAB peptidoglycans, and it is different from the structure of other tested species. Additionally, this bacterium is characterized by a unique process among bacteria—O-acetylation of peptidoglycan [66]—which has an impact on *L. plantarum* autolysis. O-acetylation of N-acetylglucosamine (GlcNAc) inhibits the N-acetylglucosaminidase Acm2 (which is required for the ultimate step of cell separation of daughter cells), while O-acetylation of N-acetylmuramic acid (MurNAc) has been shown to activate autolysis through the activity of the N-acetylmuramoyl-L-alanine amidase LytH [68]. It is possible that acrylamide interacts with the mentioned enzymes (amidases) and hence influences cell division and separation. In our study, we observed that in the presence of AA, the *L. plantarum* morphology was changed, i.e., the percentage of cells in pairs or chains increased. It is worth mentioning that in *L. plantarum*, almost all the mDAP side chains are amidated. Defects of mDAP amidation in the *L. plantarum* mutant strain strongly affect the growth and cell morphology, causing filamentation and long-chain formation, suggesting that mDAP amidation may play a critical role in controlling the septation process [69]. Further studies are needed to explain whether acrylamide interacts with the amidation of mDAP or the activity of muralytic amidases. It is also possible that the presence of AA in low-carbon and low-nitrogen medium induces the synthesis of other amidases necessary for acrylamide degradation to acrylic acid and ammonia, but also able to cleave the amide bound in mDAP, influencing cell morphology.

The impact of acrylamide on LAB morphology should also be discussed in terms of the importance of bacterial aggregation on their functioning. First of all, bacterial aggregation (auto-aggregation) may facilitate biofilm formation by favoring bacterial attachment to surfaces or other microbes (co-aggregation). It also implicates better survival of LAB in the gut. Some studies indicate that biofilms are a stable point in a biological cycle that includes initiation, maturation, maintenance, and dissolution. According to O'Toole et al. [70], microbe development involves changes in form and function that play prominent roles in the life cycle of the organism, and biofilm formation is a prominent part of the lifestyle of microbes. Moreover, bacteria seem to initiate the development of biofilm in response to specific environmental conditions, such as nutrient availability. It has been proposed that the starvation response pathway can be subsumed as a part of the overall biofilm development cycle [70]. Secondly, when growing in biofilm, organisms become more resistant to higher deliverable levels of antibiotics or other antimicrobial compounds compared to single "suspended" cells [71]. The last matter is that aggregation and co-aggregation among bacteria are important in the prevention of colonization of surfaces by pathogens. It has been proved that some lactic acid bacteria are also able to control biofilm formation by pathogens and can, therefore, prevent the colonization of food-borne pathogens [72]. It is true, for example, for some *Lactobacillus plantarum* strains showing an aggregation phenotype [73].

5. Conclusions

In conclusion, we can assume that the tested strains of lactic acid bacteria found in the human digestive tract or in fermented milk drinks are tolerant to high concentrations of acrylamide (up to 1 g/mL). Some show better growth in medium with AA than in medium with limited carbon and nitrogen sources, suggesting the possibility that they use AA for their own metabolism. Of course, in the digestive tract, especially in the initial sections of the intestine, there is sufficient availability of easily digestible food, but the possibility of using AA is beneficial for both the lactic acid bacteria and the human in whose intestine the LAB resides.

Moreover, we can assume that eating AA-containing products with a properly functioning microbiota will be less harmful to human organs than previously thought. It is also good information for producers of food (e.g., yogurt) with the addition of AA-containing ingredients, such as roasted coffee, almond or nuts, muesli, baked biscuits, or cornflakes because it should not negatively affect the microorganisms necessary for their production.

Author Contributions: Conceptualization, K.P. and A.D.-C.; methodology, K.P., T.T., and A.D.-C.; formal analysis, K.P., T.T., and A.D.-C.; investigation, K.P.; resources, A.D.-C.; writing—original draft preparation, K.P., T.T., and A.D.-C.; writing—review and editing, K.P. and A.D.-C.; visualization, K.P. and T.T.; supervision, A.D.-C.; project administration, A.D.-C.; funding acquisition, A.D.-C. All authors have read and agreed to the published version of the manuscript.

Funding: This research was supported by financial means on science in the years 2017–2020 as the research project 2016/21/B/BN9/01171 funded by the National Science Center (Krakow, Poland).

Conflicts of Interest: The authors declare no conflict of interest.

References

1. IARC. Acrylamide. In *Some Industrial Chemicals. IARC Monographs on Evaluation of Carcinogenic Risks to Humans*; World Health Organization, International Agency for Research on Cancer: Lyon, France, 1994; Volume 60, pp. 389–433.
2. Duda-Chodak, A.; Wajda, Ł.; Tarko, T.; Sroka, P.; Satora, P. A review of the interactions between acrylamide, microorganisms and food components. *Food Funct.* **2016**, *7*, 1282–1295. [CrossRef] [PubMed]
3. Shipp, A.; Lawrence, G.; Gentry, R.; McDonald, T.; Bartow, H.; Bounds, J.; Macdonald, N.; Clewell, H.; Allen, B.; Van Landingham, C. Acrylamide: Review of toxicity data and dose-response analyses for cancer and noncancer effects. *Crit. Rev. Toxicol.* **2006**, *36*, 481–608. [CrossRef] [PubMed]
4. Wei, Q.; Li, J.; Li, X.; Zhang, L.; Shi, F. Reproductive toxicity in acrylamide-treated female mice. *Reprod. Toxicol.* **2014**, *46*, 121–128. [CrossRef]
5. Parzefall, W. Minireview on the toxicity of dietary acrylamide. *Food Chem. Toxicol.* **2008**, *46*, 1360–1364. [CrossRef] [PubMed]
6. Capuano, E.; Fogliano, V. Acrylamide and 5-hydroxymethylfurfural (HMF): A review on metabolism, toxicity, occurrence in food and mitigation strategies. *LWT Food Sci. Technol.* **2011**, *44*, 793–810. [CrossRef]
7. Erkekoglu, P.; Baydar, T. Acrylamide neurotoxicity. *Nutr. Neurosci* **2014**, *17*, 49–57. [CrossRef]
8. Besaratinia, A.; Pfeifer, G.P. DNA adduction and mutagenic properties of acrylamide. *Mutat. Res.* **2005**, *580*, 31–40. [CrossRef]
9. Wang, R.S.; McDaniel, L.P.; Manjanatha, M.G.; Shelton, S.D.; Doerge, D.R.; Mei, N. Mutagenicity of acrylamide and glycidamide in the testes of big blue mice. *Toxicol. Sci.* **2010**, *117*, 72–80. [CrossRef]
10. Virk-Baker, M.K.; Nagy, T.R.; Barnes, S.; Groopman, J. Dietary acrylamide and human cancer: A systematic review of literature. *Nutr. Cancer* **2014**, *66*, 774–790. [CrossRef]

11. Al Karim, S.; El Assouli, S.; Ali, S.; Ayuob, N.; El Assouli, Z. Effects of low dose acrylamide on the rat reproductive organs structure, fertility and gene integrity. *Asian Pac. J. Reprod.* **2015**, *4*, 179–187. [CrossRef]
12. Von Tungeln, L.S.; Churchwell, M.I.; Doerge, D.R.; Shaddock, J.G.; McGarrity, L.J.; Heflich, R.H.; Gamboa da Costa, G.; Marques, M.M.; Beland, F.A. DNA adduct formation and induction of micronuclei and mutations in B6C3F1/Tk mice treated neonatally with acrylamide or glycidamide. *Int. J. Cancer* **2009**, *124*, 2006–2015. [CrossRef] [PubMed]
13. Hashimoto, K.; Tanii, H. Mutagenicity of acrylamide and its analogues in *Salmonella typhimurium*. *Mutat. Res.* **1985**, *158*, 129–133. [CrossRef]
14. Tsuda, H.; Shimizu, C.S.; Taketomi, M.K.; Hasegawa, M.M.; Hamada, A.; Kawata, K.M.; Inui, N. Acrylamide; induction of DNA damage, chromosomal aberrations and cell transformation without gene mutations. *Mutagenesis* **1993**, *8*, 23–29. [CrossRef] [PubMed]
15. Starostina, N.G.; Lusta, K.A.; Fikhte, B.A. Morphological and physiological changes in bacterial cells treated with acrylamide. *Eur. J. Appl. Microbiol. Biotechnol.* **1983**, *18*, 264–270. [CrossRef]
16. Kwolek-Mirek, M.; Zadrag-Tęcza, R.; Bednarska, S.; Bartosz, G. Yeast *Saccharomyces cerevisiae* devoid of Cu, Zn-superoxide dismutase as a cellular model to study acrylamide toxicity. *Toxicol. In Vitro* **2010**, *25*, 573–579. [CrossRef] [PubMed]
17. Sharma, M.; Sharma, N.N.; Bhalla, T.C. Amidases: Versatile enzymes in nature. *Rev. Environ. Sci. Biotechnol.* **2009**, *8*, 343–366. [CrossRef]
18. Wang, C.C.; Lee, C.-M. Isolation of the acrylamide denitrifying bacteria from a wastewater treatment system manufactured with polyacrylonitrile fiber. *Curr. Microbiol.* **2007**, *55*, 339–343. [CrossRef]
19. Ciskanik, L.M.; Wilczek, J.M.; Fallon, R.D. Purification and characterization of an enantioselective amidase from *Pseudomonas chlororaphis* B23. *Appl. Environ. Microbiol.* **1995**, *61*, 998–1003. [CrossRef]
20. Buranasilp, K.; Charoenpanich, J. Biodegradation of acrylamide by *Enterobacter aerogenes* isolated from wastewater in Thailand. *J. Environ. Sci. (China)* **2011**, *23*, 396–403. [CrossRef]
21. Sathesh-Prabu, C.; Thatheyus, A.J. Biodegradation of acrylamide employing free and immobilized cells of *Pseudomonas aeruginosa*. *Int. Biodeterior. Biodegrad.* **2007**, *60*, 69–73. [CrossRef]
22. Clamens, T.; Rosay, T.; Crépin, A.; Grandjean, T.; Kentache, T.; Hardouin, J.; Bortolotti, P.; Neidig, A.; Mooij, M.; Hillion, M.; et al. The aliphatic amidase AmiE is involved in regulation of *Pseudomonas aeruginosa* virulence. *Sci. Rep.* **2017**, *7*, 41178. [CrossRef] [PubMed]
23. Shukor, M.Y.; Gusmanizar, N.; Azmi, N.A.; Hamid, M.; Ramli, J.; Shamaan, N.A.; Syed, M.A. Isolation and characterization of an acrylamide-degrading *Bacillus cereus*. *J. Environ. Biol.* **2009**, *30*, 57–64. [PubMed]
24. Nawaz, M.S.; Khan, A.A.; Seng, J.E.; Leakey, J.E.; Siitonen, P.H.; Cerniglia, E. Purification and characterization of an amidase from an acrylamide-degrading *Rhodococcus* sp. *Appl. Environ. Microbiol.* **1994**, *60*, 3343–3348. [CrossRef] [PubMed]
25. Nawaz, M.S.; Khan, A.A.; Bhattacharayya, D.; Siitonen, P.H.; Cerniglia, C.E. Physical, biochemical, and immunological characterization of a thermostable amidase from *Klebsiella pneumoniae* NCTR 1. *J. Bacteriol.* **1996**, *178*, 2397–2401. [CrossRef]
26. Syed, S.A.; Ahmad, S.A.; Kusnin, N.; Shukor, M.Y. Purification and characterization of amidase from acrylamide-degrading bacterium *Burkholderia* sp. strain DR.Y27. *Afr. J. Biotechol.* **2012**, *11*, 329–336. [CrossRef]
27. Corthésy-Theulaz, I.; Porta, N.; Pringault, E.; Racine, L.; Bogdanova, A.; Kraehenbuhl, J.-P.; Blum, A.L.; Michetti, P. Adhesion of *Helicobacter pylori* to polarized T84 human intestinal cell monolayers is pH dependent. *Infect. Immun.* **1996**, *64*, 3827–3832. [CrossRef]
28. Lippolis, R.; Siciliano, R.A.; Mazzeo, M.F.; Abbrescia, A.; Gnoni, A.; Sardanelli, A.M.; Papa, S. Comparative secretome analysis of four isogenic *Bacillus clausii* probiotic strains. *Proteome Sci.* **2013**, *11*, 28. [CrossRef]
29. Mesnage, S.; Chau, F.; Dubost, L.; Arthur, M. Role of N-acetylglucosaminidase and N-acetylmuramidase activities in *Enterococcus faecalis* peptidoglycan metabolism. *J. Biol. Chem.* **2008**, *283*, 19845–19853. [CrossRef]
30. van Vliet, A.H.; Stoof, J.; Poppelaars, S.W.; Bereswill, S.; Homuth, G.; Kist, M.; Kuipers, E.J.; Kusters, J.G. Differential regulation of amidase- and formamidase-mediated ammonia production by the *Helicobacter pylori* Fur repressor. *J. Biol. Chem.* **2003**, *278*, 9052–9057. [CrossRef]
31. Bury-Moné, S.; Skouloubris, S.; Dauga, C.; Thiberge, J.M.; Dailidiene, D.; Berg, D.E.; Labigne, A.; De Reuse, H. Presence of active aliphatic amidases in *Helicobacter* species able to colonize the stomach. *Infect. Immun.* **2003**, *71*, 5613–5622. [CrossRef]

32. Vermassen, A.; Leroy, S.; Talon, R.; Provot, C.; Popowska, M.; Desvaux, M. Cell wall hydrolases in bacteria: Insight on the diversity of cell wall amidases, glycosidases and peptidases toward peptidoglycan. *Front. Microbiol.* **2019**, *10*, 331. [CrossRef] [PubMed]
33. Krajmalnik-Brown, R.; Ilhan, Z.E.; Kang, D.W.; DiBaise, J.K. Effects of gut microbes on nutrient absorption and energy regulation. *Nutr. Clin. Pract.* **2012**, *27*, 201–214. [CrossRef] [PubMed]
34. Ongol, M.P. Lactic acid bacteria in health and disease. *Rwanda J. Health Sci.* **2012**, *1*, 39–50.
35. George, F.; Daniel, C.; Thomas, M.; Singer, E.; Guilbaud, A.; Tessier, F.J.; Revol-Junelles, A.M.; Borges, F.; Foligné, B. Occurrence and dynamism of lactic acid bacteria in distinct ecological niches: A multifaceted functional health perspective. *Front. Microbiol.* **2018**, *27*, 2899. [CrossRef] [PubMed]
36. Vieco-Saiz, N.; Belguesmia, Y.; Raspoet, R.; Auclair, E.; Gancel, F.; Kempf, I.; Drider, D. Benefits and inputs from lactic acid bacteria and their bacteriocins as alternatives to antibiotic growth promoters during food-animal production. *Front. Microbiol.* **2019**, *10*, 57. [CrossRef] [PubMed]
37. Ali, A.A. Beneficial role of lactic acid bacteria in food preservation and human health: A review. *Res. J. Microbiol.* **2010**, *5*, 1213–1221. [CrossRef]
38. Masood, M.I.; Qadir, M.I.; Shirazi, J.H.; Khan, I.U. Beneficial effects of lactic acid bacteria on human beings. *Crit. Rev. Microbiol.* **2011**, *37*, 91–98. [CrossRef]
39. Colombo, M.; Castilho, N.P.A.; Todorov, S.D.; Nero, L.A. Beneficial properties of lactic acid bacteria naturally present in dairy production. *BMC Microbiol.* **2018**, *18*, 219. [CrossRef]
40. Najjari, A.; Amairi, H.; Chaillou, S.; Mora, D.; Boudabous, A.; Zagorec, M.; Ouzari, H. Phenotypic and genotypic characterization of peptidoglycan hydrolases of *Lactobacillus sakei*. *J. Adv. Res.* **2016**, *7*, 155–163. [CrossRef]
41. García-Cano, I.; Rocha-Mendoza, D.; Ortega-Anaya, J.; Wang, K.; Kosmerl, E.; Jiménez-Flores, R. Lactic acid bacteria isolated from dairy products as potential producers of lipolytic, proteolytic and antibacterial proteins. *Appl. Microbiol. Biotechnol.* **2019**, *103*, 5243–5257. [CrossRef]
42. Serrano-Niño, J.C.; Cavazos-Garduño, A.; González-Córdova, A.F.; Vallejo-Córdoba, B.; Hernández-Mendoza, A.; García, H.S. In vitro study of the potential protective role of *Lactobacillus* strains by acrylamide binding. *J. Food Saf.* **2014**, *34*, 62–68. [CrossRef]
43. Serrano-Niño, J.C.; Cavazos-Garduño, A.; Cantú-Cornelio, F.; González-Córdova, A.F.; Vallejo-Córdoba, B.; Hernández-Mendoza, A.; García, H.S. In vitro reduced availability of aflatoxin B1 and acrylamide by bonding interactions with teichoic acids from *Lactobacillus* strains. *LWT Food Sci. Technol.* **2015**, *64*, 1334–1341. [CrossRef]
44. Rivas-Jimenez, L.; Ramírez-Ortiz, K.; González-Córdova, A.F.; Vallejo-Cordoba, B.; Garcia, H.S.; Hernandez-Mendoza, A. Evaluation of acrylamide-removing properties of two *Lactobacillus* strains under simulated gastrointestinal conditions using a dynamic system. *Microbiol. Res.* **2016**, *190*, 19–26. [CrossRef] [PubMed]
45. Schabacker, J.; Schwend, T.; Wink, M. Reduction of acrylamide uptake by dietary proteins in a Caco-2 gut model. *J. Agric. Food Chem.* **2004**, *52*, 4021–4025. [CrossRef]
46. Hamzalıoğlu, A.; Gökmen, V. Investigation of the reactions of acrylamide during in vitro multistep enzymatic digestion of thermally processed foods. *Food Funct.* **2015**, *6*, 108–113. [CrossRef]
47. Keramat, J.; LeBail, A.; Prost, C.; Soltanizadeh, N. Acrylamide in foods: Chemistry and analysis. A Review. *Food Bioprocess Technol.* **2011**, *4*, 340–363. [CrossRef]
48. Mojska, H.; Gielecińska, I.; Szponar, L.; Ołtarzewski, M. Estimation of the dietary acrylamide exposure of the Polish population. *Food Chem. Toxicol.* **2010**, *48*, 2090–2096. [CrossRef]
49. FDA Survey 2015. Survey Data on Acrylamide in Food. Available online: https://www.fda.gov/food/chemicals/survey-data-acrylamide-food (accessed on 19 March 2020).
50. Friedman, M.; Levin, C.E. Review of methods for the reduction of dietary content and toxicity of acrylamide. *J. Agric. Food Chem.* **2008**, *56*, 6113–6140. [CrossRef]
51. Dominici, L.; Moretti, M.; Villarini, M.; Vannini, S.; Cenci, G.; Zampino, C.; Traina, G. In vivo antigenotoxic properties of a commercial prebiotic supplement containing bifidobacterial. *Int. J. Probiotics Prebiotics* **2011**, *6*, 179–186.
52. Blom, H.; Baardseth, P.; Sundt, T.W.; Slinde, E. Lactic acid fermentation reduces acrylamide formed during production of fried potato products. *Asp. Appl. Biol.* **2009**, *97*, 67–74.

53. Nachi, I.; Fhoula, I.; Smida, I.; Ben Taher, I.; Chouaibi, M.; Jaunbergs, J.; Bartkevics, V.; Hassouna, M. Assessment of lactic acid bacteria application for the reduction of acrylamide formation in bread. *LWT* **2018**, *92*, 435–441. [CrossRef]
54. Rul, F. Yogurt. Microbiology, Organoleptic Properties and Probiotic Potential. In *Fermented Foods, Part II: Technological Interventions*, 1st ed.; Ray, R.C., Montet, D., Eds.; CRC Press: Boca Raton, FL, USA, 2017; pp. 418–450.
55. Liu, M.; Bayjanov, J.R.; Renckens, B.; Nauta, A.; Siezen, R.J. The proteolytic system of lactic acid bacteria revisited: A genomic comparison. *BMC Genomics* **2010**, *11*, 36. [CrossRef] [PubMed]
56. Dalca, S.H.; Şimşek, Ö.; Gursoy, O.; Yilmaz, Y. Selection of autolytic lactic acid bacteria as potential adjunct cultures to accelerate ripening of white-brined cheeses. *Mljekarstvo* **2018**, *68*, 320–330. [CrossRef]
57. Pang, X.-Y.; Cui, W.-M.; Liu, L.; Zhang, S.-W.; Lv, J.-P. Gene knockout and overexpression analysis revealed the role of N-acetylmuramidase in autolysis of *Lactobacillus delbrueckii* subsp. bulgaricus Ljj-6. *PLoS ONE* **2014**, *9*, e104829. [CrossRef]
58. Baba, T.; Schneewind, O. Targeting of muralytic enzymes to the cell division site of Gram-positive bacteria: Repeat domains direct autolysin to the equatorial surface ring of *Staphylococcus aureus*. *EMBO J.* **1998**, *17*, 4639–4646. [CrossRef] [PubMed]
59. Yang, D.C.; Tan, K.; Joachimiak, A.; Bernhardt, T.G. A conformational switch controls cell wall remodelling enzymes required for bacterial cell division. *Mol. Microbiol.* **2012**, *85*, 768–781. [CrossRef] [PubMed]
60. Sánchez-Puelles, J.M.; Sanz, J.M.; García, J.L.; García, E. Cloning and expression of gene fragments encoding the cholinebinding domain of pneumococcal murein hydrolases. *Gene* **1990**, *89*, 69–75. [CrossRef]
61. Joris, B.; Englebert, S.; Chu, C.P.; Kariyama, R.; Daneo-Moore, L.; Shockman, G.D.; Ghuysen, J.M. Modular design of the *Enterococcus hirae* muramidase-2 and *Streptococcus faecalis* autolysin. *FEMS Microbiol. Lett.* **1992**, *70*, 257–264. [CrossRef] [PubMed]
62. Schleifer, K.H.; Kandler, O. Peptidoglycan types of bacterial cell walls and their taxonomic implications. *Bacteriol. Rev.* **1972**, *36*, 407–477. [CrossRef]
63. Shockman, G.D.; Höltje, J.-V. Microbial peptidoglycan (murein) hydrolases. *New Compr. Biochem.* **1994**, *27*, 131–166. [CrossRef]
64. Sánchez-Puelles, J.M.; Ronda, C.; García, J.L.; García, P.; López, R.; García, E. Searching for autolysin functions. Characterization of a pneumococcal mutant deleted in the lytA gene. *Eur. J. Biochem.* **1986**, *158*, 289–293. [CrossRef] [PubMed]
65. Schirner, K.; Marles-Wright, J.; Lewis, R.J.; Errington, J. Distinct and essential morphogenic functions for wall- and lipo-teichoic acids in *Bacillus subtilis*. *EMBO J.* **2009**, *28*, 830–842. [CrossRef] [PubMed]
66. Chapot-Chartier, M.; Kulakauskas, S. Cell wall structure and function in lactic acid bacteria. *Microb. Cell Fact.* **2014**, *13*, S9. [CrossRef] [PubMed]
67. Zhang, D.; Liu, W.; Li, L.; Zhao, H.-Y.; Sun, H.-Y.; Meng, M.-H.; Zhang, S.; Shao, M.-L. Key role of peptidoglycan on acrylamide binding by lactic acid bacteria. *Food Sci. Biotechnol.* **2017**, *26*, 271–277. [CrossRef]
68. Bernard, E.; Rolain, T.; Courtin, P.; Guillot, A.; Langella, P.; Hols, P.; Chapot-Chartier, M.P. Characterization of O-acetylation of N-acetylglucosamine: A novel structural variation of bacterial peptidoglycan. *J. Biol. Chem.* **2011**, *286*, 23950–23958. [CrossRef] [PubMed]
69. Bernard, E.; Rolain, T.; Courtin, P.; Hols, P.; Chapot-Chartier, M.P. Identification of the amidotransferase AsnB1 as being responsible for meso-diaminopimelic acid amidation in *Lactobacillus plantarum* peptidoglycan. *J. Bacteriol.* **2011**, *193*, 6323–6330. [CrossRef] [PubMed]
70. O'Toole, G.; Kaplan, H.B.; Kolter, R. Biofilm formation as microbial development. *Annu. Rev. Microbiol.* **2000**, *54*, 49–79. [CrossRef] [PubMed]
71. Vergères, P.; Blaser, J. Amikacin, ceftazidime, and flucloxacillin against suspended and adherent *Pseudomonas aeruginosa* and *Staphylococcus epidermidis* in an in vitro model of infection. *J. Infect. Dis.* **1992**, *165*, 281–289. [CrossRef]
72. Gómez, N.C.; Ramiro, J.M.; Quecan, B.X.; de Melo Franco, B.D. Use of potential probiotic lactic acid bacteria (LAB) biofilms for the control of *Listeria monocytogenes*, *Salmonella* Typhimurium, and *Escherichia coli* O157:H7 Biofilms Formation. *Front. Microbiol.* **2016**, *7*, 863. [CrossRef]

73. García-Cayuela, T.; Korany, A.M.; Bustos, I.; Gómez de Cadiñanos, L.P.; Requena, T.; Peláez, C.; Martínez-Cuesta, M.C. Adhesion abilities of dairy *Lactobacillus plantarum* strains showing an aggregation phenotype. *Food Res. Int.* **2014**, *57*, 44–50. [CrossRef]

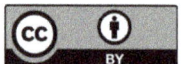

© 2020 by the authors. Licensee MDPI, Basel, Switzerland. This article is an open access article distributed under the terms and conditions of the Creative Commons Attribution (CC BY) license (http://creativecommons.org/licenses/by/4.0/).

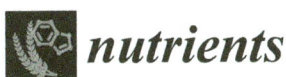

Article

Biological Activity of New Cichoric Acid–Metal Complexes in Bacterial Strains, Yeast-Like Fungi, and Human Cell Cultures In Vitro

Agata Jabłońska-Trypuć *, Urszula Wydro, Elżbieta Wołejko, Grzegorz Świderski and Włodzimierz Lewandowski

Division of Chemistry, Biology and Biotechnology, Faculty of Civil Engineering and Environmental Sciences, Białystok University of Technology, Wiejska 45E Street, 15-351 Białystok, Poland; u.wydro@pb.edu.pl (U.W.); e.wolejko@pb.edu.pl (E.W.); g.swiderski@pb.edu.pl (G.Ś.); w.lewandowski@pb.edu.pl (W.L.)
* Correspondence: a.jablonska@pb.edu.pl; Tel.: +48-797-995-971; Fax: +48-85-746-9015

Received: 22 November 2019; Accepted: 4 January 2020; Published: 6 January 2020

Abstract: Cichoric acid (CA) belongs to the group of polyphenols, which occurs in a variety of plant species and it is characterized by anticancer, antibacterial, and antiviral properties. Selected polyphenols have the ability to combine with metal ions to form chelate complexes that reveal greater biological activity than free compounds. In order to study possible antimicrobial and anticancer effect of CA and its complexes with copper(II)/zinc(II)/nickel(II)/cobalt(II) we decided to conduct cytotoxicity tests to estimate the most effective concentrations of tested compounds. The results of the presented study demonstrated, for the first time, that the treatment with newly synthesized CA-metal complexes has anticancer and antimicrobial effects, which were examined in seven different cell lines: MCF-7, MDA-MB-231, and ZR-75-1 breast cancer cell lines, A375 melanoma cell line, DLD-1 cell line, LN-229 cell line, FN cell line; five bacterial strains: *Escherichia coli*, *Pseudomonas aeruginosa*, *Staphylococcus epidermidis*, *Proteus vulgaris*, *Lactobacillus rhamnosus*, yeast *Sacchcaromyces boulardii*, and pathogenic yeast-like fungi *Candida albicans*. The presented study indicates that CA-metal complexes could be considered as a potential supplementary tool in anticancer therapy, however, because of their possible toxic activity on fibroblasts, they should be used with caution. Some of the tested complexes have also preservative properties and positive influence on normal non-pathogenic microorganisms, which was demonstrated in selected microbial strains, therefore they may serve as food preservatives of natural origin with cytoprotective properties.

Keywords: cichoric acid; metal complexes; cytotoxicity; cancer; bacterial strains; fungi; human cell culture

1. Introduction

Cichoric acid belongs to the group of polyphenols and according to its chemical formula it is a dicaffeyltartaric acid, a tartaric acid ester of two caffeic acids (a hydroxycinnamic acid). Because of its biological properties it is a very promising natural compound, which occurs in a variety of plant species such as *Cichorium intybus* L., *Ocimum basilicum* L., *Bidens tripartita* L., *Crepis capillaris* L. Wallr., *Lactuca sativa* L., *Taraxacum officinale* F.H. Wigg., *Cucurbita pepo* L., *Equisetum* hybrids, *Borago officinalis* L., *Posidonia oceanica* L. Delile, *Rabdosia rubescens*, and *Echinacea purpurea* [1]. According to the literature data cichoric acid plays an important role in plant defense against different diseases caused by viruses, bacteria, fungi, nematodes, and insects [2,3]. A variety of phenolics, including cichoric acid, are being investigated for their possible human health benefits. Cichoric acid (CA) is one of the polyphenol compounds with strong antioxidant capacities. It also exhibits free radical scavenger properties, antiviral and phagocyte promoting activity, and it protects selected structural proteins, such as collagen, against free radical damage [4]. CA has many biological activities including anti-inflammatory, antiatherosclerotic, and antidiabetic properties, which were confirmed in mouse models. Animal diabetes models indicated that CA significantly influenced insulin sensitivity, glucose tolerance, mitochondrial function, and hyperglycemia in obese mice [5–7].

Among the tested substances of natural origin, the ones that can be used in food as preservatives or pharmaceutical industry are the most popular. This is important in the context of the negative effects of drugs on human health and the increasing resistance of microorganisms to commercially available drugs and preservatives [1,8]. In addition, commonly used food preservatives such as nitrates, sodium benzoate, or monosodium glutamate may have potentially harmful effects on human health. Therefore, new alternatives that are easily accessible, safe for humans, and exhibiting antimicrobial activity are highly desirable in food industry and pharmacy. *Candida albicans*, *Escherichia coli*, *Proteus vulgaris*, *Pseudomonas aeruginosa*, and *Staphylococcus epidermidis* are examples of pathogen indicators that determine food quality and safety [8].

However, to date, a direct effect of metal complexes of CA on human cancer cells, normal healthy cells, and bacterial strains have not been investigated. Considering the stability of polyphenols, it is usually higher after binding them to a metal ion [5,9]. Also anticancer activity of metal complexes is widely used in therapy of different types of cancer; however, the utility of metal-polyphenols complexes as anticancer agents is yet to be fully realized, especially regarding some of the polyphenols such as cichoric acid [9].

According to the literature data, selected polyphenols have the ability to combine with metal ions to form chelate complexes that reveal greater biological activity than free compounds [10–12]. Out of all ions, copper seems very interesting and promising because of its biological importance and properties. It is essential in the photosynthesis process and respiration and it consists of an active center of many enzymes [13,14]. Therefore copper was one of the metals subjected to our research to determine biological activity of its complexes with CA. In complexes with fisetin–polyphenolic compound from the group of isoflavonoids, it revealed high antibacterial and antifungal activity [14]. On the other hand copper complexed with resveratrol acts as a factor, which promotes fragmentation of nuclear DNA in human cells [15]. Oleuropein, which is a non-flavonoid polyphenol, shows copper complexing properties and these copper–oleuropein complexes are probably involved in the toxic activity of analyzed polyphenolic compounds towards neuroblastoma cells, depending on their copper level [16]. The other important and biologically active metal ion which forms chelate complexes with polyphenolic compounds is zinc. Dias K et al. suggested that the combination of zinc with resveratrol enhances antioxidant activity of the polyphenolic compound [17]. The flavonoid derivative kaempferol in 1:1 coordination with Zn(II) increased phenol acidity of plant polyphenols. It may explain the very important and unique function of Zn(II) as a biologically active antioxidative compound and may help in designing new metal–polyphenol complex-based drugs derived from naturally occurring bioactive molecules [18].

Antioxidative, anti-inflammatory, and neuroprotective properties of polyphenols have been known for many years, but the discovery of their complexes with selected metals changed the course of medical chemistry and toxicology. In 2010 it was found out that complexes of biochanin with nickel(II) and copper(II) have antiviral, anticancer, and antioxidative properties [19]. Quercetin, which has in its structure hydroxyl groups capable of forming complexes with metal ions, chelates metals via 3' or and 4' phenolic group. Cobalt(II)–quercetin complexes have higher antioxidant activity than the free compound [20,21].

Our research group has shown in recent years that CA exhibits cytoprotective activity against Doxorubicin induced oxidative stress in human skin fibroblasts [22]. Furthermore we have shown that polyphenol–metal complexes exhibit better biological and antioxidative properties than free polyphenols [23]. Therefore, in order to study possible antimicrobial and anticancer effects of CA and its complexes with selected metals we decided to conduct a cytotoxicity tests to estimate the most effective concentrations of tested compounds.

2. Materials and Methods

2.1. Chemical Synthesis

2.1.1. Sample Preparation

All reagents were from Sigma–Aldrich. Sodium salt of CA was prepared as follows: 9.96 mg of cichoric acid (MW = 474,371 g/mol) was weighed, i.e., 0.021 mmol, and dissolved in 0.42 mL NaOH solution at a concentration of 0.1 M. Deionized water (2 mL) was added to the mixture. The solution was stirred in a water bath at 50 °C to dissolve the acid. The molar ratio of ligand:metal was 1:2. The solution was allowed to evaporate slowly and the precipitate was air-dried at 30 °C.

The copper(II)/zinc(II)/nickel(II)/cobalt(II) complexes were prepared in the following way: 19.92 mg of cichoric acid was dissolved in 0.84 mL NaOH (0.1 M). Then 2 mL of deionized water and water solutions containing 0.084 mmol of copper(II), zinc(II), nickel(II), and cobalt(II) chlorides were added to the mixtures. The solutions were mixed with the use of a shaker for 2 hours at room temperature. In the obtained mixture, the molar ratio of sodium salt of cichoric acid to the transition metal cation was 1:2. After several days a precipitate occurred which was filtered from the solution on filter paper and washed with deionized water until the residual chlorides were washed out. The precipitate was air-dried at 30 °C. The yield of the synthesis processes was about 70–85%. Table 1 presents the results of elemental analysis. The sodium salt was dihydrated, while the complexes of copper, zinc, cobalt, and nickel were tetrahydrated.

Table 1. Elemental analysis for metal complexes with cichoric acid.

Empirical Formula	Yield	%H (Theoret)	%C (Theoret)	%H (Exp)	%C (Exp)
$[C_{22}O_{12}H_{16}Zn_2] \cdot 4H_2O$	70–75%	3.60	39.59	3.69	39.80
$[C_{22}O_{12}H_{16}Ni_2] \cdot 4H_2O$	70–80%	3.67	40.41	3.56	39.76
$[C_{22}O_{12}H_{16}Cu_2] \cdot 4H_2O$	70%	3.62	39.81	3.57	39.13
$[C_{22}O_{12}H_{16}Co_2] \cdot 4H_2O$	70–75%	3.67	40.38	3.59	40.05

2.1.2. FTIR (Fourier Transform Infrared) Study

The FTIR spectra were recorded with an Alfa (Bruker) spectrometer within the range of 400–4000 cm^{-1}. Samples in the solid state were measured in KBr matrix pellets. FT-Raman spectra of solid samples were recorded in the range of 400–4000 cm^{-1} with a MultiRam (Bruker) spectrometer.

2.1.3. Calculations

To calculate the optimized structures quantum-mechanical methods were used: density functional (DFT) hybrid method B3LYP with non-local correlation provided by Lee–Young–Parr expression and HF (Hartree–Fock). All calculations were carried out with functional base 6-311++G(d,p). Calculations were performed using the Gaussian 09 (Frisch et al., 2009) package [24]. Experimental spectra were interpreted in terms of HF method calculations. Theoretical wavenumbers were scaled according to the formula: $\nu_{scaled} = 0.89 \cdot \nu_{calculated}$ for HF/6-311++G(d,p) level.

2.1.4. Job's Study

The composition of complexes in aqueous solutions was determined by the Job's method. Chloride solutions of $CoCl_2$, $CuCl_2$, $ZnCl_2$, and $NiCl_2$ were prepared at concentrations of 0.01 M by dissolving the appropriate weight of metal chloride salts in deionized water. A solution of CA (0.1 M) was prepared by dissolving a sample of acid in 50 mL of Tris HCl buffer (pH = 7.2). To the 10 mL flasks, 5 mL of the CA solution was added, followed by the addition of a metal chloride solution in the range of 10 to 200 μL. Then the solutions were filled to 10 mL with Tris HCl buffer. The solutions were mixed and left for 1 hour. Then, the absorption spectra of the analyzed solutions in the UV range (190–400 nm) were recorded. The measurements were taken on a HACH 5000 DR spectrophotometer.

2.2. Toxicological Studies

2.2.1. Reagents

Dulbecco's modified Eagle's medium (DMEM), containing glucose at 4.5 mg/mL (25 mM) with Glutamax and Leibovitz's L-15 medium with Glutamax, penicillin, streptomycin, trypsin–EDTA, FBS (Fetal Bovine Serum) Gold, and PBS (Phosphate Buffer Saline) (without Ca and Mg) were provided by Gibco (San Diego, CA, USA). RPMI-1640 medium with high glucose and with L-glutamine was provided by ATCC. Cell Titer-Glo™ 2.0 Assay was provided by Promega, Madison, WI, USA.

2.2.2. Microbial Strains

Escherichia coli (ATCC 25922), *Pseudomonas aeruginosa* (ATCC 27853), *Staphylococcus epidermidis* (ATCC 12228), *Candida albicans* (ATCC 10231), *Saccharomyces boulardii*, and *Lactobacillus rhamnosus* (ATCC 53103) were obtained from the American Type Culture Collection (Manassas, VA, USA). *Proteus vulgaris* (PCM 2269) strain was purchased from Polish Collection of Microorganisms (PCM, Wroclaw, Poland). Strains of bacteria and fungi were selected for antimicrobial tests. *E. coli*, *P. aeruginosa*, *P. vulgaris* (Gram negative bacteria), *S. epidermidis*, *L. rhamnosus* (Gram-positive bacteria), and *C. albicans* and *S. boulardii* (fungi) were grown overnight in Mueller Hinton II Broth at 37 °C (*E. coli*, *P. vulgaris* and *S. epidermidis*, *L. rhamnosus*, *S. boulardii*) and 27 °C (*P. aeruginosa* and *C. albicans*). Next day, the overnight cultures were diluted in fresh MH II Broth to obtain 10^8 CFU/mL (CFU—colony forming units). For the antimicrobial activity, the inoculum of the tested bacteria reached the final concentration value of 10^6 CFU/mL, while the inoculum of *C. albicans* and *S. boulardii* were about 10^4 CFU/mL.

2.2.3. Cell Culture

The effect of CA and its metal complexes were examined in MCF-7, MDA-MB-231, and ZR-75-1 breast cancer cell lines, A375 melanoma cell line, DLD-1 cell line, LN-229 cell line, and FN cell line, which were obtained from American Type Culture Collection (ATCC). MCF-7 cells, A-375 melanoma cell line, LN-229 glioblastoma cell line, and FN fibroblasts cell line were maintained in DMEM supplemented with 10% FBS, penicillin (100 U/mL), and streptomycin (100 μg/mL) at 37 °C in a humidified atmosphere of 5% CO_2 in air. ZR-75-1 cells and DLD-1 colorectal adenocarcinoma cell line were maintained in RPMI-1640 supplemented with 10% FBS, penicillin (100 U/mL), and streptomycin (100 μg/mL) at 37 °C in a humidified atmosphere of 5% CO_2 in air. MDA-MB-231 cells were maintained in Leibovitz's L-15 medium supplemented with 10% FBS, penicillin (100 U/mL), and streptomycin (100 μg/mL) at 37 °C in a humidified atmosphere.

MCF-7 cells, MDA-MB-231 cells, ZR-75-1 cells, A-375 cells line, DLD-1 cells, LN-229 cells, and FN cells (2×10^4 cells/ml) in 200 μL of culture medium were incubated without and with the test compounds in tissue culture treated white 96-well plates for the Cell Titer Glo™ 2.0 Assay. The cytotoxicity was estimated for CA and its complexes at concentration of 50 μM, 100 μM, 200 μM, 300 μM, 400 μM, and 500 μM.

2.2.4. CA and Its Metal Complexes Antimicrobial Activity

Initially, two-fold microdilutions of analyzed compounds in a liquid growth media (MH II Broth) in 96 well-plates were prepared. Next, the indicator fungi (concentration of 10^4 CFU/mL) and bacteria strain (concentration of 10^6 CFU/mL) suspensions were added into each well of a 96 well-plate, and then incubated for 24 h at 37 °C (*E. coli*, *P. vulgaris*, *S. epidermidis*, *L. rhamnosus*, and *S. boulardii*) and 27 °C (*P. aeruginosa and C. albicans*). The final concentrations of CA and its complexes in each well were: 800 μM, 400 μM, 200 μM, 100 μM, and 50 μM.

Cell viability of tested microorganisms treated with CA and its metal complexes were estimated using the BacTiter-Glo™ (Promega, Madison, WI, USA) according to the manufacturer's instruction. In brief, the assay uses a thermostable luciferase to enable reaction conditions that produce a stable "glow-type" luminescent signal while simultaneously inhibiting endogenous enzymes released during cell lysis. The homogenous assay procedure involves addition of a single reagent directly to cells cultured in serum-supplemented medium. Luminescence was measured with a GloMax®-Multi Microplate Multimode Reader. The cytotoxicity of CA and its complexes with metals was expressed a relative cell viability (%) in relation to un-treated control. The study was performed in triplicate in order to ensure that consistent results were obtained.

2.2.5. Estimation of CA and Its Metal Complexes Cytotoxicity

To measure CA and metal complexes cytotoxicity CellTiter-Glo™ 2.0 Assay (Promega) was used. The measurement was conducted according to manufacturer's protocol. Luminescence was measured with a GloMax®-Multi Microplate Multimode Reader. The study was performed in triplicate taken to ensure consistent results were obtained.

2.2.6. Statistical Analysis

All data are given as mean values ±SD (standard deviation). Differences between treatments and untreated control human cells were analyzed by one-way ANOVA, followed by Dunnett's procedure for multiple comparisons. Significant effects are represented by $p \leq 0.05$ (*), $p \leq 0.01$ (**), $p \leq 0.001$ (***). To compare the means for treatments and tested cell lines two-way analysis of variance (ANOVA) followed by the Tukey test were applied. Significance was considered when $p \leq 0.05$. Cluster analysis was used to the group the examined elements (individual microorganisms treated with metal, CA and its complexes with metal) into similar categories. Two-way joining method of clustering was applied.

3. Results

3.1. Chemical Synthesis Results

Composition and Structure of Examined Complexes

Elemental analysis showed that the metals Zn(II), Cu(II), Ni(II), and Co(II) are complexed with cichoric acid in a 2:1 molar ratio (metal:ligand) (Table 1). All complexes were hydrated and contained 4 water molecules. The yield of the synthesis oscillated around 70%–80% (based on the synthesis of complexes three times).

The composition of the complexes in aqueous solutions was determined using the Job's method for pH = 7.2. The analysis showed that in aqueous solutions cichoric acid complexes with metals in a molar ratio of 1:2. Figure 1 presents UV spectra for aqueous solutions of cichoric acid with copper (II) ions (mixed in molar ratios from 5:1 to 1:5) measured in a Tris–HCl buffer solution with pH = 7.2. Figure 2 shows the dependence of the maximum absorbance of a copper complex with cichoric acid depending on the composition of the complex. Similar results were noted for the remaining studied metal complexes with cichoric acid.

The type of metal ligand coordination was determined based on spectroscopic data analysis (FTIR). The spectra of cichoric acid and metal complexes were recorded in the KBr matrix, and theoretically calculated for the optimized structure of the acid, sodium salt, and copper complex.

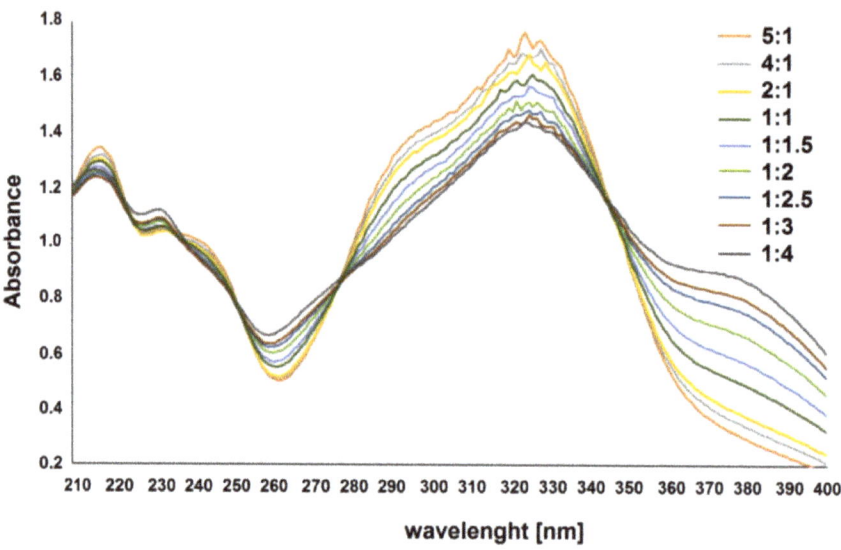

Figure 1. Absorption spectra of cichoric acid in the presence of various amounts of copper in Tris–HCl buffer pH 7.2 (different types of lines are labeled with a molar ratio of cichoric acid:metal 5:1–1:5).

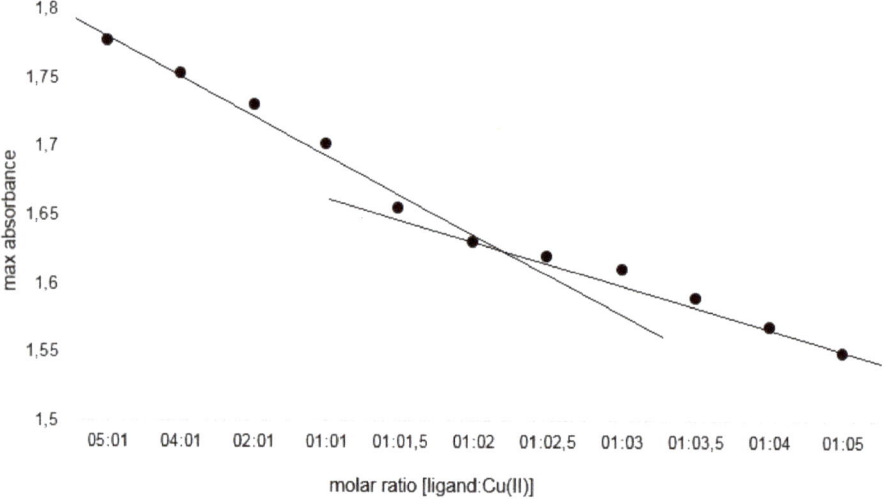

Figure 2. Absorbance as a function of [cichoric acid]: [copper] molar ratio at 320 nm.

In the spectrum of the acid the bands at 1746 and 1716 cm^{-1} were interpreted as vibrations of the carboxyl group of the tartaric acid fragment present in the cichoric acid molecule. After binding the metal ion to the ligand, these bands disappeared, which indicates that the metal is bound to the cichoric acid through the carboxylate group of the tartaric acid. In the spectra of the sodium salt and complexes, characteristic wide bands originating from vibrations of the carboxylate anion appeared. The bands derived from the stretching vibrations of the symmetric carboxylate anion $\nu_{sym}COO^-$ were identified: at the wavenumbers: 1385 cm^{-1} IR and 1381 cm^{-1} Raman in sodium salt, 1384 cm^{-1} IR in the copper complex, 1385 cm^{-1} IR in the nickel complex, 1384 cm^{-1} IR in the zinc complex, and 1385 cm^{-1} IR in the complex cobalt, and stretching asymmetric ν_{as}COO: at the wavenumbers: 1626 cm^{-1} IR in sodium salt, 1626 cm^{-1} IR in the copper complex, 1630 cm^{-1} IR in the nickel complex, 1629 cm^{-1} IR in the zinc complex, and 1605 cm^{-1} IR in the cobalt complex (Table 2). In the spectra of complexes intense bands assigned to the symmetric bending in-plane (β_sCOO$^-$) occurred: at the wavenumbers: at 853 cm^{-1} IR and 860 cm^{-1} Raman in sodium salt, 868 cm^{-1} in the copper complex, 851 cm^{-1} in the nickel complex, 853 cm^{-1} in the zinc complex, and 851 cm^{-1} in the cobalt complex, and asymmetric bending β_{as}COO$^-$: at 521 cm^{-1} IR in sodium salt, 521 cm^{-1} in the copper complex, 520 cm^{-1} in the nickel complex, 520 cm^{-1} in the zinc complex, and 521 cm^{-1} in the cobalt complex (Table 2). On the basis of the position of the ν_{as}COO$^-$ and ν_sCOO$^-$ bands in the IR spectra of the studied complexes compared to the position of these bands in the sodium salt, it was found that the bidentate chelation coordination mode is present in the copper and cobalt complexes (Figure 3) and monodentate for nickel and zinc complex (Figure 4) ($\Delta\nu$COO$^-$ of the complexes < $\Delta\nu$COO$^-$ of the sodium salt; $\Delta\nu$COO$^-$ means the difference between the wavenumber of the bands assigned to the asymmetric and symmetric vibration of the carboxylate anion).

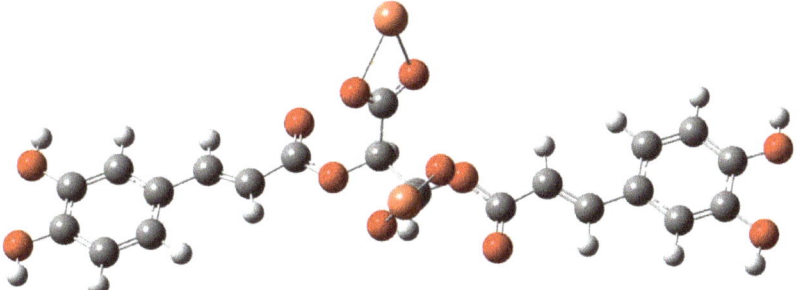

Figure 3. The propoedl structures of copper and cobalt cichoriate structures.

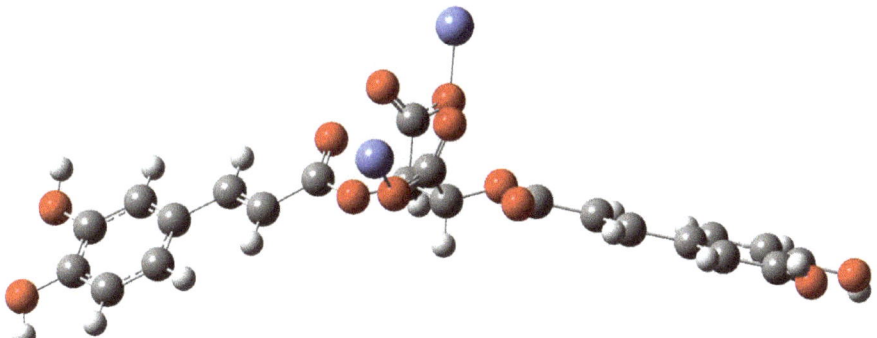

Figure 4. The proposed structures of nickel and zinc cichoriate structures.

Table 2. Wavenumbers (cm^{-1}), intensities, and assignments of bands occurring in the IR (Infrared) (KBr and HF –Hartree-Fock method) and Raman spectra of cichoric acid, sodium salt, and 3D metal complexes.

Cichoric Acid				Sodium Salt				Complexes						Assignments
Experimental		Theoretical		Experimental		Theoretical		Copper			Nickel	Zinc	Cobalt	
IR	Raman	HF	Int	IR	Raman	HF	Int	Exp IR	HF	Int	Exp IR	Exp IR	Exp IR	
1746 m		1809	331.95											ν_{as}COOH$_{tart}$
1716 s		1797	512.19											ν_{as}COOH$_{tart}$
1682 s	1681 s	1744	18.96	1699 s	1703 w	1735	7.47	1721 s	1736	9.23	1698 s	1692 m		νC=O$_{caff}$; νC=C$_{alkaff}$
1624 s	1627 vs	1742	697.97			1732	686.64		1731	669.21				νC=O$_{caff}$; νC=C$_{alkaff}$
				1626 vs		1580	1255.35	1626 s	1570	1105.71	1630 s	1629 vs	1605 s	ν_{as}COO$^-$
				1385 s	1381 vw	1447	204.62	1384 m	1446	185.54	1385 m	1384 s	1385 m	ν_sCOO$^-$
				853 w	860 vw	870	18.44	868 w	871	10.97	851 w	853 w	851 m	β_sCOO$^-$
						869	8.1		869	20.35				β_sCOO$^-$
698 vw	699 vw	739	2.12			746	3.41		745	4.05	698 w	695 m		γCOOH
680 w	685 vw	727	4.36	688 w		727	1.11		726	2.16	691 m		685 m	def$_{ring}$, γCOOH
				521 w		539	40.51	521 m	536	39.39	520 m	520 m	521 m	β_{as}COO$^-$
						472	39.33		471	46.44				β_{as}COO$^-$
504 w	504 vw	517	7.63											γO-H$_{caff}$

ν-stretching vibrations, β-bending in-plane, γ-bending out-of-plane, def$_{ring}$-deformation of the ring in-plane, s-symmetric oscillations, as-asymmetric oscillations, caff-caffeic acid, tart-tartaric acid.

3.2. Toxicological Studies Results

3.2.1. Antibacterial and Antifungal Activity of CA and Its Metal Complexes

Figures 5 and 6 show the influence of CA and its complexes with selected metals on all tested microbial and fungal strains. In all analyzed concentrations, *P. aeruginosa* incubation with CA–Co complex leads to statistically significant decreases in cell viability. The lowest tested concentration of CA–Co complex of 50 µM caused a decrease of approximately 50% after 24 h treatment. At higher concentrations of CA–Co complex, i.e., from 200 µM to 800 µM, decreases in cell viability by approximately 97% as compared to the control untreated cells were observed. Similar effects were noticed in the case of CA–Co treatments in *S. epidermidis* and *P. vulgaris*, in which all applied concentrations caused decreases in relative cell viability in *S. epidermidis* from 40% at 50 µM to 80% at 800 µM and *P. vulgaris* from 20% at 50 µM to 70% at 400 µM. In turn, using the lowest concentration of CA–Co complex caused an increase in relative cell viability of *E. coli* of approx. 20%.

At all investigated treatments, the CA–Cu and CA–Ni complexes resulted in a decrease in cell viability in both *S. epidermidis* and *P. vulgaris*. The CA–Cu complex in all analyzed concentrations caused an increase in *P. aeruginosa* viability by approximately 50% as compared to the control untreated cells. The treatment of *E coli* with CA–Cu and CA–Ni did not cause any significant decreases in relative cell viability at lower tested concentrations. The decrease was observed only at 800 µM in relative cell viability by about 40% and 50% respectively. After introducing CA–Ni and CA–Zn complexes on *P. aeruginosa* we observed a decrease in cell viability with simultaneous increase in concentrations used. In the case of *S. epidermidis*, at lower tested concentrations of CA–Zn complex (50 and 100 µM) there was an increase in the viability by about 7%, while at other concentrations, i.e., from 200 to 800 µM a decrease by approximately 15% at 200 µM, 20% at 400 µM, and 25% at 800 µM was observed. The highest concentration of CA–Zn complex caused over 20% decline in *E. coli* cell viability, whereas lower concentrations stimulated cell viability by nearly 60% after 24 h incubation.

The application of CA and its complexes with selected metals on *C. albicans* caused a decrease in relative cell viability after 24 h. The highest (800 µM) concentration of CA complexed with selected metals caused a decrease in relative cell viability by approximately 60% for CA–Zn, 80% for CA–Cu, and 95% for CA–Co and CA–Ni as compared to the control untreated cells. In CA–Cu and CA–Zn, the lowest analyzed concentration did not cause any significant changes in relative cell viability, since it achieved the value of approximately 3% (Figure 5).

The application of CA on nonpathogenic microorganisms such as *L. rhamnosus* and *S. bouldardii* caused an increase in relative cell viability in *L. rhamnosus* by approximately 26% at 50 µM and 12% at 100 µM and in *S. bouldardii* by approximately 34% at 50 µM, 14% at 100 µM, and 4% at 200 µM. After introducing CA–Zn complexes on *L. rhamnosus* an increase in relative cell viability from 40% at 50 µM to 10% at 200 µM was observed, while in *S. bouldardii* a decrease in relative cell viability from 29% at 50 µM to 40% at 800 µM was noticed. *L. rhamnosus* incubation with CA–Co complexes lead to decreases in cell viability after 24 h treatment as compared to the control untreated cells. In turn, using the 50 µM CA–Co and CA–Cu complex caused an increase in relative cell viability of *S. bouldardii* by approximately 18%. Similar effects were noticed in the case of CA–Cu and CA–Ni complexes, i.e., by approximately 30% in *L. rhamnosus*.

Summarizing, cytotoxic effect of tested compounds on selected microorganisms decreases in the following sequence:

C. albicans: Ca–Co > Ca–Ni > Ca–Cu > Ca–Zn > CA
E. coli: CA–Co > CA–Cu > CA > CA–Ni > CA–Zn
P. vulgaris: CA–Ni > CA–Co > CA–Cu > CA–Zn > CA
P. aeruginosa: CA–Co > CA–Zn > CA > CA–Ni > CA–Cu
S. epidermidis: CA–Co > CA–Cu > CA–Ni > CA > CA–Zn.

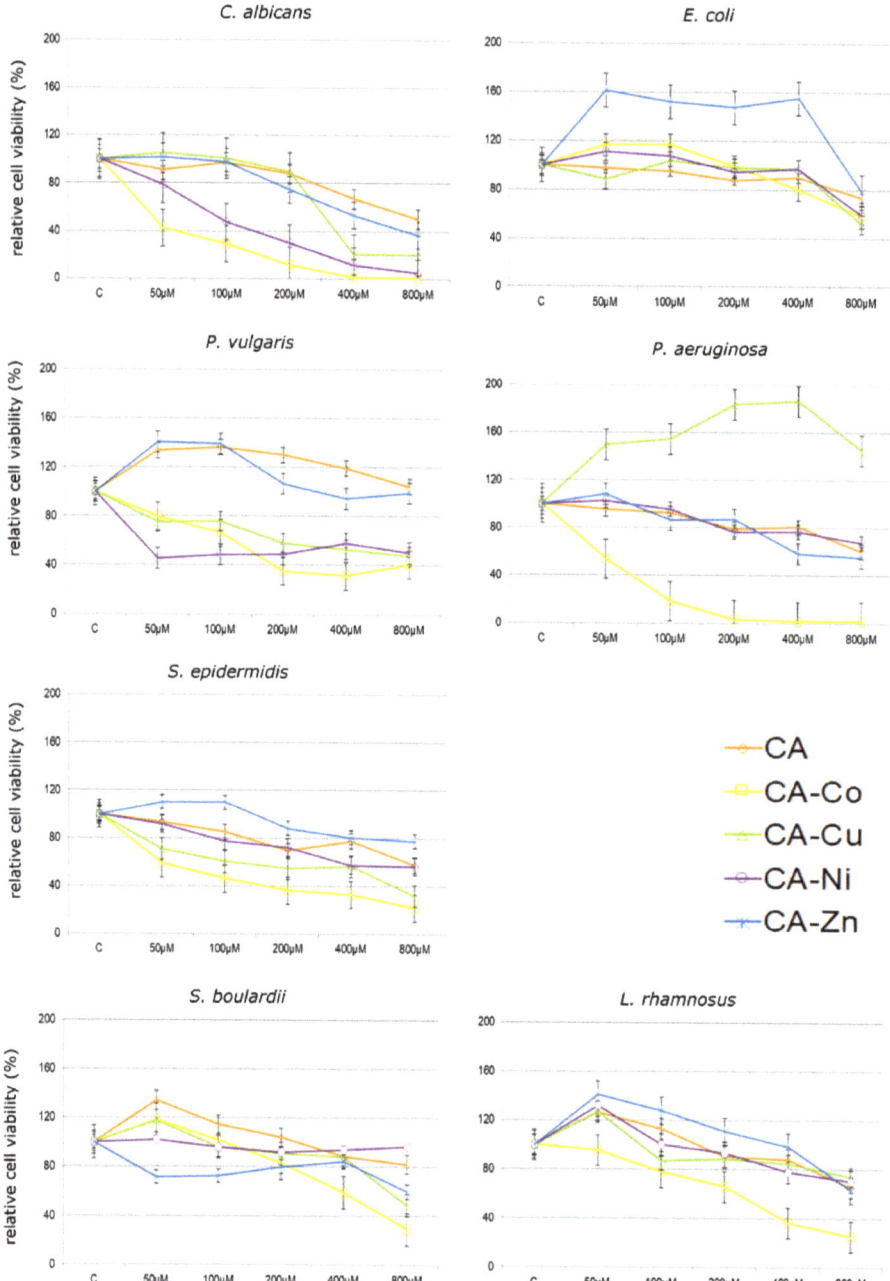

Figure 5. Cytotoxicity of cichoric acid (CA) and its complexes with Co (CA–Co), Cu (CA–Cu), Ni (CA–Ni) and Zn (CA–Zn) on fungi (*C. albicans* and *S. boulardii*) and bacteria strains (*E. coli*, *P. vulgaris*, *P. aeruginosa*, *S. epidermidis*, *L. rhamnosus*) expressed as relative cell viability (%) as compared to non-treated control (C). Each value on the graph is the mean of three independent experiments and error bars show the standard deviation (SD).

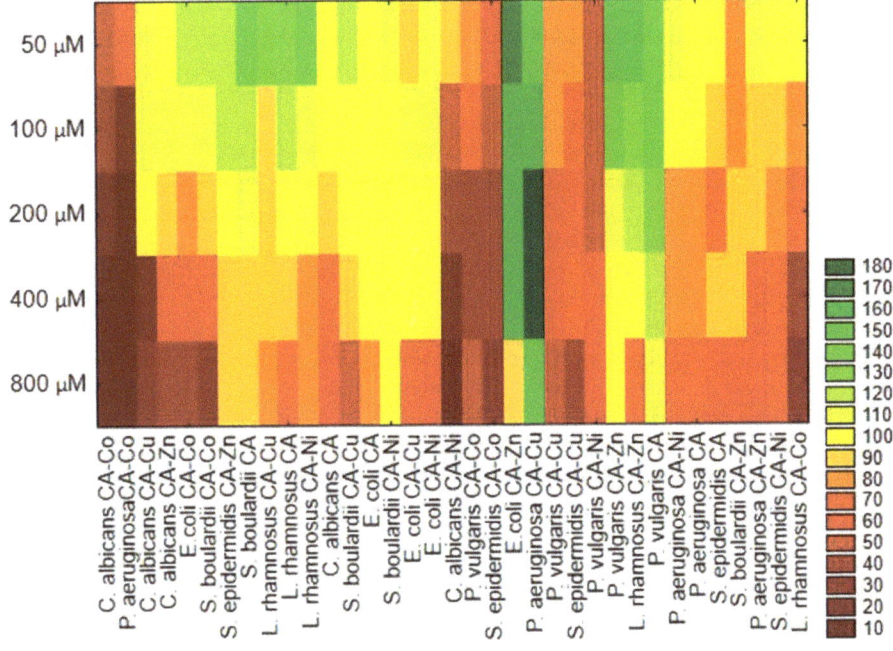

Figure 6. Cluster analysis for relative fungi and bacteria cells viability (%) after treatment of CA and its complexes with metals.

Based on resulted of cluster analysis (Figure 6), we can distinguish the groups that contain microorganisms with similar sensitivity/resistance to individuals treatments. For example, the similar highest inhibitory effect was observed for *C. albicans*, *P. aeruginosa*, and *S. epidermidis* treatment with the CA–Co complex. On the other hand, the similar stimulatory effects for *E. coli* treated with CA–Zn, *P. aeruginosa* with CA–Cu, and *P. vulgaris* with CA and CA–Zn were noted.

3.2.2. Cytotoxicity of Analyzed Compounds in Human Cancerous and Non-Cancerous Cells

As shown in Figure 7 both CA and its complexes with selected metals exert cytotoxic effect in all tested cell lines. In the LN-229 glioblastoma cell line incubation with especially CA–Co complexes in all analyzed concentrations leads to statistically significant decreases in cell viability. Even the lowest tested concentration of CA–Co complexes—50 µM—caused a decrease by about 60% after 24 h treatment and by about 70% after 48 h treatment. A similar effect was observed in the case of CA–Zn treatment in both incubation times. The lowest analyzed concentration caused a decrease in relative cell viability by about 50% after 24 h and 48 h treatment. Higher concentrations of CA–Zn complex caused more than 90% decline in LN-229 cells viability. CA treatment did not cause any significant decreases in relative cell viability in LN-229 cell line. DLD-1 colorectal adenocarcinoma cells treated with CA and CA–metal complexes also exhibited statistically significant decreases in relative cell viability. An effect comparable with the LN-229 cell line was observed. CA complexed with Co already in the lowest concentration caused almost 50% decline in DLD-1 cell viability after 24 h incubation. Ca complexed with Zn in both analyzed incubation times caused statistically significant decreases in cell viability in all tested concentrations. The most inhibitory effect on cell viability was noticed for CA–Co and CA–Zn complexes causing decreases higher than 90%. In the case of CA–Zn complex all of the analyzed concentrations, except 50 µM, caused decline in cell viability. The influence of CA on the DLD-1 cell line was more significant that on the LN-229 cell line; however we did observe significant effects only in higher concentrations such as 300 µM. In the A-375 melanoma cell line CA–metal complexes also caused significant decreases in cell viability. Co, Zn, and Cu complexes were characterized by the greater inhibitory activity towards melanoma cells. After 48 h treatment, the CA–Zn complex in the lowest concentration of 50 µM caused a decrease by about 95% in relative cell viability. Cytotoxicity assay revealed also that statistically significant changes in cell number were observed in analyzed breast cancer cell lines, especially in the MCF-7 cell line after 48 h treatment. CA–metal complexes were more cytotoxic to breast cancer cells than free cichoric acid. An especially active compound was CA–Zn complex in 200 µM, 400 µM, and 500 µM concentration. In the MDA-MB-231 cell line we did observe only slight significant changes in cell viability under the influence of tested compounds. Only the CA–Co complex in 400 µM concentration after 48 h treatment caused significant changes in cell viability. In the ZR-75-1 cell line CA–Cu and CA–Zn were especially active in 400 µM and 500 µM concentrations. In fibroblasts, which represent normal, healthy cells, significant declines in cell viability were observed. Only free CA exhibited stimulatory activity against fibroblasts. It caused insignificant increases in relative cell viability in the concentration range 50 µM to 300 µM. Higher concentrations such as 400 µM and 500 µM inhibited cell proliferation by about 20% as compared to control untreated cells.

Summarizing, the influence of CA and CA-metal complexes on cancerous and non-cancerous cells is depicted in Figure 8. Presented results are shown as a percentage of live cells compared to control, untreated cells set at 100 percent, with no regard both to the concentration of CA or to the concentration of CA-metal complexes. The differences in relative cell viability are especially easily visible in CA–metal complexes. In case of CA treatment, significant changes and differences between analyzed cell lines were observed after 48 h incubation. From the presented graph it can be deducted that every analyzed CA–metal complex, without considering concentration, caused decrease in cell viability in three cancer cell lines: A-375, DLD-1, and LN-229. Interestingly, breast cancer cell lines, especially MDA-MB-231 and MCF-7, were more resistant to CA–metal complexes as compared to other cancer cell lines and to ZR-75-1 breast cancer cell line. Unfortunately, CA–metal complexes, especially CA–Ni and CA–Co after 48 h incubation, were cytotoxic to fibroblasts, which represent normal healthy cell lines. Free CA did not exhibit toxicity against fibroblasts and after 48 h treatment it was toxic to the MCF-7 cell line. In every tested concentration, except for free CA, after 48 h treatment the level of viable cells did not exceed 100% control untreated cells.

Summarizing, cytotoxic effect of tested compounds on selected human cancerous and non-cancerous cell lines decreases in the following sequence:

LN-229: CA–Zn > CA–Co > CA–Ni > CA–Cu > CA
DLD–1: CA–Zn > CA–Cu > CA–Co > CA–Ni > CA
A–375: CA–Zn > CA–Co > CA–Cu > CA–Ni > CA
MCF–7: CA–Zn > CA–C > CA–Ni > CA–Cu > CA
MDA–MB–231: CA–Zn > CA–Co > CA–Cu > CA–Ni > CA
ZR–75–1: CA–Cu > CA–Zn > CA–Ni > CA–Co > CA
FN: CA–Ni > CA–Co > CA–Cu > CA–Zn > CA

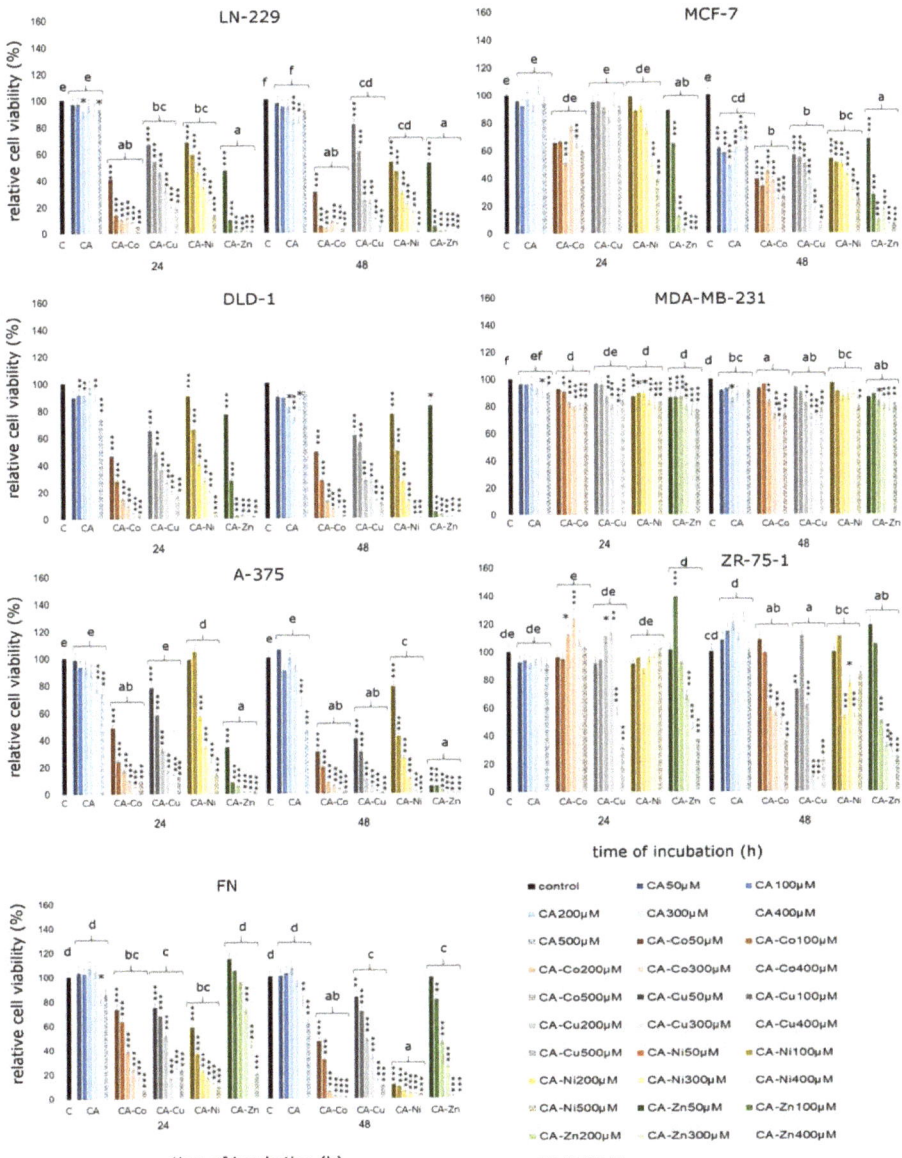

Figure 7. Cell viability results for MCF-7, MDA-MB-231, ZR-75-1, A375, DLD-1, LN-229, and FN cell lines exposed to different concentrations of CA and CA complexed with metals (Cu, Zn, Co, Ni) for 24 h and 48 h calculated as a percentage of control, untreated cells. Each value on the graph is the mean of three independent experiments and error bars show the standard deviation (SD). * $p < 0.05$, ** $p < 0.01$, and *** $p < 0.001$ represent significant effects between treatments and control followed by a Dunnett's test.

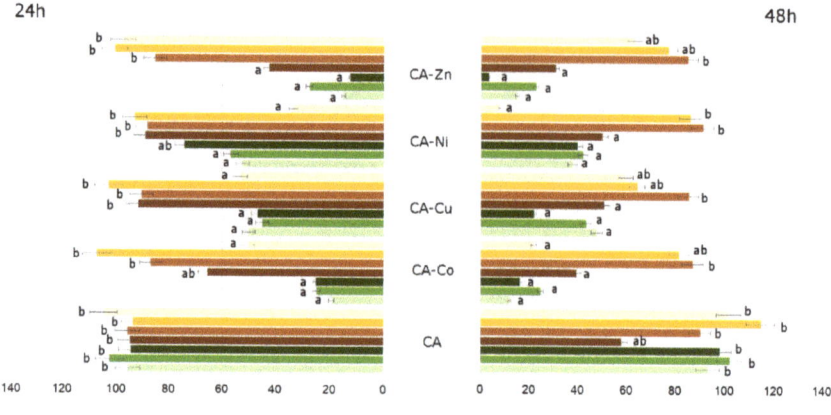

Figure 8. The viability of LN-229, DLD-1, A-375, FN, MCF-7, MDA-MB-231, and ZR-75-1 cell lines treated with different concentrations of CA and CA–metal (Cu, Zn, Ni, Co) complexes for 24 and 48 h. The results represent means for pooled triplicate values from three independent experiments. Significant alterations are expressed relative to control untreated cells (marked with asterisks). Statistical significance was considered if * $p < 0.05$.

4. Discussion

Cichoric acid, due to its numerous beneficial biological properties, is a valuable product of natural origin. Literature data indicate its immunostimulatory and antiviral activity, and the capacity of stimulating the effect of phagocytosis in vitro and in vivo. In addition, CA inhibits hyaluronidase activity, which is a key enzyme in the course of bacterial infection [25]. In the present study we examined the effect of CA and its complexes with metals against foodborne pathogenic microorganisms such as *E. coli*, *P. vulgaris*, *P. aeruginosa*, *S. epidermidis*, and *C. albicans* as well as nonpathogenic microorganisms like *L. rhamnosus* and *S. boulardii*. In literature, there are limited numbers of studies about the influence of CA on bacteria or fungi. However, several data indicate that polyphenolic acids have antibacterial and antifungal properties against foodborne pathogens [26–28]. Furthermore, it has been reported that chemical complexes with selected heavy metals such as Co, Cu, Zn, and Ni may improve antibacterial and antifungal potential [29].

According to obtained results, antimicrobial effect varies depending on studied microorganism as well as on applied agent. Generally, CA complexed with Co was the strongest antibacterial and antifungal compound, whereas the least efficient in reducing tested bacteria and fungi viability were CA and CA–Zn complexes. Inhibitory or stimulatory effects of studied compounds on individual bacterial strains and fungi may be explained by the different structure of cell membranes, as reported by many authors [30,31]. Gram-negative bacteria are generally most resistant to antibacterial compounds due to the presence of the outer cell membrane. In Gram-negative bacteria the molecules are transported through the outer lipopolysaccharide membrane rich in porins, which significantly hinder the penetration of antibacterial agents. Our data indicate that free CA exhibited a similar impact against *S. epidermidis* (Gram-positive) and *P. aeruginosa* (Gram-negative). These results are not consistent with previous studies reporting that polyphenolic acids have a higher antibacterial potential against Gram-positive than Gram-negative bacteria [28]. However, research conducted by Cueva et al. showed that selected phenolic compounds (e.g., gallic acid, caffeic acid) may inhibit the growth of both Gram-positive (*S. aureus*) and Gram-negative bacteria (*P. aeruginosa*), which is in agreement with our results regarding to CA [32]. Kavak and Kacec (2019) also drew similar conclusions in study about arbutin (polyphenols extracted from *Pyrus elaeagrifolia*), which was an effective antibacterial agent against *Bacillus cereus* (Gram-positive), *Staphylococcus aureus* (Gram-positive), and *Escherichia coli* (Gram-negative) [30]. According to Mokhtar et al. antimicrobial properties of some polyphenolic acids may be associated with irreversible changes in the structure and properties of the bacteria cell membrane [8]. These compounds may cause changes in hydrophobicity and the formation of local ruptures or pores resulting in leakage of cell components. Furthermore, polyphenols can destroy the bacteria membrane proteins and disrupt bacterial metabolic processes [33]. In addition, Lou et al. (2015) showed that phenolic acids like p-coumaric acid may increase membrane permeability as well as may bind to genomic DNA and disrupt major processes such as replication, transcription, and translation [34].

In the present study we tested antifungal properties of free CA. It was found that CA inhibited fungi cell growth by approximately 20% as compared to control. It has been reported the transfer of molecules is associated with the ultrastructure of the chitin wall, membrane ergosterols, and genetic material. Therefore, a complex structure of fungal cell walls could hinder the transport of antifungal agents [31].

In our research free cichoric acid was not effective in reducing the tested microorganisms' growth. The maximum inhibitory effect of CA (20%) was observed for *S. epidermidis*, *C. albicans*, and *P. aeruginosa*. As reported by Prasad et al. and Świslocka et al. (poli)phenolic compounds are characterized by low antimicrobial activity as compared to their combinations with other molecules [23,35]. In our research we proposed determining the antimicrobial properties of one from polyphenol acids, cichoric acid, in combination with metals such as Co, Cu, Ni, and Zn. Antimicrobial and antifungal properties of metal ions have been known and explored for many years [36]. The antimicrobial activity of the metal ions is linked with the cell membrane destabilization and disruption of the bacterial membrane permeability. Whereas the antifungal effect of the metal ions is mainly due to the disorder of ergosterol biosynthesis. The application of metal ions alone as a preservative agent or drug compound is problematic because they exhibit cytotoxic activity to human cells. The combination of metal ions and CA may be a promising strategy to obtain antimicrobial agent safety for humans.

In our study, among examined complexes, CA–Zn exhibited the weakest antimicrobial effect, especially against *L. rhamnosus*, *E. coli*, and *P. vulgaris*, when complex CA–Co is characterized by the strongest inhibitory effect against the all of tested microorganism with the exception of *E. coli* and *S. boulardii*. Gałczyńska et al. pointed the fact that Co and Cu-based complexes have an antibacterial and antifungal effect [37]. These properties depend on the mechanism of transport through the bacterial/fungal cell membrane and more precisely, through Ca^{2+} channels in cellular membranes.

In addition, it should be noted that, the transport of a substance into a bacterial cell depends on the relationship between the individual metals. For example Co may have antagonistic effect against Fe(III). As a result of interaction of Co with a siderophore (pyoverdine) which is produced by *P. aeruginosa*, decrease in ferric ion availability for bacteria cells may be observed. This phenomenon could be connected with the highest CA–Co toxicity observed for *P. aeruginosa*. In our study *C. albicans* appears to be the most sensitive on CA–Co and CA–Ni treatments. Castillo et al. indicate that chemical complexes with Co and Cu have better antimicrobial effect as compared to those containing zinc [38]. In our study, the similar results for CA–Cu were obtained for *C. albicans*, *E. coli*, *P. vulgaris*, and *S. epidermidis*. The probable cytotoxicity effect of metal complexes against bacteria and fungi may be connected with metal complex–membrane components interaction. The study by Lv et al. showed that ergosterol present in *C. albicans* cell membrane together with numerous proteins creates lipid rafts, which are responsible for hyphae morphogenesis, polarization, and membrane fusion during endocytosis [39]. Therefore, treatment of cells with antifungal agents may result in the destruction of lipid rafts in filamentation and thus disrupt the synthesis of ergosterol and hyphae. In turn, antibacterial ability of metal complexes with CA may be connected with changes in membrane properties such as its rigidity and permeability due to membrane protein destruction [33].

The previous studies have indicated that the antimicrobial capacity of polyphenolic compounds depends on their properties and structure. As reported by Murcia et al., antibacterial and antifungal responses to treatments may due to different lipophilic properties and dipole moments of examined complexes [40]. Moreover, research conducted by Wu et al. (2013) demonstrated that antimicrobial ability is associated with a negative correlation between the relative hydrophobicity and the numbers of hydroxyl groups in some polyphenolic compounds (flavonoids) [33].

Phenolic compounds, such as cichoric acid, consist of a group of compounds of natural plant origin with significant and proved antioxidant activity. They prevent many diseases, including cancer, and cardiovascular and neurodegenerative diseases, mainly by reducing oxidative stress [41–43]. Polyphenolic compounds can prevent oxidative stress by inhibiting ROS (Reactive Oxygen Species), but on the other hand they may also act as a prooxidant mainly in the presence of transition metals. Prooxidant activity of polyphenolic compounds is conditioned by many factors, including high concentration of polyphenolic compound, high pH, and the presence of transition metals, such as Cu and Fe [44,45]. Two of the above mentioned factors are especially important—an acidic pH and the number of hydroxyls in aromatic rings. The solubility and stability of reduced forms of transition metals is determined by acidic pH of the solution and the higher number of hydroxyl substitutions, mainly in *ortho* position, determines stronger prooxidant properties [46].

Among trace minerals, chromium, cobalt, selenium, iron, manganese, molybdenum, copper, and zinc can be mentioned. Some of them, particularly transition metal ions such as copper, are involved in oxidative reactions in the presence of other compounds, such as polyphenols [47]. One of the most important microelements is copper, which plays an important role in various physiological functions. In cancer cells its concentration is significantly higher than in normal cells, which subsequently makes them less resistant to the prooxidant activity of polyphenols [48,49]. It is in accordance with our results indicating that copper complexed with cichoric acid significantly decreases relative cell viability in every analyzed cell line except for MCF-7 after 24 h incubation. We observed that CA complexed with Cu as compared to free CA caused significantly higher declines in cell viability. It is in agreement with literature data indicating that in the presence of copper prooxidant activity of polyphenols is supposed to progress through the generation of a high level of ROS. It is well known that cancer cells generate oxidative stress, which stimulates their proliferation, but significantly high level of ROS and RNS (Reactive Nitrogen Species) may cause cancer cell damage and death. In the presence of Cu and polyphenols such as CA, cancer cells produce large amount of free radicals which cause DNA damage and apoptosis in cancer cells. The vast majority of studies regarding possible prooxidant activity of polyphenols were conducted in vitro and in the presence of copper as a catalyzer of oxidative reactions [47].

Obtained results indicate that the most biologically active compound was CA complexed with Zn. It was especially cytotoxic against melanoma, colorectal adenocarcinoma, and glioblastoma cell lines. Although, according to the literature data zinc is rather an antioxidant, its overdoses may result in prooxidant activity [50]. Borovansky et al. indicated that melanoma cells are uniquely susceptible to increases of certain divalent metal salts, for example Zn(II). They demonstrated that compounds containing zinc in their structure may induce melanoma cell death at concentrations several times lower than those that are lethal to melanocytes [51]. We observed that zinc complexed with CA was very effective in decreasing relative melanoma cell viability even at lower analyzed concentrations. In fact, the CA–Zn complex was the most efficient from all the analyzed complexes. It could be related with the high susceptibility of melanoma to Zn activity, which was also mentioned by Farmer et al. [52].

Similar results were observed for Ni and Co complexes with CA. Both of them are essential trace elements for the human body, but scarce data is available on the cytotoxic and prooxidant activity of Co and Ni in the presence of natural antioxidants such as polyphenolic compounds. Chen et al. indicated that Ni complexes with polyphenolic ligands exhibited three times stronger responses than a parent compound in the human colon carcinoma cell line (SW620) and the lowest IC_{50} values against the human breast carcinoma cell line (MDA-MB-435) [19]. Our results indicated statistically significant response in MDA-MB-231 breast cancer cell line viability observed as a decrease in analyzed parameter especially after 24 h treatment with CA–Ni complexes. Chen et al. noticed also that anti-proliferative activities of polyphenol–metal complexes were stronger than cisplatin, which was used as a positive control in this experiment. Nickel complexes with CA, similarly as in the case of CA–Zn complexes, were significantly efficient against melanoma, colorectal adenocarcinoma, and glioblastoma cell lines, as compared to three analyzed breast cancer cell lines, which were more resistant to studied compounds. Song et al. suggested that affinity of Ni complexes to DNA may play an important role in determining their anticancer activity [53]. It is possible that complexes synthesized in our laboratory also act through inducing alterations in the DNA structure. However, even though literature data indicate that complexes of polyphenols with selected metals are selective towards cancerous cells over normal cells, we observed different effects. In normal healthy fibroblasts CA–metal complexes exhibited a significant toxicity level as compared to control untreated cells and as compared to free CA. Similarly, as we have shown in our previous work, CA has positive influence on normal healthy cells, stimulating their proliferation and decreasing oxidative stress level, even in the presence of strong prooxidants [22].

According to Baile et al. the most effective are copper complexes where pyridine-type ligands (pyridine, bipyridine, phenanthroline, etc.) are present and such where copper(I) ion is coordinated to phosphine ligands. Copper complexes exhibit an excellent antiproliferative effects in cancer cells, which may result from their ability to generate reactive oxygen species [4]. Our results are also in accordance with the other literature data indicating that cichoric acid has a strong growth inhibitory effect against cancer cells resulting from pro-apoptotic effect [54]. We observed that the addition of metals significantly enhanced antiproliferative activity of CA, therefore we conclude that CA–metal complexes have higher efficacy than free polyphenol compound. Literature data showed that daily consumption of *Echinacea*, which is a main source of CA, may be a prophylactic and attenuates leukemia studied in mouse models [55]. In conclusion, the most significant response for CA and CA–metal complexes treatment among three breast cancer cell lines we observed in MCF-7 and ZR-75-1 cell lines. In the MDA-MB-231 cell line we didn't observe any significant changes as compared to control untreated cells. In general, among all tested cancer cell lines, breast cancer cells were more resistant to studied compounds that the other types of cancer cells.

Although cichoric acid reveals many beneficial properties and its complexes with selected metals exhibit anticancer and antibacterial properties, it should be mentioned that according to the literature data bioavailability of hydroxycinnamic acids is rather low. Majority of studies regarding hydroxycinnamic acids bioavailability are focused in caffeic acid and chlorogenic acid. The definition of bioaccessibility consists mainly of the estimation of relative amounts of compound which could be released from the food matrix during digestion and could be available for absorption. Literature data indicate that cichoric acid is characterized by rather low bioaccessibility, which is very low in the mouth and stomach steps, but it recovers during the intestinal digestion phase, probably because of the pH changes [56].

Complexing drugs with metals is a well-known and common procedure that has been gaining more and more attention in recent years. Complexing some therapeutic compounds, such as polyphenols, can improve their physicochemical and pharmacological properties or reduce their potential side effects. In general, phenolic compounds are often and effectively used to form chelate complexes with various metal ions [57,58].

5. Conclusions

In conclusion, the results of the presented study demonstrated, for the first time, that the treatment with newly synthesized CA-metal complexes has anticancer and antimicrobial effects, which was demonstrated in seven different cell lines, five bacterial strains, and pathogenic yeast-like fungi *C. albicans* and yeast *S. boulardii*. The presented study indicates that CA–metal complexes could be potentially effective supplementary tools in anticancer therapy; however they should be used with caution and their activity should be analyzed in other normal healthy cell lines. This is due to their potentially toxic action in fibroblast cells. They have also preservative properties and positive influence on normal non-pathogenic microorganisms, which was demonstrated in selected microbial strains, therefore they may serve as food preservatives of natural origin with cytoprotective properties. There is a huge amount of research and literature data on the anti-tumor effects of polyphenolic compounds. However, although complexing these compounds with selected metals significantly improves their anti-cancer activity, the amount of research conducted on complexes of polyphenols with metals is much smaller. Moreover, none of these complexes have yet entered the phase of clinical trials. This may be due to many problems caused by the presence of a metal ion; among others, an important problem is the stability of such compounds and their solubility in physiological solvents. Therefore, further studies are necessary to determine the mechanisms by which the analyzed compounds affect a reduction in viability of tumor cells and in normal cells, and cells of bacterial and fungal origins.

Author Contributions: A.J.-T.—corresponding author; wrote the paper; planned experiments; performed experiments on human cell lines; analyzed the data. U.W.—planned and performed bacterial and fungal experiments; statistical analysis; analyzed the data. E.W.—planned and performed bacterial and fungal experiments; analyzed the data. G.Ś.—planned and performed chemical analysis; analyzed the data. W.L.—analyzed the data. All authors have read and agreed to the published version of the manuscript.

Funding: This work was financially supported by National Science Centre, Poland, under the research project number 2015/17/B/NZ9/03 581.

Conflicts of Interest: The authors declare no conflict of interest. Compliance with ethical standards: The manuscript does not contain clinical studies or patient data.

References

1. Lee, J.; Scagel, C. Chicoric acid: Chemistry, distribution, and production. *Front. Chem.* **2013**, *1*, 40. [CrossRef] [PubMed]
2. Nishimura, H.; Satoh, A. Antimicrobial and nematicidal substances from the root of chicory (Cichorium intybus). *Allelochem. Biol. Control Plant Pathog. Dis.* **2006**, *2*, 177–180.
3. Cheynier, V.; Comte, G.; Davies, K.M.; Lattanzio, V.; Martens, S. Plant phenolics: Recent advances on their biosynthesis, genetics, and ecophysiology. *Plant Physiol. Biochem.* **2013**, *72*, 1–20. [CrossRef]
4. Barnes, J.; Anderson, L.A.; Gibbons, S.; Phillipson, J.D. Echinacea species (Echinacea angustifolia (DC.) Hell., Echinacea pallida (Nutt.) Nutt., Echinacea purpurea (L.) Moench): A review of their chemistry, pharmacology and clinical properties. *J. Pharm. Pharmacol.* **2005**, *57*, 929–954. [CrossRef] [PubMed]
5. Kim, J.S.; Lee, H.; Jung, C.H.; Lee, S.J.; Ha, T.Y.; Ahn, J. Chicoric acid mitigates impaired insulin sensitivity by improving mitochondrial function. *Biosci. Biotechnol. Biochem.* **2018**, *82*, 1197–1206. [CrossRef]
6. Zhu, D.; Zhang, X.; Niu, Y.; Diao, Z.; Ren, B.; Li, X.; Liu, Z.; Liu, X. Cichoric acid improved hyperglycaemia and restored muscle injury via activating antioxidant response in MLD-STZ-induced diabetic mice. *Food Chem. Toxicol.* **2017**, *107*, 138–149. [CrossRef]
7. Tsai, K.L.; Kao, C.L.; Hung, C.H.; Cheng, Y.H.; Lin, H.C.; Chu, P.M. Chicoric acid is a potent anti-atherosclerotic ingredient by anti-oxidant action and anti-inflammation capacity. *Oncotarget* **2017**, *8*, 29600–29612. [CrossRef]
8. Mokhtar, M.; Ginestra, G.; Youcefi, F.; Filocamo, A.; Bisignano, C.; Riazi, A. Antimicrobial Activity of Selected Polyphenols and Capsaicinoids Identified in Pepper (Capsicum annuum L.) and Their Possible Mode of Interaction. *Curr. Microbiol.* **2017**, *74*, 1253–1260. [CrossRef]
9. Smith, N.A.; Sadler, P.J. Photoactivatable Metal Complexes: From Theory to Applications in Biotechnology and Medicine. *Philos. Trans. R. Soc. A* **2013**, *371*, 20120519. [CrossRef]
10. Sanna, D.; Ugone, V.; Lubinu, G.; Micera, G.; Garribba, E. Behavior of the potential antitumor V(IV)O complexes formed by flavonoid ligands. 1. Coordination modes and geometry in solution and at the physiological pH. *J. Inorg. Biochem.* **2014**, *140*, 173–184. [CrossRef]
11. Sanna, D.; Ugone, V.; Pisano, L.; Serra, M.; Micera, G.; Garribba, E. Behavior of the potential antitumor V(IV)O complexes formed by flavonoid ligands. 2. Characterization of sulfonate derivatives of quercetin and morin, interaction with the bioligands of the plasma and preliminary biotransformation studies. *J. Inorg. Biochem.* **2015**, *153*, 167–177. [CrossRef] [PubMed]
12. Sanna, D.; Ugone, V.; Fadda, A.; Micera, G.; Garribba, E. Behavior of the potential antitumor V(IV)O complexes formed by flavonoid ligands. 3. Antioxidant properties and radical production capability. *J. Inorg. Biochem.* **2016**, *161*, 18–26. [CrossRef] [PubMed]

13. Leone, A.; Mercer, J.F.B. *Copper Transport and Its Disorders, Molecular and Cellular Aspects*; Springer Science & Business Media: Berlin/Heidelberg, Germany, 1999; Volume 448, ISBN 978-1-4613-7204-2.
14. Łodyga-Chruscińska, E.; Pilo, M.; Zucca, A.; Garribba, E.; Klewicka, E.; Rowińska-Żyrek, M.; Symonowicz, M.; Chruściński, L.; Cheshchevik, V.T. Physicochemical, antioxidant, DNA cleaving properties and antimicrobial activity of fisetin-copper chelates. *J. Inorg. Biochem.* **2018**, *180*, 101–118. [CrossRef] [PubMed]
15. Hadi, S.M.; Ullah, M.F.; Azmi, A.S.; Ahmad, A.; Shamim, U.; Zubair, H.; Khan, H.Y. Resveratrol mobilizes endogenous copper in human peripheral lymphocytes leading to oxidative DNA breakage: A putative mechanism for chemoprevention of cancer. *Pharm. Res.* **2010**, *27*, 979–988. [CrossRef]
16. Capo, C.R.; Pedersen, J.Z.; Falconi, M.; Rossi, L. Oleuropein shows copper complexing properties and noxious effect on cultured SH-SY5Y neuroblastoma cells depending on cell copper content. *J. Trace Elem. Med. Biol.* **2017**, *44*, 225–232. [CrossRef]
17. Dias, K.; Nikolaou, S. Does the combination of resveratrol with Al (III) and Zn (II) improve its antioxidant activity? *Nat. Prod. Commun.* **2011**, *6*, 1673–1676. [CrossRef]
18. Xu, Y.; Qian, L.L.; Yang, J.; Han, R.M.; Zhang, J.P.; Skibsted, L.H. Kaempferol Binding to Zinc(II), Efficient Radical Scavenging through Increased Phenol Acidity. *J. Phys. Chem. B* **2018**, *122*, 10108–10117. [CrossRef]
19. Chen, X.; Tang, L.J.; Sun, Y.N.; Qiu, P.H.; Liang, G.J. Syntheses, characterization and antitumor activities of transition metal complexes with isoflavones. *J. Inorg. Biochem.* **2010**, *104*, 379–384. [CrossRef]
20. Bravo, A.; Anacona, J.R. Metal complexes of the flavonoid quercetin: Antibacterial properties. *Transit. Met. Chem.* **2001**, *26*, 20–23. [CrossRef]
21. Zhou, J.; Wang, L.; Wang, J.; Tang, N. Synthesis, characterization, antioxidative and antitumor activities of solid quercetin rare earth(III) complexes. *J. Inorg. Biochem.* **2001**, *83*, 41–48. [CrossRef]
22. Jabłońska-Trypuć, A.; Krętowski, R.; Kalinowska, M.; Świderski, G.; Cechowska-Pasko, M.; Lewandowski, W. Possible Mechanisms of the Prevention of Doxorubicin Toxicity by Cichoric Acid—Antioxidant Nutrient. *Nutrients* **2018**, *10*, 44. [CrossRef] [PubMed]
23. Świsłocka, R.; Regulska, E.; Karpińska, J.; Świderski, G.; Lewandowski, W. Molecular Structure and Antioxidant Properties of Alkali Metal Salts of Rosmarinic Acid. Experimental and DFT Studies. *Molecules* **2019**, *24*, 2645. [CrossRef] [PubMed]
24. Frisch, M.; Trucks, G.W.; Schlegel, H.B.; Scuseria, G.E.; Robb, M.A.; Cheeseman, J.R.; Scalmani, G.; Barone, V.; Mennucci, B.; Petersson, G.A. *Gaussian 09, Revision A. 02*; Gaussian Inc.: Wallingford, CT, USA, 2009.
25. Kuban-Jankowska, A.; Sahu, K.K.; Gorska, M.; Tuszynski, J.A.; Wozniak, M. Chicoric acid binds to two sites and decreases the activity of the YopH bacterial virulence factor. *Oncotarget* **2016**, *7*, 2229–2238. [CrossRef] [PubMed]
26. Campos, F.M.; Couto, J.A.; Hogg, T.A. Influence of phenolic acids on growth and inactivation of Oenococcus oeni and Lactobacillus hilgardii. *J. Appl. Microbiol.* **2003**, *94*, 167–174. [CrossRef]
27. Wu, Y.; Bai, J.; Zhong, K.; Huang, Y.; Qi, H.; Jiang, Y.; Gao, H. Antibacterial Activity and Membrane-Disruptive Mechanism of 3-p-trans-Coumaroyl-2-hydroxyquinic Acid, a Novel Phenolic Compound from Pine Needles of Cedrus deodara, against Staphylococcus aureus. *Molecules* **2016**, *21*, 1084. [CrossRef]
28. Qin, F.; Yao, L.; Lu, C.; Li, C.; Zhou, Y.; Su, C.; Chen, B.; Shen, Y. Phenolic composition, antioxidant and antibacterial properties, and in vitro anti-HepG2 cell activities of wild apricot (Armeniaca Sibirica L. Lam) kernel skins. *Food Chem. Toxicol.* **2019**, *129*, 354–364. [CrossRef]
29. Faheim, A.A.; Abdou, S.N.; El-Wahab, Z.H.A. Synthesis and characterization of binary and ternary complexes of Co(II), Ni(II), Cu(II) and Zn(II) ions based on 4-aminotoluene-3-sulfonic acid. *Spectrochim. Acta Part A Mol. Biomol. Spectrosc.* **2013**, *105*, 109–124. [CrossRef]
30. Kavak, D.D.; Kecec, S. Extraction of phenolic antioxidants from Pyrus elaeagrifolia Pallas: Process optimization, investigation of the bioactivity and β-glucuronidase inhibitory potential. *J. Food Meas. Charact.* **2019**, *13*, 2894–2902. [CrossRef]
31. EL Moussaoui, A.; Zahra Jawhari, F.; Almehdi, A.M.; Elmsellem, H.; Fikri Benbrahim, K.; Bousta, D.; Bari, A. Antibacterial, antifungal and antioxidant activity of total polyphenols of Withania frutescens.L. *Bioorg. Chem.* **2019**, *93*, 103337. [CrossRef]
32. Cueva, C.; Mingo, S.; Munoz-Gonzalez, I.; Bustos, I.; Requena, T.; del Campo, R.; Martın-Alvarez, P.J.; Bartolome, B.; Moreno-Arribas, M.V. Antibacterial activity of wine phenolic compounds and oenological extracts against potential respiratory pathogens. *Lett. Appl. Microb.* **2012**, *54*, 557–563. [CrossRef]

33. Wu, T.; He, M.; Zang, X.; Ying, Z.; Qiu, T.; Pan, S.; Xu, X.A. structure–activity relationship study of flavonoids as inhibitors of E. coli by membrane interaction effect. *Biochim. Biophys. Acta* **2013**, *1828*, 2751–2756. [CrossRef] [PubMed]
34. Lou, Z.; Wang, H.; Rao, S.; Sun, J.; Ma, C.; Li, J. p-coumaric acid kills bacteria through dual damage mechanisms. *Food Control* **2012**, *25*, 550–554. [CrossRef]
35. Prasad, V.G.N.V.; Krishna, B.V.; Swamy, P.L.; Rao, T.S.; Rao, G.S. Antibacterial synergy between quercetin and polyphenolic acids against bacterial pathogens of fish. *Asian Pac. J. Trop. Dis.* **2014**, *4*, 326–329. [CrossRef]
36. Anh, H.T.P.; Huang, C.; Huang, C. Intelligent Metal-Phenolic Metallogels as Dressings for Infected Wounds. *Sci. Rep.* **2019**, *9*, 11562. [CrossRef] [PubMed]
37. Gałczyńska, K.; Ciepluch, K.; Madej, Ł.; Kurdziel, K.; Maciejewska, B.; Drulis-Kawa, Z.; Węgierek-Ciuk, A.; Lankoff, A.; Arabski, M. Selective cytotoxicity and antifungal properties of copper(II) and cobalt(II) complexes with imidazole-4-acetate anion or 1-allylimidazole. *Sci. Rep.* **2019**, *9*, 9777. [CrossRef] [PubMed]
38. Castillo, K.F.; Bello-Vieda, N.J.; Nuñez-Dallos, N.G.; Pastrana, H.F.; Celis, A.M.; Restrepo, S.; Hurtado, J.J.; Ávila, A.G. Metal complex derivatives of azole: A study on their synthesis, characterization, and antibacterial and antifungal activities. *J. Braz. Chem. Soc.* **2016**, *27*, 2334–2347. [CrossRef]
39. Lv, Q.; Yan, L.; Jiang, Y. The synthesis, regulation, and functions of sterols in Candida albicans: Well-known but still lots to learn. *Virulence* **2016**, *7*, 649–659. [CrossRef]
40. Murcia, R.A.; Leal, S.M.; Roa, M.V.; Nagles, E.; Muñoz-Castro, A.; Hurtado, J.J. Development of Antibacterial and Antifungal Triazole Chromium(III) and Cobalt(II) Complexes: Synthesis and Biological Activity Evaluations. *Molecules* **2018**, *13*, 23. [CrossRef]
41. Saitta, M.; Curto, S.L.; Salvo, F.; Di Bella, G.; Dugo, G. Gas chromatographic–tandem mass spectrometric identification of phenolic compounds in Sicilian olive oils. *Anal. Chim. Acta* **2002**, *466*, 335–344. [CrossRef]
42. Pham-Huy, L.A.; He, H.; Pham-Huy, C. Free radicals, antioxidants in disease and health. *Int. J. Biomed. Sci.* **2008**, *4*, 89–96.
43. Rangel-Huerta, O.D.; Pastor-Villaescusa, B.; Aguilera, C.M.; Gil, A. A systematic review of the efficacy of bioactive compounds in cardiovascular disease: Phenolic compounds. *Nutrients* **2015**, *29*, 5177–5216. [CrossRef] [PubMed]
44. Park, E.J.; Pezzuto, J.M. Flavonoids in cancer prevention. *Anti-Cancer Agents Med. Chem.* **2012**, *12*, 836–851. [CrossRef] [PubMed]
45. Prochazkova, D.; Bousova, I.; Wilhelmova, N. Antioxidant and prooxidant properties of flavonoids. *Fitoterapia* **2011**, *82*, 513–523. [CrossRef]
46. Hider, R.C.; Liu, Z.D.; Khodr, H.H. Metal chelation of polyphenols. *Methods Enzymol.* **2001**, *335*, 190–203. [PubMed]
47. Eghbaliferiz, S.; Iranshahi, M. Prooxidant Activity of Polyphenols, Flavonoids, Anthocyanins and Carotenoids: Updated Review of Mechanisms and Catalyzing Metals. *Phytother. Res.* **2016**, *30*, 1379–1391. [CrossRef]
48. Watanabe, T.; Kiron, V.; Satoh, S. Trace minerals in fish nutrition. *Aquaculture* **1997**, *151*, 185–207. [CrossRef]
49. Azmi, A.S.; Bhat, S.H.; Hadi, S. Resveratrol–Cu (II) induced DNA breakage in human peripheral lymphocytes: Implications for anticancer properties. *FEBS Lett.* **2005**, *579*, 3131–3135. [CrossRef]
50. Ahmadi, M.; Pup, M.; Olariu, L.; Vermean, H.; Prejbeanu, R. Manganese and zinc overdose-risk of oxidative stress appearance. *Rev. Chim.* **2008**, *59*, 982–985.
51. Borovansky, J.; Blasko, M.; Siracky, J.; Schothorst, A.A.; Smit, N.P.M.; Pavel, S. Cytotoxic interactions of Zn2+ in vitro: Melanoma cells are more susceptible than melanocytes. *Melanoma Res.* **1997**, *7*, 449–453. [CrossRef]
52. Farmer, P.J.; Gidanian, S.; Shahandeh, B.; Di Bilio, A.J.; Tohidian, N.; Meyskens, F.L., Jr. Melanin as a target for melanoma chemotherapy: Pro-oxidant effect of oxygen and metals on melanoma viability. *Pigment Cell Res.* **2003**, *16*, 273–279. [CrossRef]
53. Song, Y.; Yang, P.; Yang, M.; Kang, J.; Qin, S.; Lü, B.; Wang, L. Spectroscopic and voltammetric studies of the cobalt (II) complex of Morin bound to calf thymus DNA. *Transit. Met. Chem.* **2003**, *28*, 712–716. [CrossRef]
54. Baile, M.B.; Kolhe, N.S.; Deotarse, P.P.; Jain, A.S.; Kulkarni, A.A. Metal Ion Complex -Potential Anticancer Drug- A Review. *IJPRR* **2015**, *4*, 59–66.
55. Miller, S.C. Echinacea: A miracle herb against aging and cancer? Evidence in vivo in mice. *Evid. Based Complement. Altern. Med.* **2005**, *2*, 309–314. [CrossRef] [PubMed]

56. Lee, H.J.; Cha, K.H.; Kim, C.Y.; Nho, C.W.; Pan, C.H. Bioavailability of hydroxycinnamic acids from Crepidiastrum denticulatum using simulated digestion and Caco-2 intestinal cells. *J. Agric. Food Chem.* **2014**, *23*, 5290–5295. [CrossRef] [PubMed]
57. Ronconi, L.; Sadler, P. Using coordination chemistry to design new Medicines. *Coord. Chem. Rev.* **2007**, *251*, 1633–1648. [CrossRef]
58. Pereira, R.M.; Andrades, N.E.; Paulino, N.; Sawaya, A.C.; Eberlin, M.N.; Marcucci, M.C.; Favero, G.M.; Novak, E.M.; Bydlowski, S.P. Synthesis and characterization of a metal complex containing naringin and Cu, and its antioxidant, antimicrobial, antiinflammatory and tumor cell cytotoxicity. *Molecules* **2007**, *12*, 1352–1366. [CrossRef] [PubMed]

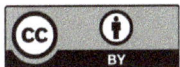

© 2020 by the authors. Licensee MDPI, Basel, Switzerland. This article is an open access article distributed under the terms and conditions of the Creative Commons Attribution (CC BY) license (http://creativecommons.org/licenses/by/4.0/).

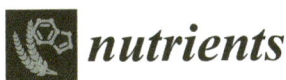

Article

Soluble Extracts from Chia Seed (*Salvia hispanica* L.) Affect Brush Border Membrane Functionality, Morphology and Intestinal Bacterial Populations In Vivo (*Gallus gallus*)

Bárbara Pereira da Silva [1], Nikolai Kolba [2], Hércia Stampini Duarte Martino [1], Jonathan Hart [2] and Elad Tako [2,*]

1. Department of Nutrition and Health, Federal University of Viçosa, Viçosa 36570000, Minas Gerais, Brazil; barbarapereira2805@gmail.com (B.P.d.S.); hercia72@gmail.com (H.S.D.M.)
2. USDA-ARS, Robert W. Holley Center for Agriculture and Health, Cornell University, Ithaca, NY 14853, USA; nikolai.kolba@ars.usda.gov (N.K.); jjh16@cornell.edu (J.H.)
* Correspondence: elad.tako@ars.usda.gov or et79@cornell.edu; Tel.: +1-607-255-5434

Received: 6 August 2019; Accepted: 20 September 2019; Published: 14 October 2019

Abstract: This study assessed and compared the effects of the intra-amniotic administration of various concentrations of soluble extracts from chia seed (*Salvia hispanica* L.) on the Fe and Zn status, brush border membrane functionality, intestinal morphology, and intestinal bacterial populations, in vivo. The hypothesis was that chia seed soluble extracts will affect the intestinal morphology, functionality and intestinal bacterial populations. By using the *Gallus gallus* model and the intra-amniotic administration approach, seven treatment groups (non-injected, 18 Ω H_2O, 40 mg/mL inulin, non-injected, 5 mg/mL, 10 mg/mL, 25 mg/mL and 50 mg/mL of chia seed soluble extracts) were utilized. At hatch, the cecum, duodenum, liver, pectoral muscle and blood samples were collected for assessment of the relative abundance of the gut microflora, relative expression of Fe- and Zn-related genes and brush border membrane functionality and morphology, relative expression of lipids-related genes, glycogen, and hemoglobin levels, respectively. This study demonstrated that the intra-amniotic administration of chia seed soluble extracts increased ($p < 0.05$) the villus surface area, villus length, villus width and the number of goblet cells. Further, we observed an increase ($p < 0.05$) in zinc transporter 1 (ZnT1) and duodenal cytochrome b (Dcytb) proteins gene expression. Our results suggest that the dietary consumption of chia seeds may improve intestinal health and functionality and may indirectly improve iron and zinc intestinal absorption.

Keywords: intra amniotic (in ovo) administration; zinc gene expression; iron gene expression; brush border membrane functional genes; intestinal bacterial populations; villus surface area

1. Introduction

Micronutrient deficiency affects approximately two billion people worldwide. Iron (Fe) and zinc (Zn) deficiencies are the most prevalent, affecting approximately 45% and 17%, respectively, of the world population [1–3]. Both mineral deficiencies are more prevalent in Africa, South East Asia and Latin America [4,5]. Among the dietary factors that contribute to Fe and Zn deficiencies is their low bioavailability due to dietary potential inhibitors, such as phytic acid and phenolic compounds [2,6,7]. Dietary Fe and Zn deficiencies affect normal cell division and differentiation, as well as growth and development, impair physical and cognitive development, and increase the risk of infection [4,7,8].

We have previously established the *Gallus gallus* as a model to assess dietary Fe and Zn bioavailability [9–15]. In addition, this experimental model presents a complex gut microbiota [16], as the phylum level was shown to be similar to humans [17,18]. Further, the intra amniotic administration method has been widely used and demonstrates the potential prebiotic effects of soluble fibers from beans, chickpeas, lentil and wheat, with demonstrated effects on the intestinal functionality, morphology, and microbial populations [10,13,15].

Prebiotics are dietary substrates that selectively promote the proliferation and/or activity of health-promoting bacterial populations in the colon [19,20]. The soluble extracts are obtained by the isolation process of the prebiotics of the food matrix and are composed for the most part of soluble fiber. The most commonly used prebiotics, as inulin, raffinose and stachyose, are dietary fibers with a well-investigated and proven ability to promote the abundance of intestinal bacterial populations, which may provide additional health benefit to the host [21]. It is known that soluble extracts are responsible for improving gastrointestinal motility [22,23], intestinal functionality and intestinal morphology [10,13,24,25], and improving mineral absorption [10,26]. Recent Studies have shown that the consumption of plant seed origin soluble extracts can up regulate the gene expression of brush border membrane (BBM) proteins that contribute to the digestion and absorption of nutrients, such as sucrase-isomaltase, aminopeptidase and sodium glucose cotransporter-1 [10,11,13]. Further, soluble extracts can positively affect intestinal health by increasing mucus production, goblet cell number, goblet cell diameter, villus surface area, villus height, villus width, and crypt depth [10,13,15,27,28]. These functional and morphological effects appears to occur due to the increased motility of the digestive tract by the soluble extracts, leading to hyperplasia and/or hypertrophy of muscle cells [29]. In addition, plant origin soluble extract (with high fiber content and, therefore, potential prebiotic properties) administration may act, directly or indirectly, as a factor that increases iron and zinc bioavailability [30–32]. This event occurs due the lower intestine (colon) fiber fermentation process and the bacterial production of short-chain fatty acids (SCFAs) that reduce the intestinal pH, inhibiting the growth of potentially pathogenic bacterial populations and increasing the solubility and, therefore, the absorption of minerals [10,26]. The SCFAs can increase the proliferation of epithelial cells, which, in return, increases the absorptive surface area, which contributes to the absorption of dietary minerals [33]. Also, it was previously shown that the consumption of soluble extracts has a synergistic effect, as it promotes the metabolic interactions within the gastrointestinal microbial community via the production of organic acids, which provide an acidic environment in the colon, indirectly suppressing the growth of pathogens [34].

The use of iron- and zinc-rich foods may be a good strategy aimed to reduce the prevalence of iron and zinc deficiencies, respectively. Chia (*Salvia hispanica* L.) is an herbaceous plant with good nutritional and functional value with high concentrations of bioactive compounds such as dietary fiber and minerals, including iron and zinc [35]. Although iron and zinc are present in high concentrations, it is important to take into account the bioavailability of these minerals [36]. In the present study, chia was chosen as the soluble extract source, since the consumption of chia bacame extensively common worldwide, and specifically consumed with increasing amounts in Mexico, Argentina, Chile, New Zealand, Japan, USA, Canada and Australia [37], as in some of these geographical regions (e.g., South America), dietary Fe and Zn deficiencies are a major health concern [4,5]. Thus, the primary objective of this study was to assess the effects of the intra-amniotic administration of chia soluble extracts with a putative prebiotic effect on Fe and Zn status and brush border membrane functionality, in vivo. A secondary objective was to evaluate the effects of the tested extracts on intestinal bacterial populations. The third objective was to evaluate the effects of the chia soluble extracts on intestinal morphology. We hypothesized that the chia soluble extracts will affect the intestinal morphology, functionality and bacterial populations.

2. Material and Methods

2.1. Sample Preparation

Chia seeds (*Salvia hispanica* L.) grown in the state of Mato Grosso (Brazil) were used for this study. To obtain the flour, the seeds were ground up in three replicates, using a knife mill (Marconi Equipment,

Algodoal, Brazil), to a particle size of 850 μm. Subsequently, chia flour was packed in polyethylene aluminum bags and stored in a freezer (−20 °C) until analysis.

2.2. Polyphenols Analysis

2.2.1. Chia Sample Preparation

A volume of 5 mL of methanol:water (50:50 *v/v*) was added to 0.5 g of chia flour. The resulting slurry was vortexed for 1 min before incubation in a 24 °C sonication water bath for 20 min at room temperature. Samples were again vortexed and placed on a rocker at room temperature for 60 min before centrifuging at 4000× *g* for 15 min. Supernatants were filtered with a 0.2 μm PTFE syringe filter and stored at −20 °C for later use.

2.2.2. Liquid Chromatography–Mass Spectrometry (LC-MS) Analysis

Extracts and standards were analyzed by an Agilent 1220 Infinity Liquid Chromatograph (LC; Agilent Technologies, Inc., Santa Clara, CA, USA) coupled to an Advion expressionL® compact mass spectrometer (CMS; Advion Inc., Ithaca, NY, USA). Ten-microliter samples were injected and passed through an XBridge Shield RP18 3.5 μm 2.1 × 100 mm column (Waters, Milford, MA, USA) at 0.6 mL/min. The column was temperature-controlled at 40 °C. The mobile phase consisted of ultra-pure water with 0.1% formic acid (solvent A) and acetonitrile with 0.1% formic acid (solvent B). Polyphenols were eluted using linear gradients of 94.0 to 84.4% A in 1.50 min, 84.4 to 81.5% A in 2.25 min, 81.5 to 77.0% A in 6.25 min, 77.0 to 55.0% in 1.25 min, 55.0 to 46.0% in 2.25 min, 46.0 to 94.0% in 2.25 min and hold at 94.0% A for 2.25 min for a total run time of 18 min. From the column, the flow was directed into a variable wavelength Ultraviolet (UV) detector set at 280 nm. The flow was then directed into the source of an Advion expressionL® CMS, and Electrospray ionization (ESI) mass spectrometry was performed in the negative ionization mode using selected ion monitoring with a scan time of 200 ms. The capillary temperature and voltages were 250 °C and 180 volts, respectively. The ESI source voltage and gas temperature were 2.5 kilovolts and 250 °C, respectively. The desolvation gas flow was 240 L/h. Advion Mass Express™ software (Advidon, Ithaca, USA) was used to control the LC and compact mass spectrometers (CMS) instrumentation and data acquisition. Individual polyphenols were identified and confirmed by comparison of *m/z* and LC retention times with authentic standards. The analysis of MS and UV data was performed using Advion Data Express™ software (Advidon, Ithaca, USA).

2.3. Extraction of Soluble Extracts from Chia

The extraction of prebiotics was performed according to Tako et al. [14], Hou et al. [13] and Pacific et al. [10]. Chia flour samples were dissolved in distilled water (50 g/L) (60 °C, 60 min) and centrifuged at 3000 rpm (4 °C) for 25 min, and then the supernatant was collected. The supernatant was then dialyzed (MWCO 12–14 kDa) (48 h) against distilled water. The dialysate was collected and lyophilized to yield a fine off-white powder [12].

2.4. Phytate, Dietary Fiber, Iron and Zinc Analysis in Chia Seeds and Chia Extract

Dietary phytic acid (phytate)/total phosphorous was measured as phosphorus released by phytase and alkaline phosphatase, according to manufacturer's instructions (*n* = 5) (K-PHYT 12/12. Megazyme International, Bray, Ireland). The determination of total fiber and soluble and insoluble fractions was performed by the enzymatic-gravimetric method according to AOAC [38], using enzymatic hydrolysis for a heat-resistant amylase, protease and amyloglucosidase (Total dietary fiber assay Kiyonaga, Sigma®, Kawasaki, Japan). For the determination of iron and zinc, chia seed and chia extract (0.5 g) were treated with 3.0 mL of a 60:40 HNO_3 and $HClO_4$ mixture in a Pyrex glass tube and left overnight to destroy organic matter. The analyses were performed using an inductively coupled plasma atomic emission spectrometer (ICP-AES) (Thermo iCAP 6500 series, Thermo Jarrell Ash Corp., Franklin, MA, USA) [12,28].

2.5. Animals and Design

Cornish-cross fertile broiler eggs ($n = 105$) were obtained from a commercial hatchery (Moyer's chicks, Quakertown, PA, USA). The eggs were incubated under optimal conditions at the Cornell University Animal Science poultry farm incubator. All animal protocols were approved by the Cornell University Institutional Animal Care and Use committee (ethic approval code: 2007-0129).

Intra Amniotic Administration

Lyophilized soluble extracts were diluted in 18 Ω H_2O and for sample osmolarity determination (≤320 OSM). At 17 days of embryonic incubation, eggs containing viable embryos were weighed and divided into 7 groups ($n = 15$). All treatment groups were assigned eggs of a similar weight frequency distribution. Each group was then injected with the specified solution (1 mL per egg), using a 21 gauge needle into the amniotic fluid, which was identified by candling. The 7 groups were assigned as follows: (1) non-injected; (2) 18 Ω H_2O; (3) inulin (40 mg/mL); (4) chia seed extract 0.5% (5 mg/mL); (5) chia seed extract 1% (10 mg/mL); (6) chia seed extract 2.5%; (7) chia seed extract 5% (50 mg/mL). After the injections, the holes were sealed with cellophane tape and the eggs were placed in hatching baskets. Immediately after hatch (21 days), the chicks were euthanized by CO_2 exposure and their small intestine, blood, pectoral muscle, cecum and liver were collected.

2.6. Iron and Zinc Content in Serum and Liver

Liver (0.5 g) and serum (50 µL) were treated with 3.0 mL of a 60:40 HNO_3 and $HClO_4$ mixture in a Pyrex glass tube and were incubated overnight. The mixture was then heated to 120 °C for two hours and 0.25 mL of 40 µg/g Yttrium was added as an internal standard. Next, the temperature of the heating block was raised to 145 °C for 2 h. Then, for 10 min, the temperature of the heating block was raised to 190 °C. The cooled samples were then diluted to 20 mL, vortexed and transferred into autosampler tubes to be analyzed via inductively coupled plasma atomic emission spectrometer (ICP-AES). (Thermo Jarrell Ash Corp., Franklin, MA, USA) [12,28].

2.7. Isolation of Total RNA from Duodenum and Liver

Total RNA was extracted from 30 mg of the proximal duodenal tissue or liver tissue ($n = 10$) using Qiagen RNeasy Mini Kit (RNeasy Mini Kit, Qiagen Inc., Valencia, CA, USA) according to the manufacturer's protocol. Total RNA was eluted in 50 µL of RNase-free water. All steps were carried out under RNase-free conditions. RNA was quantified by absorbance at A 260/280 and the integrity of the 18S ribosomal RNAs was verified by 1.5% agarose gel electrophoresis followed by ethidium bromide staining. RNA was stored at −80 °C.

2.8. Real Time Polymerase Chain Reaction (RT-PCR)

To create the cDNA, a 20 µL reverse transcriptase (RT) reaction was completed in a BioRad C1000 touch thermocycler using the Improm-II Reverse Transcriptase Kit (Catalog #A1250; Promega, Madison, WI, USA). The concentration of cDNA obtained was determined by measuring the absorbance at 260 and 280 nm using an extinction coefficient of 33 (for single stranded DNA). Genomic DNA contamination was assessed by a real-time RT-PCR assay for the reference gene samples [12].

2.9. Primer Design

The primers used in the real-time qPCR were designed based on 13 gene sequences from the Genbank database, using Real-Time Primer Design Tool software (IDT DNA, Coralvilla, IA, USA). The sequences and the description of the primers used in this work are summarized in Table 1.

The specificity of the primers was tested by performing a BLAST search against the genomic National Center for Biotechnology Information (NCBI) database. The *Gallus gallus* primer 18S rRNA was designed as a reference gene. Results obtained from the qPCR system were used to normalize those obtained from the specific systems as described below.

Table 1. The sequences of the primers used in this study.

Analyte	Forward Primer (5′–3′)	Reverse Primer (5′–3′)	Base Pair	GI Identifier
DMT1	TTGATTCAGAGCCTCCCATTAG	GCGAGGAGTAGGCTTGTATTT	101	206597489
Ferroportin	CTCAGCAATCACTGGCATCA	ACTGGGCAACTCCAGAAATAAG	98	61098365
Dcytb	CATGTGCATTCTCTTCCAAAGTC	CTCCTTGGTGACCGCATTAT	103	20380692
Hepcidin *	GAGCAAGCCATGTCAAGATTTC	GTCTGGGCCAAGTCTGTTATAG	132	8056490
ZnT1	GGTAACAGAGCTGCCTTAACT	GGTAACAGAGCTGCCTTAACT	105	54109718
SI	CCAGCAATGCCAGCATATTG	CGGTTTCTCCTTACCACTTCTT	95	2246388
AP	CGTCAGCCAGTTTGACTATGTA	CTCTCAAAGAAGCTGAGGATGG	138	45382360
SGLT1	GCATCCTTACTCTGTGGTACTG	TATCCGCACATCACACATCC	106	8346783
LPL *	TGCTCAGATGCCCTACAAAG	TCTCGTCTAGAGTGCCATACA	119	396219
CEL *	ATGCTGCTGACATCGACTAC	TTCTGAAGTGGACGGTTGATAG	97	417165
18S rRNA *	GCAAGACGAACTAAAGCGAAAG	TCGGAACTACGACGGTATCT	100	7262899

DMT1, Divalent metal transporter 1; Dcytb, Duodenal cytochrome b; Znt 1, Zinc transporter 1; SI, Sucrose isomaltase; AP, Amino peptidase; SGLT1, Sodium-Glucose transport protein 1; LPL, Lipoprotein lipase; CEL, Carboxyl ester lipase; 18S rRNA, 18S Ribosomal subunit. * liver analyses.

2.10. Real-Time qPCR Design

All procedures were conducted as previously described [10–13]. The specific primers that were used are shown in Table 1.

2.11. Collection of Microbial Samples and Intestinal Content DNA Isolation

The cecum contents were removed under sterile conditions, placed into a sterile tube containing 9 mL of Phosphate buffered saline (PBS) and homogenized by vortexing with glass beads for 3 min [27,39]. All procedures were conducted as previously described [10–14].

2.12. Primer Design and PCR Amplification of Bacterial 16S rDNA

Primers for *Lactobacillus*, *Bifidobacterium*, *Clostridium* and *Escherichia coli* were used [16,39]. The universal primers were designed with the invariant region in the 16S rRNA of bacteria and were used as internal standards. The proportions of each bacterial group are presented. The PCR products were loaded on 2% agarose gel stained with ethidium bromide and quantified by Quantity One 1-D analysis software (Bio-Rad, Hercules, CA, USA) [12]. The evaluation of the relative abundance of each examined bacterium was conducted as previously described [10–14].

2.13. Glycogen Analysis

At hatch, the pectoral muscle (20 mg) was collected for glycogen analysis. The tissue samples were homogenized in 8% perchloric acid, and glycogen concentration was determined as previously described [40]. After homogenization, the samples were centrifuged at 12,000 rpm at 4 °C for 15 min. The supernatant was removed, and 1.0 mL of petroleum ether was added. After mixing, the petroleum ether fraction was removed, and samples from the bottom layer were transferred to a new tube containing 300 µL of color reagent. All samples were read at a wavelength of 450 nm in an ELISA reader and the amount of glycogen was calculated according to a standard curve. The amount of glycogen present in pectoral sample was determined by multiplying the weight of the tissue by the amount of glycogen per 1 g of wet tissue.

2.14. Morphological Examination

As previously described [10,41], liver and intestine samples were collected at the conclusion of this study. Samples were fixed in 4% (v/v) buffered formaldehyde, dehydrated, cleared, and embedded in paraffin. Serial sections of 5 μm were obtained and were deparaffinized in xylene, rehydrated in a different concentration of alcohol, stained with hematoxylin/eosin or Alcian Blue/Periodic acid-Schiff, and examined by light microscopy. The following variables were measured in the intestine: villus height, villus width, depth of crypts, goblet cell number and goblet cell diameter in each segment, performed with a light microscope using EPIX XCAP software (Standard version, Olympus, Waltham, MA, USA). Four segments for each biological sample and five biological samples per treatment group were used. Villi height was measured using the lamina propria as the base; villi width, depth of the crypt and the number of goblet cell were measured per side of a longitudinal section through the villus; goblet cell size was measured as the diameter of the goblet cells (μm^2). Villi surface area was calculated from the villus height and width at half height as according to Uni et al. [42]. For the Alcian Blue and Periodic acid-Schiff stain, the segments were only counted for the types of goblet cells in the villi epithelium, goblet cells within the crypts and the mucus layer thickness. Goblet cells were enumerated on 10 villi/sample, and the means were utilized for statistical analysis. The liver was stained with hematoxylin-esoin (H&E) for standard microscopy and visualized using the same light microscope. Mean adipocyte diameter was determined by random, utilizing the EPIX XCAP software (standard version, Olympus, Waltham, MA, USA), by enumerating 10 adipocytes/segment/sample, and the means were utilized for statistical analysis.

2.15. Statistical Analysis

All values are expressed as the means and standard deviations. Experimental treatments for the in ovo assay were arranged in a completely randomized design. The results were analyzed by ANOVA. For significant "p-value", post hoc Duncan test was used to compare test groups. Statistical analysis was carried out using SPSS version 20.0 software (IBM, Armonk, USA). The level of significance was established at $p < 0.05$.

3. Results

3.1. Concentration of Iron, Zinc, Phytic Acid and Dietary Fiber and the Phytate:Iron Ratio in Chia Flour and in Chia Extract

The iron and zinc concentrations, insoluble fiber content, phytic acid and the phytate:iron ratio were higher ($p < 0.05$) in the chia seed compared to the chia extract (Table 2). However, the content of soluble fiber was significantly greater ($p < 0.05$) in the chia extract relative to chia seed.

Table 2. Concentration of iron, zinc, dietary fiber and phytic acid in chia flour and in chia extract.

Treatment Group	Iron (μg/g)	Zinc (μg/g)	Insoluble Fiber (g/100g)	Soluble Fiber (g/100g)	Phytic Acid (g/100g)	Phytic Acid: Iron Ratio
Chia seed	110.25 ± 4.97 [a]	57.82 ± 0.40 [a]	34.67 ± 1.84 [a]	4.01 ± 0.21 [b]	0.71 ± 0.02 [a]	5.47 [a]
Chia extract	41.46 ± 0.89 [b]	31.29 ± 0.89 [b]	23.53 ± 1.74 [b]	19.68 ± 0.76 [a]	0.08 ± 0.00 [b]	1.60 [b]

Values are the means ± SEM, $n = 5$. [a,b] Treatment groups not indicated by the same letter are significantly different ($p < 0.05$).

3.2. Polyphenol Profile in Chia Flour

The concentration of the five most prevalent polyphenolic compounds found in chia is presented in Table 3. Chia presented high concentrations of rosmarinic acid and rosmarinyl glucoside. In addition, we observed the presence of ferulic acid, caffeic acid and protocatechuic acid.

Table 3. Polyphenol profile present in chia flour.

Polyphenolic Compounds	Mean Peak Area (mAU-min/10⁶)
Rosmarinic acid	42.30 ± 1.90
Rosmarinyl glucoside	57.70 ± 0.02
Ferulic acid	1.19 ± 0.06
Caffeic acid	0.76 ± 0.38
Protocatechuic acid	0.21 ± 0.03

Values are the means ± SEM, $n = 10$. mAU: milli absorbance unit; min: minutes.

3.3. In Ovo Assay (Gallus Gallus Model)

3.3.1. Hb Concentration

The Hb values were significantly ($p < 0.05$) higher in the "2.5% chia" extract treatment group compared to the 18 Ω H$_2$O and non-inject group. The other treatments did not differ from each other (Table 4).

Table 4. Blood hemoglobin (Hb) concentrations (g/dL).

Treatment Group	Hb (g/dL)
Non-injected	5.93 ± 0.00 [b]
18 Ω H$_2$O	5.52 ± 1.49 [b]
Inulin	7.76 ± 1.16 [a,b]
0.5% Chia	7.08 ± 1.16 [a,b]
1.0% Chia	9.51 ± 1.34 [a,b]
2.5% Chia	10.41 ± 1.37 [a]
5.0% Chia	10.06 ± 2.48 [a,b]

Values are the means ± SEM, $n = 10$. [a,b] Treatment groups not indicated by the same letter are significantly different ($p < 0.05$).

3.3.2. Iron and Zinc Concentration in Liver and Serum

As shown in Table 5, there were no significant ($p > 0.05$) differences in liver iron concentration and serum zinc concentration between treatment groups. However, "1% chia" extract treatment increased ($p < 0.05$) the zinc liver content compared to non-inject treatment. In addition, we observed that "5% chia" extract treatment showed a lower ($p < 0.05$) serum iron concentration when compared to the 18 Ω H$_2$O and inulin groups. In general, different concentrations of chia extract did not affect iron and zinc concentrations in liver and serum.

Table 5. Iron and zinc concentrations (ppm).

Treatment Group	Liver		Serum	
	Iron (μg/g)	Zinc (μg/g)	Iron (μg/g)	Zinc (μg/g)
Non-injected	35.28 ± 2.52 [a]	14.77 ± 1.26 [b]	3.14 ± 0.25 [a,b,c]	0.001 ± 0.000 [a]
18 Ω H$_2$O	41.00 ± 3.24 [a]	16.10 ± 1.57 [a,b]	4.04 ± 0.52 [a,b]	0.002 ± 0.000 [a]
Inulin	40.92 ± 3.32 [a]	16.39 ± 2.43 [a,b]	4.24 ± 0.96 [a]	0.001 ± 0.000 [a]
0.5% Chia	35.57 ± 3.16 [a]	18.45 ± 1.13 [a,b]	2.99 ± 0.44 [a,b,c]	0.002 ± 0.000 [a]
1.0% Chia	43.17 ± 4.08 [a]	21.63 ± 2.59 [a]	2.36 ± 0.24 [a,b]	0.003 ± 0.001 [a]
2.5% Chia	33.52 ± 1.67 [a]	16.60 ± 1.41 [a,b]	3.23 ± 0.63 [a,b,c]	0.001 ± 0.000 [a]
5.0% Chia	35.88 ± 2.81 [a]	17.87 ± 2.52 [a,b]	1.59 ± 0.29 [c]	0.002 ± 0.000 [a]

Values are the means ± SEM, $n = 10$. [a,b,c] Treatment groups not indicated by the same letter are significantly different ($p < 0.05$).

3.3.3. Gene Expression of Fe- and Zn-Related Genes

The gene expression of DMT1 was lower ($p < 0.05$) in the group treated with 2.5% chia soluble extract compared to the inulin and 18 Ω H$_2$O groups (Figure 1). However, other various concentrations of chia soluble extract did not affect the expression of DMT1 ($p > 0.05$). The relative expression of DcytB and hepcidin was significantly up-regulated ($p < 0.05$) in the 1%, 2.5% and 5% chia extract. The groups treated with 1%, 2.5% and 5% chia extract showed lower ($p > 0.05$) ferroportin gene expression compared to the 18 Ω H_2O injected group. However, no differences ($p > 0.05$) were observed between chia treatment groups. The relative expression of ZnT1 was significantly up-regulated ($p < 0.05$) in the 1%, 2.5% and 5% chia extract.

	DMT1	DcytB	Ferroportin	Hepcidin	ZnT1	AP	SGLT-1	SI	CEL	LpL
Non injected	bc 1.86±0.035	c 8.10±0.130	ab 16.91±0.347	ab 0.94±0.004	b 9.05±0.377	b 2.79±0.056	bc 1.82±0.034	b 4.33±0.069	b 0.90±0.000	ab 0.78±0.005
18 Ω H_2O	a 2.11±0.054	c 8.30±0.136	a 18.27±0.502	a 0.94±0.003	b 9.73±0.180	a 3.05±0.082	a 1.96±0.051	ab 4.56±0.036	b 0.90±0.000	ab 0.78±0.005
5% Inulin	ab 2.05±0.054	c 8.30±0.136	ab 16.84±0.462	a 0.94±0.002	b 8.77±0.375	ab 2.93±0.080	ab 1.91±0.053	ab 4.38±0.090	b 0.89±0.002	ab 0.78±0.004
0.5% Chia	abc 2.02±0.039	c 6.47±0.133	ab 16.92±0.529	a 0.94±0.005	b 10.33±0.239	ab 2.86±0.064	abc 1.88±0.036	ab 4.45±0.066	b 0.90±0.004	ab 0.79±0.005
1% Chia	abc 2.01±0.029	a 9.04±0.129	b 16.63±0.449	bc 0.93±0.005	a 13.00±0.225	ab 2.69±0.048	abc 1.87±0.027	ab 4.53±0.040	b 0.89±0.002	ab 0.78±0.003
2.5% Chia	c 1.93±0.021	b 9.08±0.185	c 16.55±0.671	a 0.92±0.002	a 12.12±0.496	b 2.79±0.039	c 1.70±0.020	b 4.34±0.079	a 0.91±0.005	b 0.77±0.006
5% Chia	abc 2.00±0.020	a 9.94±0.229	b 16.24±0.239	a 0.92±0.005	a 13.22±0.649	b 2.86±0.031	abc 1.06±0.019	a 4.58±0.066	b 0.90±0.004	a 0.79±0.004

Figure 1. Effect of the intra-amniotic administration of experimental solutions on intestinal and liver gene expression. Values are the means ± SEM, $n = 10$. $^{a-c}$ Per gene, treatments groups not indicated by the same letter are significantly different ($p < 0.05$). DMT1, Divalent metal transporter 1; Dcytb, Duodenal cytochrome b; ZnT1, Zinc transporter 1; AP, Amino peptidase; SGLT1, Sodium-Glucose transport protein 1; SI, Sucrase isomaltase; CEL, Carboxyl ester lipase; LpL, Lipoprotein lipase.

3.3.4. Gene Expression of BBM Functional Proteins

The gene expression of aminopeptidase (AP), sodium-glucose transport protein 1 (SGLT1) and sucrase isomaltase (SI) are used as biomarkers of brush border membrane digestive and absorptive functions. AP and SGLT1 gene expression did not differ ($p > 0.05$) between groups treated with chia extract. However, the gene expression of SI was higher ($p < 0.05$) in "5% chia" extract treatment group compared to the "2.5% chia" extract treatment group (Figure 1).

3.3.5. Gene Expression of Lipids Metabolism Protein

The gene expressions of carboxyl ester lipase (CEL) and lipoprotein lipase (LpL) are used as biomarkers of lipid metabolism. As shown in Figure 1, the "2.5% chia" extract treatment group presented higher ($p > 0.05$) CEL expression compared to the control groups. However, the gene expression of LpL did not differ between chia extract groups and control groups ($p < 0.05$).

3.3.6. Cecum-to-Body-Weight Ratio

As shown in Figure 2, the chia soluble extract treatment groups showed a higher ($p < 0.05$) cecum weight (B) and cecum weight/body weight ratio (C) compared to control groups ($p < 0.05$). However, no significant difference ($p > 0.05$) was observed in body weight (A) among treatment groups and controls.

A
B
C
Body Weight (g)
Cecum Weight (g)
Cecum Weight/Body Weight Ratio (%)
Non-inject
18Ω H20
Inulin
0.5% Chia
1% Chia
2.5% Chia
5% Chia

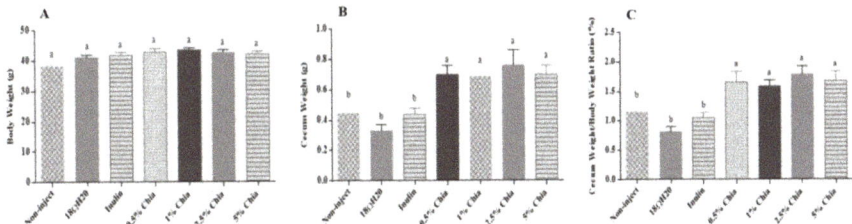

Figure 2. The effect of chia on the: (**A**) body weight; (**B**) cecum weight; and (**C**) cecum weight/body weight ratio (%). Values are the means ± SEM $n = 15$. ^{a,b} Within a column, means without a common letter are significantly different ($p < 0.05$).

3.3.7. Microbial Analysis

As shown in Figure 3, the relative abundance of both *Bifidobacterium* and *Lactobacillus* genera, increased ($p < 0.05$) in the "0.5% chia" treatment, relative to the 18 Ω H_2O group and non-injected group. The "5% chia" treatment group showed a lower ($p < 0.05$) concentration of these bacterial populations compared to the other groups. The relative abundance of *E. coli* significantly decreased ($p < 0.05$) in the 1%, 2.5% and 5% chia extract treatment groups compared to the control groups. The relative abundance of *Clostridium* was significantly ($p < 0.05$) lower in the non-inject group, 18 Ω H_2O group and "5% chia" treatment group. These results suggest that a lower concentration of chia extract may positively affect gut health.

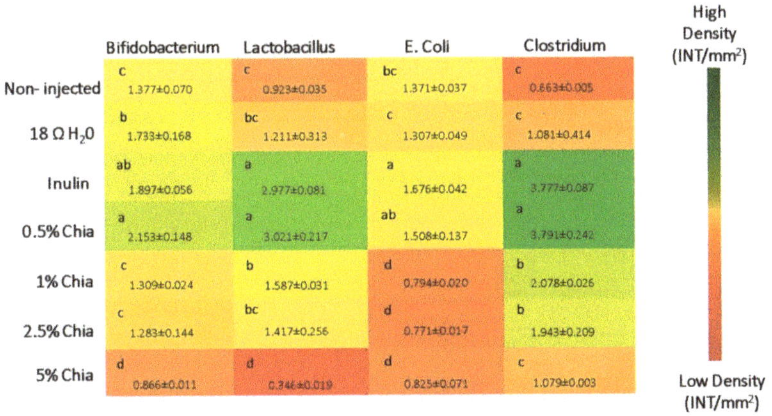

Bifidobacterium
Lactobacillus
E. Coli
Clostridium
Non- injected
c 1.377±0.070
c 0.923±0.035
bc 1.371±0.037
c 0.663±0.005
18 Ω H2O
b 1.733±0.168
bc 1.211±0.313
c 1.307±0.049
c 1.081±0.414
Inulin
ab 1.897±0.056
a 2.977±0.081
a 1.676±0.042
a 3.777±0.087
0.5% Chia
a 2.153±0.148
a 3.021±0.217
ab 1.508±0.137
a 3.791±0.242
1% Chia
c 1.309±0.024
b 1.587±0.031
d 0.794±0.020
b 2.078±0.026
2.5% Chia
c 1.283±0.144
bc 1.417±0.256
d 0.771±0.017
b 1.943±0.209
5% Chia
d 0.866±0.011
d 0.346±0.019
d 0.825±0.071
c 1.079±0.003
High Density (INT/mm2)
Low Density (INT/mm2)

Figure 3. Genera- and species-level bacterial populations (AU) from cecal contents measured on the day of hatch. Values are the means ± SEM, $n = 10$. $^{a\text{–}d}$ Per bacterial category, treatment groups not indicated by the same letter are significantly different.

3.3.8. Glycogen Analysis

No significant difference was observed in pectoral muscle glycogen content between groups (Table 6, $p > 0.05$).

Table 6. Concentration of glycogen in pectoral muscle.

Treatment Group	Glycogen Concentration (mg/g)
Non-injected	0.17 ± 0.04 [a]
18 Ω H_2O	0.21 ± 0.05 [a]
Inulin	0.29 ± 0.06 [a]
0.5% Chia	0.13 ± 0.03 [a]
1.0% Chia	0.31 ± 0.06 [a]
2.5% Chia	0.26 ± 0.08 [a]
5.0% Chia	0.29 ± 0.15 [a]

Values are the means ± SEM, $n = 10$. [a] Treatment groups not indicated by the same letter are significantly different ($p < 0.05$).

3.3.9. Morphometric Data for Villi, Depth of Crypts and Goblet Cell

The villus surface areas, villi length, width and the number of goblet cells were significantly ($p < 0.05$) higher in all chia extract treatment groups compare to controls (Tables 7 and 8), indicating that soluble extracts from chia had a positive effect on intestinal development, through the proliferation of enterocytes, and the increased number in mucus-producing cells. However, there were no significant ($p > 0.05$) differences in crypt depth and mucus layer width between treatment groups. Further, all chia extract treatments increased ($p < 0.05$) the diameter of goblet cells compared to controls. In relation to the types of goblet cells observed (acidic, neutral, mixed), we can note that the administration of 2.5% chia soluble extracts reduced ($p < 0.05$) the number of neutrals goblet cells compared to the control groups. In addition, the administration of 2.5% and 5% chia soluble extracts increased ($p < 0.05$) the number of acidic goblet cells, whereas the administration of 1% and 2.5% chia extract caused an increase ($p < 0.05$) in mixed goblet cells, compared to controls. In relation to the types of goblet cells in the crypt epithelium, the administration of 0.5% chia soluble extract increased ($p < 0.05$) the number of neutrals goblet cells compared to controls. In addition, the administration of 2.5% chia extracts increased ($p < 0.05$) the number of mixed goblet cells compared to controls. The number of acid goblet cells did not differ ($p > 0.05$) between groups (Figure 4). No significant differences between treatment groups were measured in fat cell diameter ($p > 0.05$, Figure 5).

Table 7. Effect of the intra-amniotic administration of experimental solutions on the duodenal small intestinal villus and crypt.

Treatment Group	Villus Surface Area (mm²)	Villus Length (μM)	Villus Width (μM)	Depth of Crypts (μM)	Mucus Layer Width (μM)
Non-injected	170.29 ± 5.33 [c]	248.64 ± 2.83 [c]	43.26 ± 0.42 [c]	12.76 ± 0.10 [a]	2.21 ± 0.27 [a]
18 Ω H_2O	127.13 ± 8.16 [c]	204.30 ± 3.40 [d]	39.24 ± 0.37 [d]	12.60 ± 0.09 [a]	2.32 ± 0.15 [a]
Inulin	130.00 ± 9.42 [c]	208.90 ± 3.63 [d]	41.20 ± 0.56 [c,d]	13.01 ± 0.10 [a]	2.36 ± 0.1 [a]
0.5% Chia	237.53 ± 7.98 [b]	323.85 ± 3.51 [b]	46.42 ± 0.40 [b]	12.49 ± 0.08 [a]	2.41 ± 0.25 [a]
1.0% Chia	234.78 ± 7.36 [b]	298.82 ± 2.43 [b]	49.70 ± 0.51 [b]	13.08 ± 0.09 [a]	2.22 ± 0.10 [a]
2.5% Chia	264.95 ± 2.74 [b]	334.44 ± 5.62 [b]	50.15 ± 0.57 [b]	12.83 ± 0.10 [a]	2.20 ± 0.13 [a]
5.0% Chia	343.93 ± 9.38 [a]	374.47 ± 5.50 [a]	58.18 ± 0.59 [a]	12.71 ± 0.11 [a]	2.15 ± 0.14 [a]

Values are the means ± SEM, $n = 5$. [a–d] Treatment groups not indicated by the same letter are significantly different ($p < 0.05$).

Table 8. Effect of the intra-amniotic administration of experimental solutions on the goblet cells.

Treatment Group	Goblet Cell Diameter (μM)	Total Goblet Cell Number (Unit)	Villus Goblet Cell Number (Unit)			Crypts Goblet Cell Number (Unit)		
			Neutral	Acid	Mixed	Neutral	Acid	Mixed
Non-injected	4.20 ± 0.03 [c]	21.23 ± 0.24 [c]	2.50 ± 0.33 [a,b]	8.77 ± 0.23 [b]	9.11 ± 0.33 [c]	0.01 ± 0.00 [b]	10.36 ± 0.57 [a]	0.47 ± 0.15 [c]
18 Ω H_2O	4.10 ± 0.03 [c]	20.18 ± 0.26 [c]	2.14 ± 0.24 [b]	8.05 ± 0.74 [c]	9.62 ± 0.47 [c]	0.10 ± 0.00 [b]	9.69 ± 0.55 [a]	1.64 ± 0.16 [a]
Inulin	4.89 ± 0.06 [b]	24.88 ± 0.20 [b]	3.90 ± 0.99 [a]	8.67 ± 0.48 [b]	11.02 ± 1.02 [b,c]	0.01 ± 0.00 [b]	10.32 ± 0.36 [a]	0.43 ± 0.14 [c]
0.5% Chia	5.48 ± 0.03 [a,b]	28.59 ± 0.32 [a]	3.63 ± 0.25 [a,b]	10.76 ± 0.71 [a,b]	14.26 ± 0.51 [a]	0.46 ± 0.12 [a]	10.02 ± 0.91 [a]	0.89 ± 0.06 [b,c]
1.0% Chia	5.36 ± 0.05 [a,b]	29.19 ± 0.29 [a]	2.07 ± 0.17 [b]	11.43 ± 0.61 [a,b]	15.55 ± 0.71 [a]	0.09 ± 0.05 [b]	9.65 ± 1.05 [a]	1.30 ± 0.11 [a,b]
2.5% Chia	5.61 ± 0.02 [a]	29.61 ± 0.40 [a]	1.63 ± 0.16 [c]	13.70 ± 1.53 [a]	13.72 ± 1.35 [a]	0.05 ± 0.02 [b]	9.45 ± 0.49 [a]	1.45 ± 0.30 [a]
5.0% Chia	5.42 ± 0.06 [a,b]	29.91 ± 0.39 [a]	2.55 ± 0.43 [a,b]	13.13 ± 1.35 [a]	13.20 ± 1.51 [a,b]	0.18 ± 0.06 [a,b]	9.88 ± 0.13 [a]	0.82 ± 0.21 [b,c]

Values are the means ± SEM, $n = 5$. [a–c] Treatment groups not indicated by the same letter are significantly different ($p < 0.05$).

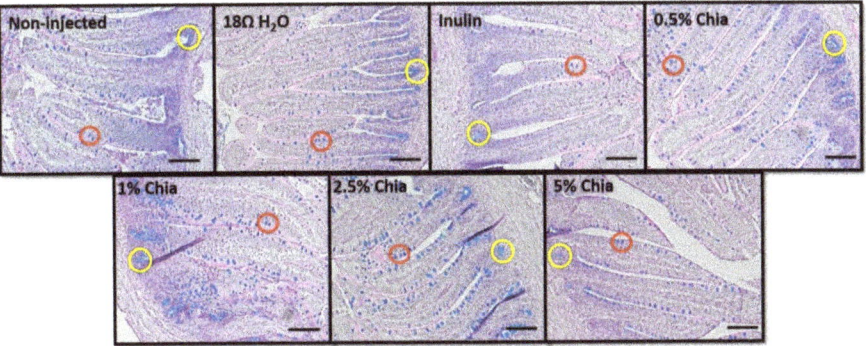

Figure 4. Representations of the intestinal morphology of each treatment group are shown (Alcian Blue and Periodic acid-Schiff Stain). The yellow circles indicate crypts within the villi and the red circles indicate goblet cells on the villi. Bar = 50 μm.

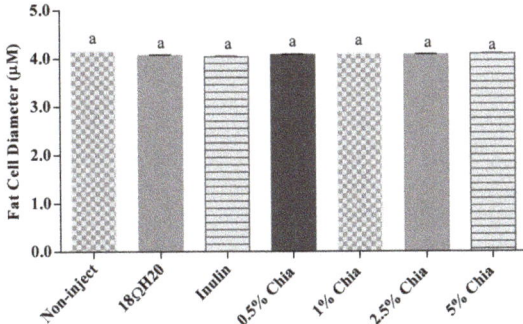

Figure 5. Fat cell diameter. Values are the means ± SEM, $n = 5$. [a] Treatment groups not indicated by the same letter are significantly different.

3.3.10. Hepatic Morphometric Measurement

As shown in Figure 4, no significant differences were observed in hepatic fat cell diameter between all treatment groups ($p > 0.05$).

4. Discussion

Chia is a good source of dietary fiber, which was demonstrated to have a beneficial effect on intestinal health [29]. However, until now, the potential effects of soluble extracts from chia seed on the intestinal microbiota, intestinal morphology and mineral bioavailability, such as iron and zinc, were not investigated. Further, it is important to highlight that the alterations in microbiota populations, due the consumption of dietary fiber, may be associated, directly or indirectly, to the increased dietary bioavailability of iron and zinc in vulnerable populations [13,15,18,27]. The present study indicates that the in ovo administration of soluble extracts from chia seed increased the intestinal villus surface area, villi length, villi width, goblet cell number and goblet cell size (diameter), as well as cecum weight (used as biomarker of microbial presence and activity). In addition, the administration of chia seed soluble extracts up-regulated the expression of proteins related to zinc metabolism. Further, the chia soluble extract (0.5%) increased the *Bifidobacterium* and *Lactobacillus* relative abundance in cecum content.

According to our results, the hemoglobin concentration results corroborate with our findings of serum iron. We did not observe a change in liver iron concentrations, due to the short time of exposure of the soluble extracts, which was not sufficient to cause a modification in hepatic iron storage. This was in agreement with previous observations that evaluated the effects of intra-amniotic raffinose and stachyose administration on Fe status, as the results showed no significant differences in hemoglobin values between treatment groups [10]. Further, another study that assessed the effect of the intra-amniotic administration of bean soluble extracts on iron status indicated that bean extracts did not affect serum or liver iron concentrations [12]. A similar result was observed post intra-amniotic administration of wheat extracts [14]. In addition, a BBM Fe metabolism-related gene expression analysis of DcytB, DMT, ferroportin and hepcidin was conducted. DcytB is the protein responsible for reducing Fe^{3+} to Fe^{2+} in the apical membrane of the enterocyte [10,43]. DMT1 plays a key role in Fe^{2+} transport into the enterocyte, being considered the major Fe intestinal transporter [10,43], whereas ferroportin is the protein that transports Fe^{2+} from the enterocyte into the bloodstream [10,43]. In the current study, the administration of 1%, 2.5% and 5% chia soluble extract solutions up-regulated the expression of DcytB, which in return may increase the transportation of Fe by DMT1 into the enterocyte, and as previously demonstrated, this effect can potentially increase iron absorption efficiency in a long-term feed trial [12]. Further, we investigated hepcidin gene expression as the key iron-regulatory hormone that controls systemic iron homeostasis, as hepcidin is able to down regulate the expression of ferroportin [44,45]. Further, the increase in hepcidin production is stimulated by iron loading and inflammation [46,47]. In the present study, hepcidin gene expression was lower ($p < 0.05$) in the 1%, 2.5% and 5% chia soluble extract groups compared to the inulin and water groups, which suggests that in a long-term feeding trial, the dietary inclusion of chia may have a positive effect on Fe-related proteins.

ZnT1 is the only transporter of the ZnT transporters family that is localized on the enterocyte's basolateral membrane and functions by exporting cytosolic zinc into the extracellular space [48], an up-regulation in ZnT1 mRNA gene expression may occur under increased cellular zinc levels [49]. In the current study, the groups treated with chia seed soluble extract (1%, 2.5% and 5%) shown a gene expression up-regulation ($p < 0.05$) of ZnT1 compared to the other groups, although the zinc serum concentrations did not differ between experimental groups.

Previous studies demonstrated the potential beneficial effects of soluble extract from various sources and plant origin compounds (such as raffinose, stachyose, diadzein, bean, and wheat) on BBM functionality and intestinal bacterial populations [10–13,27]. In the current study, the expression of BBM functional genes (AP, SI and SGLT1) was not affected by the chia seed soluble extract administration, due to the short exposure time. However, in relation to microbial populations, there was an increasing abundance of *Lactobacillus* ($p < 0.05$), and *Bifidobacterium* ($p < 0.05$) in the cecal contents of animals received 0.5% chia soluble extracts compared to the 18 Ω H_2O and non-injected group. Further, we observed an increased abundance in *Lactobacillus* ($p < 0.05$), *Bifidobacterium* ($p < 0.05$), *E. Coli* ($p < 0.05$) and *Clostridium* ($p < 0.05$) in the cecal contents of the animals that received 0.5% chia seed soluble extracts compared to other groups treated with chia seed extract. It is important to highlight that the increase in *Lactobacillus* and *Bifidobacterium* abundance, due the consumption of dietary fiber, may further contribute, directly or indirectly, to the increased bioavailability of iron and zinc in vulnerable populations, as these bacterial genera produce short-chain fatty acids (SCFAs), which reduce the intestinal pH, and therefore, may increase mineral (as Fe and Zn) solubility and therefore absorption [50]. *Bifidobacterium* and *Lactobacillus* can break down non-digestible fiber (prebiotics), due to their 1,2-glycosidase activity, leading to greater SCFA production [16,27,39], culminating with the increase in the absorption of iron and zinc.

The morphological parameters described in the current study, including villi development parameters and the crypt depth, are used as indicators of intestinal health, functionality and development [51]. The administration of chia seed soluble extracts, regardless of the concentration used, increased all parameters related to intestinal villi. These values (villus surface area, villus length and width) were significantly higher ($p < 0.05$) in the 5.0% chia group and relative to all other groups. This can be explained by the potential increased proliferation of intestinal cells in the short term, due the presence of soluble fiber, leading to hyperplasia and/or hypertrophy of intestinal cells and potentially enhancing the absorptive and digestive capacity of the villi BBM [29]. Another explanation is that the tested extracts had potentially increased butyrate production, which may lead to enterocyte proliferation [52]. Added to these factors, the soluble extract of chia seed contains a high concentration of phenolic compounds, among them are rosmarinic acid and rosmarinyl glucoside, which present the ability to affect intestinal morphology [53], increasing the villus height, crypt depth ratio, and muscularis thickness, as observed in the study that evaluated the administration of dietary polyphenol concentrate previously performed in *Gallus gallus* [54]. The morphological results agree with our cecum weight and cecum weight/body weight ratio observations. All experimental groups showed a higher ($p >$ 0.05) cecal weight (Figure 2B) post intra-amniotic soluble extract administration, indicating, and as previously suggested, increased cecal bacterial populations activity [10,12,13]. As for crypt depth, no differences between the experimental groups were observed, since duodenal crypts require a longer time to allow cellular proliferation. However, the intestinal crypts are meager and are able to rise to the surface of the villus, increasing the number of enterocytes in intestinal villi [52]—a phenomenon that was observed in the current study. Additionally, we observed increased goblet cell number and goblet cell diameter, which suggests an increased production of mucus that coats the intestinal lumen. As previously suggested, this may increase the intestinal BBM digestive and absorptive capabilities, and may indirectly increase the bioavailability of dietary components as suggested by the effects observed on the morphometric parameters [55–57]. The increase in "acidic goblet cells", containing acidic mucin due to the administration of 2.5% and 5% chia soluble extracts, may contribute to the reduction of intestinal pH, which in the long term, may lead to increased solubilization and uptake of iron and zinc and affect intestinal microbial profile [14,39]. The increase in "acidic goblet cells" was previously observed in a study that evaluated the effects of the intra amniotic administration of carbohydrate solution (containing maltose, sucrose and dextrin) on mucin content, goblet cell development, and levels of mucin mRNA in the *Gallus gallus* small intestine [58].

In general, previous studies showed a positive effect of prebiotic administration on intestinal morphology [10,13,25,51,52], for example, the intra-amniotic administration of raffinose and stachyose increased villus surface area compared to the control [10]. Similar results were observed by Hou et al. [13], who evaluated the effect of chickpea and lentil prebiotics administration in ovo. In another study, the authors evaluated the development of morphological parameters in *Gallus gallus*, and the results showed that the administration of a synthetic prebiotic increased the villus width and crypt depth. The prebiotic had no impact on villus height, villus surface area, and muscular thickness compared to the animals that received saline solution administration [51]. Bogucka et al. [52] evaluated the effect of inulin administration on the development of the intestinal villi and the number of goblet cells in the small intestine on the 1st and the 4th day post hatch (*Gallus gallus*) and the study indicated that on day one, the villus height did not differ among experimental groups. However, the villus width, villus surface area and crypt depth were lower in the prebiotic group. On day four, the inulin group showed a lower villus width, villus surface area and crypt depth [52]. Another study that evaluated the effect of the intra aminiotic administration of wheat bran prebiotic extract indicated increased villus height, goblet cell diameter and number in all treatment groups [11]. Further, Mista et al. [25] evaluated the effect of intra amniotic administered prebiotics on the development of the small intestine (*Gallus gallus*) and found that prebiotics did not affect the villus length, but did increase the crypt depth.

The observations described in the current study suggest that dietary chia seed consumption may be an effective strategy to reduce dietary iron and zinc deficiency and to potentially improve intestinal health. Overall, the up-regulation of Zn gene expression and the DcytB-Fe metabolism protein, the increase in villus surface area, villus length, villus width, goblet cell number and goblet cell diameter as well as cecum weight suggest that chia is a promising food ingredient that may improve mineral bioavailability and intestinal morphology. Hence, long-term feeding trials assessing the dietary effects of chia are now warranted.

5. Conclusions

The intra-amniotic (in ovo) administration of chia seed soluble extracts with putative prebiotic effects improved the intestinal morphology and up-regulated Zn-related protein gene expression. Further, chia seed soluble extract administration affected the intestinal microbiota and iron-related gene expression. The current study is the first to investigate the effects of chia seed soluble extracts with a potential prebiotic effect in vivo; thus, future studies aimed to assess dietary chia seed in a long-term feeding trials should be conducted, since chia may be a viable dietary ingredient that may improve intestinal health and contribute to intestinal mineral absorption.

Author Contributions: Data curation, B.P.d.S., and E.T.; Formal analysis, B.P.d.S., N.K., and E.T.; Investigation, B.P.d.S. and E.T.; Methodology, N.K., J.H., and E.T.; Resources, H.S.D.M. and E.T.; Supervision, E.T.; Writing—original draft, B.P.d.S. and E.T.; Writing—review and editing, E.T.

Funding: This research received no external funding.

Conflicts of Interest: The authors declare no conflict of interest.

References

1. Wegmüller, R.; Bah, A.; Kendall, L.; Goheen, M.M.; Mulwa, S.; Cerami, C.; Moretti, D.; Prentice, A.M. Efficacy and safety of hepcidin-based screen-and-treat approaches using two different doses versus a standard universal approach of iron supplementation in young children in rural Gambia: A double-blind randomised controlled trial. *BMC Pediatr.* **2016**, *149*, 1–9. [CrossRef]
2. World Health Organization. *WHO Guideline: Infants and Young Children Aged 6–23 Months and Children Aged 2–12 Years for Point-of-Use Fortification of Foods Consumed by Use of Multiple Micronutrient Powders*; WHO: Geneva, Switzerland, 2016; p. 52.
3. Bailey, R.L.; West, K.P., Jr.; Black, R.E. The epidemiology of global micronutrient deficiencies. *Ann. Nutr. Metab.* **2015**, *66*, 22–33. [CrossRef] [PubMed]
4. Black, R.E.; Victora, C.G.; Walker, S.P.; Bhutta, Z.A.; Christian, P.; Onis, M.; Ezzati, M.; Grantham-McGregor, S.; Katz, J.; Martorell, R.; et al. Maternal and Child Nutrition 1 Maternal and child undernutrition and overweight in low-income and middle-income countries. *Lancet* **2013**, *382*, 3–9. [CrossRef]
5. Hess, S.Y. National Risk of Zinc Deficiency as Estimated by National Surveys. *Food Nutr. Bull.* **2017**, *38*, 3–17. [CrossRef] [PubMed]
6. Bouis, H.E.; Saltzman, A. Improving nutrition through biofortifcation: A review of evidence from HarvestPlus, 2003 through 2016. *Glob. Food Sec.* **2017**, *12*, 49–58. [CrossRef] [PubMed]
7. Tako, E.; Reed, S.; Anandaraman, A.; Beebe, S.E.; Hart, J.J.; Glahn, R.P. Studies of Cream Seeded Carioca Beans (*Phaseolus vulgaris* L.) from a Rwandan Efficacy Trial: In Vitro and In Vivo Screening Tools Reflect Human Studies and Predict Beneficial Results from Iron Biofortified Beans. *PLoS ONE* **2015**, *10*, 1–15. [CrossRef] [PubMed]
8. Wintergerst, E.S.; Maggini, S.; Hornig, D.H. Contribution of Selected Vitamins and Trace Elements to Immune Function. *Ann. Nutr. Metab.* **2007**, *51*, 301–323. [CrossRef] [PubMed]
9. Tako, E.; Rutzke, M.A.; Glahn, R.P. Using the domestic chicken (*Gallus gallus*) as an in vivo model for iron bioavailability. *Poult. Sci.* **2010**, *89*, 514–521. [CrossRef]
10. Pacifici, S.; Song, J.; Zhang, C.; Wang, Q.; Glahn, R.P.; Kolba, N.; Tako, E. Intra Amniotic Administration of Raffinose and Stachyose Affects the Intestinal Brush Border Functionality and Alters Gut Microflora Populations. *Nutrients* **2017**, *9*, 304. [CrossRef]
11. Wang, X.; Kolba, N.; Liang, J.; Tako, E. Alterations in gut microflora populations and brush border functionality following intra-amniotic administration (*Gallus gallus*) of wheat bran prebiotic extracts. *Food Funct.* **2019**. [CrossRef]
12. Dias, D.M.; Kolba, N.; Hart, J.J.; Ma, M.; Sybil, T.S.; Lakshmanan, N.; Nutti, M.R.; Martino, H.S.D.; Glahn, R.P.; Tako, E. Soluble extracts from carioca beans (*Phaseolus vulgaris* L.) affect the gut microbiota and iron related brush border membrane protein expression in vivo (*Gallus gallus*). *Food Res. Int.* **2019**, *123*, 172–180. [CrossRef] [PubMed]

13. Hou, T.; Kolba, N.; Glahn, R.P.; Tako, E. Intra-amniotic administration (*Gallus gallus*) of cicer arietinum and lens culinaris prebiotics extracts and duck egg white peptides affects calcium status and intestinal functionality. *Nutrients* **2017**, *9*, 785. [CrossRef] [PubMed]
14. Tako, E.; Glahn, R.P.; Knez, M.; Stangoulis, J.C.R. The effect of wheat prebiotics on the gut bacterial population and iron status of iron deficient broiler chickens. *Nutr. J.* **2014**, *13*, 1–10. [CrossRef] [PubMed]
15. Tako, E.; Glahn, R.P. Intra-amniotic administration and dietary inulin affect the iron status and intestinal functionality of iron-deficient broiler chickens. *Poult. Sci.* **2012**, *91*, 1361–1370. [CrossRef] [PubMed]
16. Zhu, X.Y.; Zhong, T.; Pandya, Y.; Joerger, R.D. 16S rRNA-Based Analysis of Microbiota from the Cecum of Broiler Chickens. *Appl. Environ. Microbiol.* **2002**, *68*, 124–137. [CrossRef] [PubMed]
17. Hillier, L.W.; Miller, W.; Birney, E.; Warren, W.; Hardison, R.C.; Ponting, C.P. Sequence and comparative analysis of the chicken genome provide unique perspectives on vertebrate evolution. *Nature* **2004**, *432*, 695–716.
18. Reed, S.; Neuman, H.; Moscovich, S.; Glahn, R.P.; Koren, O.; Tako, E. Chronic zinc deficiency alters chick gut microbiota composition and function. *Nutrients* **2015**, *7*, 9768–9784. [CrossRef]
19. Conlon, M.A.; Bird, A.R. The Impact of Diet and Lifestyle on Gut Microbiota and Human Health. *Nutrients* **2015**, *7*, 17–44. [CrossRef]
20. Markowiak, P.; Slizewska, K. Effects of Probiotics, Prebiotics, and Synbiotics on Human Health. *Nutrients* **2017**, *9*, 1021. [CrossRef]
21. Sarao, L.K.; Arora, M. Probiotics, prebiotics, and microencapsulation: A review. *Crit. Rev. Food Sci. Nutr.* **2017**, *57*, 344–371. [CrossRef]
22. Lindsay, J.O.; Whelan, K.; Stagg, A.J.; Gobin, P.; Al-Hassi, H.O.; Rayment, N.; Kamm, M.A.; Knight, S.C.; Forber, A. Clinical, microbiological, and immunological effects of fructo-oligosaccharide in patients with Crohn's disease. *Gut* **2006**, *55*, 348–355. [CrossRef] [PubMed]
23. Kellow, N.J.; Coughlan, M.T.; Reid, C.M. Metabolic benefits of dietary prebiotics in human subjects: A systematic review of randomised controlled trials. *Br. J. Nutr.* **2014**, *111*, 1147–1161. [CrossRef] [PubMed]
24. Berrocoso, J.D.; Kida, R.; Singh, A.K.; Kim, Y.S.; Jha, R. Effect of in ovo injection of raffinose on growth performance and gut health parameters of broiler chicken. *Poult. Sci.* **2017**, *96*, 1573–1580. [CrossRef] [PubMed]
25. Miśta, D.; Króliczewska, B.; Pecka-Kiełb, E.; Kapuśniak, V.; Zawadzki, W.; Graczyk, S.; Kowalczyk, A.; Łukaszewic, E.; Bednarczyk, M. Effect of *in ovo* injected prebiotics and synbiotics on the caecal fermentation and intestinal morphology of broiler chickens. *Anim. Prod. Sci.* **2017**, *57*, 1884–1892. [CrossRef]
26. Yeung, C.K.; Glahn, R.E.; Welch, R.M.; Miller, D.D. Prebiotics and Iron Bioavailability—Is There a Connection? *J. Food Sci.* **2005**, *70*, 88–92. [CrossRef]
27. Hartono, K.; Reed, S.; Ankrah, N.A.; Glahn, R.P.; Tako, E. Alterations in gut microflora populations and brush border functionality following intra-amniotic daidzein administration. *RSC Adv.* **2015**, *5*, 6407–6412. [CrossRef]
28. Dias, D.; Kolba, N.; Binyamin, D.; Ziv, O.; Nutti, M.R.; Martino, H.S.D.; Glahn, R.P.; Koren, O.; Tako, E. Iron Biofortified Carioca Bean (*Phaseolus vulgaris* L.)—Based Brazilian Diet Delivers More Absorbable Iron and Affects the Gut Microbiota in vivo (*Gallus gallus*). *Nutrients* **2018**, *10*, 1970. [CrossRef]
29. Silva, B.P.; Dias, D.M.; Moreira, M.E.C.; Toledo, R.C.L.; da Matta, S.L.P.; Della Lucia, C.M.; Matino, H.S.D.; Pinheiro-Sant'Ana, H.M. Chia Seed Shows Good Protein Quality, Hypoglycemic Effect and Improves the Lipid Profile and Liver and Intestinal Morphology of Wistar Rats. *Plant Foods Hum. Nutr.* **2016**, *71*, 225–230. [CrossRef]
30. Pérez-Conesa, D.; López, G.; Ros, G. Effect of Probiotic, Prebiotic and Synbiotic Follow-up Infant Formulas on Iron Bioavailability in Rats. *Food Sci. Technol. Int.* **2007**, *13*, 69–77. [CrossRef]
31. Weinborn, V.; Valenzuela, C.; Olivares, M.; Arredondo, M.; Pizarro, F. Prebiotics increase heme iron bioavailability and do not affect non-heme iron bioavailability in humans. *Food Funct.* **2017**, *8*, 1994–1999. [CrossRef]
32. Steed, H.; Macfarlane, S. Mechanisms of Prebiotic Impact on Health. *Prebiotics Probiotics Sci. Technol.* **2009**, *2*, 135–161.
33. Baye, K.; Guyot, J.; Mouquet-Rivier, C. The unresolved role of dietary fibers on mineral absorption. *Crit. Rev. Food Sci. Nutr.* **2017**, *57*, 949–957. [CrossRef] [PubMed]

34. Holscher, H.D. Dietary fiber and prebiotics and the gastrointestinal microbiota. *Gut Microbes* **2017**, *8*, 172–184. [CrossRef] [PubMed]
35. Silva, B.P.; Anunciação, P.C.; Matyelka, J.C.S.; Della Lucia, C.M.; Martino, H.S.D.; Pinheiro-Sant'Ana, H.M. Chemical composition of Brazilian chia seeds grown in different places. *Food Chem.* **2017**, *221*, 1709–1716. [CrossRef] [PubMed]
36. Jafari, S.M.; Mcclements, D.J. Nanotechnology Approaches for Increasing Nutrient Bioavailability. *Adv. Food Nutr. Res.* **2017**, *81*, 1–30. [CrossRef] [PubMed]
37. Ullah, R.; Nadeem, M.; Khalique, A.; Imran, M.; Mehmood, S.; Javid, A. Nutritional and therapeutic perspectives of Chia (*Salvia hispanica* L.): A review. *J. Food Sci. Technol.* **2016**, *53*, 1750–1758. [CrossRef]
38. AOAC-Association of Official Analytical Chemistry. *Official Methods of Analysis*; AOAC-Association of Official Analytical Chemistry: Gaithersburg, MD, USA, 2012; p. 19.
39. Tako, E.; Glahn, R.P.; Welch, R.M.; Lei, X.; Yasuda, K.; Miller, D.D. Dietary inulin affects the expression of intestinal enterocyte iron transporters, receptors and storage protein and alters the microbiota in the pig intestine. *Br. J. Nutr.* **2008**, *99*, 472–480. [CrossRef]
40. Dreiling, C.E.; Brown, D.E.; Casale, L.; Kelly, L. Muscle Glycogen: Comparison of Iodine Binding and Enzyme Digestion Assays and Application to Meat Samples. *Meat Sci.* **1987**, *20*, 167–177. [CrossRef]
41. Tako, E.; Ferket, P.R.; Uni, Z. Changes in chicken intestinal zinc exporter mRNA expression and small intestinal functionality following intra-amniotic zinc-methionine administration. *J. Nutr. Biochem.* **2005**, *16*, 339–346. [CrossRef]
42. Uni, Z.; Noy, Y.; Sklan, D. Posthatch Development of Small Intestinal Function in the Poult. *Metab. Nutr.* **1999**, *78*, 215–222. [CrossRef]
43. Andrews, N.C. A genetic view of iron homeostasis. *Semin. Hematol.* **2002**, *39*, 227–234. [CrossRef] [PubMed]
44. Sangkhae, V.; Nemeth, E. Regulation of the Iron Homeostatic Hormone Hepcidin. *Adv. Nutr.* **2017**, *8*, 126–136. [CrossRef] [PubMed]
45. Abboud, S.; Haile, D.J. A novel mammalian iron-regulated protein involved in intracellular iron metabolism. *J. Biol. Chem.* **2000**, *275*, 19906–19912. [CrossRef] [PubMed]
46. Wang, C.; Canali, S.; Bayer, A.; Dev, S.; Agarwal, A.; Babitt, J.L. Iron, erythropoietin, and inflammation regulate hepcidin in Bmp2 -deficient mice, but serum iron fails to induce hepcidin in Bmp6 -deficient mice. *Am. J. Hematol.* **2019**, 240–248. [CrossRef] [PubMed]
47. Vela, D. The Dual Role of Hepcidin in Brain Iron Load and Inflammation. *Front. Neurosci.* **2018**, *12*, 1–13. [CrossRef]
48. Hara, T.; Takeda, T.A.; Takagishi, T.; Fukue, K.; Kambe, T.; Fukada, T. Physiological roles of zinc transporters: Molecular and genetic importance in zinc homeostasis. *J. Physiol. Sci.* **2017**, *67*, 283–301. [CrossRef]
49. Langmade, S.J.; Ravindra, R.; Daniels, P.J.; Andrews, G.K. The Transcription Factor MTF-1 Mediates Metal Regulation of the Mouse ZnT1 Gene. *J. Biol. Chem.* **2000**, *275*, 34803–34809. [CrossRef]
50. Patterson, J.K.; Lei, X.G.; Miller, D.D. The Pig as an Experimental Model for Elucidating the Mechanisms Governing Dietary Influence on Mineral Absorption. *Exp. Biol. Med.* **2008**, *233*, 651–664. [CrossRef]
51. Sobolewska, A.; Elminowska-Wenda, G.; Bogucka, J.; Dankowiakowska, A.; Kułakowska, A.; Szczerba, A.; Stadnicka, K.; Szpinda, M.; Bednarczyk, M. The influence of in ovo injection with the prebiotic DiNovo® on the development of histomorphological parameters of the duodenum, body mass and productivity in large-scale poultry production conditions. *J. Anim. Sci. Biotechnol.* **2017**, *8*, 1–8. [CrossRef]
52. Bogucka, J.; Dankowiakowska, A.; Elminowska-Wenda, G.; Sobolewska, A.; Szczerba, A.; Bednarczyk, M. Effects of prebiotics and synbiotics delivered in ovo on broiler small intestine histomorphology during the first days after hatching. *Folia Biol.* **2016**, *64*, 131–146. [CrossRef]
53. Akbarian, A.; Golian, A.; Kermanshahi, H.; Farhoosh, R.; Raji, A.R. Growth performance and gut health parameters of finishing broilers supplemented with plant extracts and exposed to daily increased temperature. *Span. J. Agric. Res.* **2013**, *11*, 109–119. [CrossRef]
54. Viveros, A.; Chamorro, S.; Pizarro, M.; Arija, I.; Centeno, C.; Brenes, A. Effects of dietary polyphenol-rich grape products on intestinal microflora and gut morphology in broiler chicks. *Poult. Sci.* **2011**, *90*, 566–578. [CrossRef] [PubMed]
55. Ma, J.; Rubin, B.K.; Voynow, J.A. Mucins, Mucus, and Goblet Cells. *Chest* **2017**, *154*, 169–176. [CrossRef] [PubMed]

56. Hou, T.; Tako, E. The *in ovo* feeding administration (*Gallus gallus*)—An emerging in vivo approach to assess bioactive compounds with potential nutritional benefits. *Nutrients* **2018**, *10*, 418. [CrossRef] [PubMed]
57. Han, H.Y.; Zhang, K.Y.; Ding, X.M.; Bai, S.P.; Luo, Y.H.; Wang, J.P.; Zeng, Q.F. Effect of dietary fiber levels on performance, gizzard development, intestinal morphology, and nutrient utilization in meat ducks from 1 to 21 days of age. *Poult. Sci.* **2017**, *96*, 4333–4341. [CrossRef]
58. Smirnov, A.; Tako, E.; Ferket, P.R.; Uni, Z. Mucin gene expression and mucin content in the chicken intestinal goblet cells are affected by in ovo feeding of carbohydrates. *Poult. Sci.* **2006**, *85*, 669–673. [CrossRef]

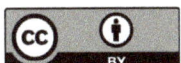

© 2019 by the authors. Licensee MDPI, Basel, Switzerland. This article is an open access article distributed under the terms and conditions of the Creative Commons Attribution (CC BY) license (http://creativecommons.org/licenses/by/4.0/).

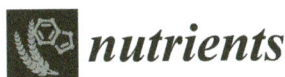

Review

Non-Dairy Fermented Beverages as Potential Carriers to Ensure Probiotics, Prebiotics, and Bioactive Compounds Arrival to the Gut and Their Health Benefits

Estefanía Valero-Cases [1], Débora Cerdá-Bernad [1], Joaquín-Julián Pastor [2] and María-José Frutos [1],*

[1] Research Group on Quality and Safety, Food Technology Department, Miguel Hernández University, 03312 Orihuela, Spain; e.valero@umh.es (E.V.-C.); dcerda@umh.es (D.C.-B.)
[2] Engineering Department, Miguel Hernández University; 03312 Orihuela, Spain; jjpastor@umh.es
* Correspondence: mj.frutos@umh.es; Tel.: +34-96-674-97-44

Received: 30 April 2020; Accepted: 28 May 2020; Published: 3 June 2020

Abstract: In alignment with Hippocrates' aphorisms "Let food be your medicine and medicine be your food" and "All diseases begin in the gut", recent studies have suggested that healthy diets should include fermented foods to temporally enhance live microorganisms in our gut. As a result, consumers are now demanding this type of food and fermented food has gained popularity. However, certain sectors of population, such as those allergic to milk proteins, lactose intolerant and strict vegetarians, cannot consume dairy products. Therefore, a need has arisen in order to offer consumers an alternative to fermented dairy products by exploring new non-dairy matrices as probiotics carriers. Accordingly, this review aims to explore the benefits of different fermented non-dairy beverages (legume, cereal, pseudocereal, fruit and vegetable), as potential carriers of bioactive compounds (generated during the fermentation process), prebiotics and different probiotic bacteria, providing protection to ensure that their viability is in the range of 10^6–10^7 CFU/mL at the consumption time, in order that they reach the intestine in high amounts and improve human health through modulation of the gut microbiome.

Keywords: intestinal microbiota; vegetable drink; fermentation; beneficial microorganisms; lactic acid bacteria; cereal; legume; pseudocereal; fruit; synbiotic

1. Introduction

Following Hippocrates' aphorism "Let food be your medicine and medicine be your food". In recent years, consumers have become more aware of the relationship between health and diet, and are now demanding healthier products with better nutritional characteristics and specific components to prevent health problems and improve their quality of life and life expectancy. This trend offers new opportunities for products with health benefits beyond basic nutrition, which meet consumer expectations and at the same time, drives the growth of the functional food market [1–3]. Nowadays, functional foods have been developed that incorporate different components with health benefits, such as bioactive compounds isolated from plants, polyunsaturated fatty acids, probiotics, prebiotics, minerals and vitamins, among others [4–7].

Twenty-five centuries ago, Hippocrates also stated that "All diseases begin in the gut" when referring to the relevance of the gastrointestinal system for human health. Currently, scientists studying the human microbiome suggest that healthy diets should include fermented foods to temporally enhance live microorganisms in our gut. The intestinal microbiota is a huge and varied collection of microorganisms. The large intestine hosts around 10^{13}–10^{14} microorganisms (almost 10 times the number of cells that make up the human body) and most consist of the bacteria phyla Firmicutes and Bacteroidetes. They play an important role in the health of the host, having effects on the regulation of energy metabolism and maturation of the immune system [8]. The administration of live probiotics maintains the balance of gut microbiota and contributes to the overall intestinal health. As a result, fermented foods have gained popularity and are highly demanded by the population [9,10]. Products with probiotics which contribute to gut health represent one of the largest and fastest growing sectors. Probiotics are defined as "live microorganisms that when are administered in an adequate amount confer a beneficial effect on the host health" [11]. Probiotics can be consumed as part of fermented foods or as dietary supplements. The most common genera that have been employed as probiotics and are available on the food market are the lactic acid bacteria (LAB) *Lactobacillus* and *Bifidobacterium*. Their species have mostly been given a generally-recognized-as-safe (GRAS) status and qualified presumption of safety (QPS) status, as their consumption does not present risks for the host's health [11–13].

A probiotic must survive during gastrointestinal digestion and adhere to the intestinal epithelium to exert its beneficial effects. The adherence ability depends on the hydrophobicity and autoaggregation capacity of the probiotic microorganisms [14]. The period of survival and residence of probiotics in the colon can be influenced by their duration and dose of probiotic, as well as by the matrix used as a carrier of the probiotics (Figure 1) [15,16].

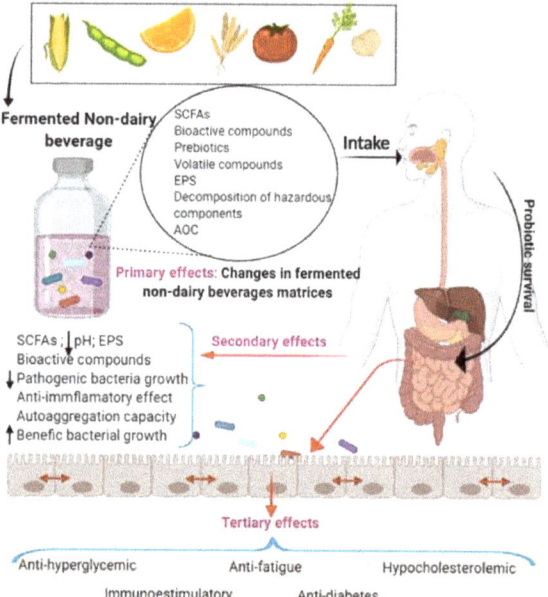

Figure 1. Summary of the beneficial effects of probiotics in different fermented non-dairy beverage matrices. Primary effects: changes in non-dairy matrices during fermentation. Secondary effects: changes in the intestinal epithelium. Tertiary effects: positive changes in health. SCFAs: short chain fatty acids; EPS: exopolysaccharides; AOC: antioxidant capacity [14–16].

Dairy foods have traditionally been used as carriers for probiotic microorganisms. Therefore, foods such as kefir, milk, yogurts, and cheese have been widely explored as dairy matrices for probiotic bacteria [17–20]. However, certain sectors of the population such as those allergic to milk proteins, those who are lactose intolerant, and those who are strictly vegetarian, cannot consume dairy products. Therefore, a need has arisen to offer consumers an alternative to fermented dairy products by exploring new non-dairy matrices as probiotics carriers [21,22]. However, the viability of probiotic microorganisms is more difficult to maintain in non-dairy matrices than in dairy matrices. The physicochemical parameters must be carefully controlled to guarantee the probiotic viability and to achieve adequate organoleptic properties (mainly aroma and flavor) that can be modified by fermentation [23]. Nevertheless, to improve the probiotic viability in non-dairy beverages, prebiotics could be used as a supplement. Prebiotics can be defined as "non-digestible food ingredients that beneficially affect the host by selectively stimulating the growth and/or activity of one of a limited number of bacteria in the colon" [24]; thus, they can improve the gut microbiome by specific beneficial bacteria fermentation in the colon. Foods or beverages that contain probiotics and prebiotics are known as synbiotic foods. Therefore, the proper selection of food matrices as potential carriers of probiotics is an essential factor to consider in the development of probiotic foods. It is important to ensure the viability of probiotics during processing and storage, in order to maintain their concentrations at high levels (10^6–10^7 colony-forming units (CFU) per mL or g of food) at the time of consumption (Figure 2). It is also essential to ensure their survival during gastrointestinal digestion, and thus a high viability of the probiotics, so that a sufficient amount reach the large intestine to exert their beneficial effects. Accordingly, this review aims to explore the potential of different fermented non-dairy beverages (legume, cereal, pseudocereal, fruit, and vegetable), as carriers of bioactive compounds (also generated during the fermentation process), prebiotics and different probiotic bacteria. This review will also examine their effectiveness in providing protection to ensure high probiotic survival during processing, storage and gastrointestinal digestion, in order to make sure that they reach the intestine in sufficient amounts to improve human health.

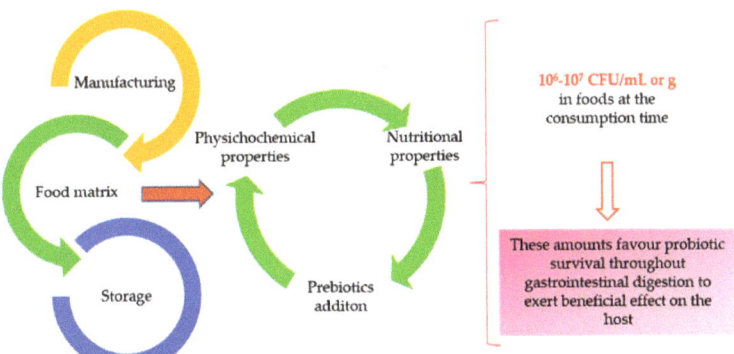

Figure 2. Important factors to be considered when assessing a fermented non-dairy beverage matrices as potential carriers for the viability of probiotic bacteria.

2. Non-Dairy Fermented Beverages as Vehicles for Bioactive Compound, Probiotic, and Prebiotic Delivery to the Gut and their Health Benefits

2.1. Fermented Legume Beverages

Several researchers have tried to produce non-dairy probiotic beverages based on legume, as a food matrix for the delivery of bioactive compounds, probiotics, or prebiotics, in order to enhance human intestinal health. Legumes are potential matrices as carriers of probiotics because they contain non-digestible oligosaccharides that can be metabolized by the microorganisms. Soybean legume (*Glycine max*, L.) is the most used since it has high quality proteins and minerals, and due to its isoflavones contents it has the potential to reduce the incidence of osteoporosis and menopausal symptoms [25]. However, due to soy allergies which affect about 0.5% of the general population, other legumes, such as chickpeas (*Cicer arietinum*, L.), are also used [26]. Chickpeas contain a high amount of resistant starch and amylose and some studies have proved that they can reduce the risks of high blood pressure and type-2 diabetes [27].

The production of soy beverages is one of the traditional unfermented food uses of soybeans. Recently, some studies have developed fermented soy drinks with probiotics, in order to improve their beneficial health properties and their flavor and texture [28]. Bedani et al. [29] prepared a soy beverage fermented with probiotic cultures and studied the viability and resistance of probiotics to simulated gastrointestinal digestion, as well as the effect of adding ingredients such as inulin as prebiotic and okara flour, which is a by-product of the soy milk industry. This study concluded that soy milk is a potential food matrix for the delivery of probiotics and prebiotics which could protect them against gastrointestinal juices. The probiotics used, *Bifidobacterium animalis* Bb-12 and *Lactobacillus acidophilus* La-5, survived at high concentrations maintaining their viability at above 8 Log CFU/mL during 28 days of storage at 4 °C with an acidic pH between 4.30 and 4.70. However, the survival was not affected by inulin and/or okara flour. In addition, during the in vitro gastrointestinal digestion, *B. animalis* Bb-12 maintained populations above 7 Log CFU/mL, but *L. acidophilus* La-5 was very sensitive and its viability was reduced, the final concentration being below 5 Log CFU/mL (the initial concentrations of both probiotics were above 8 Log CFU/mL). Therefore, soybeans could be a potential vehicle for probiotics, being able to maintain a high viability to exert their beneficial effects on human gut microbiota, although further studies are required.

Other studies have combined soy milk with cereals (sprouted wheat, barley, and pearl millet) and legumes (green gram), or with peanut milk, producing beverages with probiotic characteristics and high cell concentrations after fermentation [30,31]. Mridula and Sharma [30] analyzed fermented beverages based on soy milk combined with different cereals or legumes, such as green gram (*Vigna radiata*, L.). In the beverage based on green gram, after the fermentation at 37 °C for 8 h by *L. acidophilus* NCDC14, the probiotic count ranged from 10.36 to 11.32 Log CFU/mL with an acidity between 0.50% and 0.80% and a pH of 4.2–4.4. Besides, a high sensory acceptability score was obtained. Therefore, this fermented legume beverage might be a potential vehicle for probiotics. Santos et al. [31] developed a fermented beverage of soy and peanut milk, using these two substrates to improve the nutrient availability for probiotics. For the fermentation, six different LAB were used, including probiotic strains (*Pediococcus acidilactici* UFLA BFFCX 27.1, *Lactococcus lactis* CCT 0360, *Lactobacillus rhamnosus* LR 32, and *Lactobacillus acidophilus* LACA 4) and yeasts, in a binary culture or in co-culture. *L. acidophilus* LACA 4 and *P. acidilactici* UFLA BFFCX 27.1 reached counts above 8 Log CFU/mL after fermentation for 24 h at 37 °C and another 24 h at ±4 °C. Higher lactic acid contents were also obtained by co-culture with *Saccharomyces cerevisiae* yeast which might serve as a source of vitamin B and proteins. Therefore, a beverage based on peanuts may be a good carrier of probiotics, since it allows larger populations of the probiotic bacteria to be grown and maintained, but further studies are necessary.

There are few documented studies that have determined the effect of fermented legume beverages on modulation of the gut microbiome in either animal or humaninvestigations. Cabello-Olmo et al. [32] evaluated the impact of long-term supplementation with a non-dairy fermented beverage in the development of type-2 diabetes in rats, which is related to the host's intestinal microbiota since diabetic individuals present a characteristic intestinal microbial community. The plant-based beverage was composed of legumes and cereals such as alfalfa meal, soya flour, and barley sprouts with other minor components. It was fermented at 37 °C after the incorporation of LAB and debittered brewer's yeast, and the *Lactobacillus* genus was the most predominant. This research analyzed the fecal microbiota of rat feces collected at six months of study. The specimens had ad libitum access to food supplemented with the fermented beverages whose composition included a high level of fermentable carbohydrates. The study revealed that, at genus level, supplementation with the fermented beverage enriched the abundance of *Sutterella* which includes commensal species found in healthy humans and animals, and *Proteus*, for which there is no evidence for its function in diabetes. However some studies have suggested its role in several pathological conditions. Some *Barnesiella* species and the *Anaerococcus* genus were more numerous in the group treated with the beverage. The abundance of *Barnesiella* is related to a better glucose tolerance and important metabolic improvements, and the relative abundance of *Anaerococcus* includes many bacterial species which produce butyrate in experimental conditions. Butyrate, as well as acetate and propionate, are short-chain fatty acids (SCFAs) which produce beneficial effects on the gastrointestinal tract. SCFAs are produced by the probiotic fermentation of non-digestible carbohydrates and improve the intestinal barrier, inhibiting the development of pathogens and the production of toxic elements, and they are used by intestinal cells as colonocytes to grow [33]. Therefore, the administration of this plant-based beverage fermented with probiotics leads to an enrichment of the gut microbiota population, improving glucose metabolism and protecting against type-2 diabetes development in rats. These novel fermented beverages could be potential vehicles of probiotics, prebiotics, and/or bioactive compounds to protect against metabolic alterations of the diabetic pathology. However, further studies on microbial metabolites which are also important and responsible for gut health are required.

Another study on the effect of the intake of a soy milk beverage fermented with *Lactobacillus casei* Shirota on gut microbiota in sixty healthy premenopausal women twice a day for 8 weeks, reported that there was an increase of *Lactobacillaceae* and *Bifidobacteriaceae* levels and a decrease of *Enterobacteriaceae* and *Porphyromonadaceae* levels during the intake period. The results suggested that a daily intake of fermented soy milk beverage beneficially contributes to modulation of the gut microbiota in premenopausal healthy women [34].

Other studies have focused on the use of different legumes, such as chickpeas (*Cicer arietinum*, L.), as alternatives to soy in fermented plant-based beverages, which could be a promising carrier of probiotics. The results showed probiotic counts of about 6 Log CFU/mL after fermentation for 16 h at 42 °C, but more optimization studies are required to minimize synerisis and improve the sensory acceptability [35]. One study developed a non-dairy beverage fermented by *Lactobacilli acidophilus* probiotics using germinated and ungerminated seeds of moth bean (*Vigna aconitifolia*, L.) and cereals, obtaining promising results since the levels of microorganisms after fermentation for 6 h at 37 °C were above 8 Log CFU/mL and a good sensory acceptability was obtained [36]. The main studies that have been conducted to date on fermented legume beverages and their results are summarized in Table 1.

Table 1. Summary of fermented legume beverages as potential carriers for bioactive compound, probiotic, and prebiotic delivery to the gut.

Legume Fermented Beverage	Probiotic Bacteria	Results	Reference
Soy milk with inulin and okara flour	*L. acidophilus* La-5, *B. animalis* Bb-12	Probiotic viability above the minimum recommended after 28 days of storage, high probiotic viability after in vitro gastrointestinal digestion	Bedani et al. [29]
Soy milk with green gram	*L. acidophilus* NCDC14	High probiotic viability after fermentation, high sensory acceptability score	Mridula and Sharma [30]
Peanut-soy milk	*P. acidilactici* UFLA BFFCX 27.1, *L. lactis* CCT 0360, *L. rhamnosus* LR 32, *L. acidophilus* LACA 4	High probiotic viability after fermentation, high acid lactic contents	Santos et al. [31]
Soya flour, alfalfa meal, barley sprouts	Different LAB, mostly *Lactobacillus* genus	Enrichment of the gut microbiota population	Cabello-Olmo et al. [32]
Soy milk	*L. casei* Shirota	Beneficial modulation of the gut microbiota	Nagino et al. [34]
Chickpeas	*S. thermophilus*, *L. bulgaricus*, *L. acidophilus*	High probiotic viability after fermentation	Wang et al. [35]
Germinated and ungerminated cereals and legumes: barley, ragi, moth bean, soybean	*L. acidophilus*	High probiotic viability after fermentation, good sensory acceptability	Chavan et al. [36]

2.2. Fermented Cereal Beverages

Cereals are consumed all over the world and are considered one of the most important sources of carbohydrates, proteins, dietary fiber, minerals, and vitamins in our diet. Therefore, they are a good option among non-dairy raw materials for producing fermented beverages [37]. Oat (*Avena sativa*, L.) is a potential functional ingredient, due to its proteins, soluble fiber, and antioxidant properties, with β-glucan being the most important carbohydrate fraction because of its prebiotic properties in the gut [38]. Kedia et al. [39] investigated the prebiotic potential of oat through in vitro fermentation for

24 h with human fecal cultures. Their results showed an increase in SCFAs and beneficial intestinal bacteria such as *Enterobacteria*, and a reduction in harmful bacteria such as anaerobes and clostridia. Oat beverages fermented with different *Lactobacillus* strains have also been reported to display a high antioxidant capacity and an increase in polyphenol content with respect to non-fermented beverages. However, only fermented oat with *L. plantarum* LP09 showed an in vitro decrease in the hydrolysis index of starch (used as a measure of the glycemic index in healthy subjects). The fermentation also increased the β-glucan content. However, the soluble and insoluble fiber ratio decreased after fermentation. At the same time, the aroma and flavor were better than in the unfermented control samples [40]. Other studies have also shown that fermented oat beverages may be potential probiotic carriers. They resulted in optimization of the fermentation process and the beverage formulations, reaching high microbial levels (>10^7 CFU/mL) during production and storage, and were able to maintain the β-glucan content at the end of storage [41–45]. The viability and in vitro probiotic potential were recently investigated by Funck et al. [46] in oat beverages fermented with *L. curvatus* P99. The results showed a high probiotic viability (above 7 log CFU/mL) during 35 days of being refrigerated at 4 °C. The acceptability of the fermented beverages was good, since most consumers gave high scores for all sensory attributes evaluated. Regarding the probiotic properties, *L. curvatus* P99 showed high gastrointestinal survival and antimicrobial activity against Gram-negative and Gram-positive bacteria. Additionally, it has the capacity of auto-aggregation and of blocking the adhesion of pathogenic bacteria to gut epithelial cells. Johansson et al. [47] carried out an in vivo controlled randomized double-blind study with a rose-hip beverage supplemented with oats fermented with *L. plantarum* DSM9843 in 48 healthy adults. The group receiving the administration of 400 mL/day of this beverage for three weeks showed an increase of total fecal carboxylic acid (lactic, acetic, and propionic acid) and the probiotic bacteria were found in feces at a high concentration, indicating their survival during gastrointestinal digestion. Decreased flatulence and a softer stool consistency were also reported.

Among other cereals, rice (*Oryza sativa*, L.) is also used in the production of fermented beverages that are very popular in Asian-Pacific countries. Ghosh et al. [48] demonstrated a probiotic role of *L. fermentum* KKL1 in a fermented rice beverage. The beverages fermented at 37 °C for 4 days consecutively in anaerobic conditions showed a strong antioxidant activity; the production of glucoamylase, α-amylase and phytase (therefore, an increase of phytate bioavailability) and a mineral increase (Ca, Fe, Mg, Mn and Na). Besides, the hydrosoluble vitamin content in fermented samples was higher than in unfermented control samples such as folic acid, thiamine, ascorbic acid and pyridoxine. However, riboflavin decreased due to bacterial metabolism during fermentation. At the same time, rice was a good carrier for maintaining the *L. fermentum* KKL1 at a high concentration after gastrointestinal digestion and showed sensitivity to the antibiotics tested, except for polymyxin. Nevertheless, this strain showed a moderate cell surface hydrophobicity. Another study reported similar results in fermented rice beverages, but with different species of *Lactobacillus* bacteria, such as *L. plantarum* L7. This strain showed good in vitro characteristics, such as high survival to gastrointestinal digestion, antimicrobial activity, autoaggregation to the intestinal cell surface, and susceptibility to some antibiotics, the latter is a desirable characteristic because probiotics should not carry transmissible antibiotic-resistance genes, in order to avoid the development of new antibiotic-resistant pathogens The fermented beverages increased the lactic, succinic and acetic acids during fermentation for 6 days under anaerobic conditions at 35 °C. At the same time, increases in phytase activity and minerals (Na, Mg, Mn, Fe and Ca) were also observed. Furthermore, the fermented rice beverage presented a high antioxidant capacity [49]. Therefore, rice is a good matrix for *L. fermentum* KKL1 and *L. plantarum* L7 growth and survival in adequate concentrations. Furthermore, these bacteria played an important role in improving the functional properties of rice beverages. However, in vivo investigations are required to explore and verify their probiotic properties.

Maize (*Zea mays*, L.) is another highly consumed cereal that contains about 72% starch, 10% proteins, and 4% fiber, together with vitamin B and essential minerals [50]. Menezes et al. [51] used the *L. paracasei* LBC-81 with the yeast *S. cerevisiae* CCMA 0731 and *L. paracasei* LBC-81 with *S. cerevisiae* CCMA 0732 in combination, for the fermentation of maize beverages at 30 °C for 24 h. The results showed a high microorganism viability of above 7 Log CFU/mL during fermentation and during 28 days of refrigerated storage (4 °C). The beverages achieved a score of 5 out of 9 points for general acceptance, corresponding to the descriptor "neither dislike nor like". Lactic acid was the main organic acid produced during the fermentation time and low concentrations of acetic acid and ethanol were also detected. A total of 70 volatile compounds were identified. Although the physicochemical results presented in this study were interesting, more in vivo studies on the viability and health benefits of these microorganisms are needed.

The fermentation process can be used for the delivery of probiotic bacteria and for food detoxification. Probiotic growth in the fermented food medium reduces toxins in raw materials. Aflatoxins can suppress the activity of the human immune system, affect nutrient absorption, and induce liver cancer. This was evaluated by Wacoo et al. [52] in a modification of the traditional method of the production of the Kwete beverage (traditional African fermented maize). Kwete was produced by fermentation with *L. rhamnosus* yoba 2012 and *S. thermophilus* C106 at 30 °C for 24 h. The results showed that the beverage was stable for a month under refrigeration storage at 4 °C, with a mean pH of 3.9 and titratable acidity of 0.6%; the bacteria could also reduce the aflatoxins to undetectable levels during fermentation. The aflatoxins reduction is a novel approach to detoxification of this kind of beverage widely consumed in Africa.

The use of cereal mixtures for the development of fermented beverages has also been investigated. Rathore et al. [5] made comparisons of single and mixed cereal beverages fermented with different strains of LAB. The results of this study indicated that the organic acid production in mixed cereal substrates was lower than in the single cereal beverages. However, the microbial populations were similar for all substrates. These results are very interesting for future investigations on sensorial properties and consumer acceptance. Nevertheless, malt was the best substrate for microbial growth used as single or mixed beverages. Freire et al. [53] developed mixed beverages from rice and maize fermented with *L. acidophilus* LACA 4 and *L. pantarum* CCMA 0743 for 36 h at 37 °C and supplemented with frutooligosaccharides (FOS). The FOS were an important prebiotic for maintaining the microbial viability in high concentrations (>10^7 CFU/mL) during 28 days of refrigerated storage (4 °C). The main organic acids were lactic and acetic acid. The sensory acceptance of the beverages was good with high scores with respect to unfermented ones, indicating their high potential for the market.

Maize beverages have been shown to be a potential matrix for the growth and survival of the bacteria studied, with important changes in their composition. However, in the future, further studies focused on the identification, quantification and potential effect of bioactive compounds, as well as the modulation of intestinal microbiota, will be of great interest to elucidate the functionality of maize beverages in the human organism. A summary of the studies on fermented cereal beverages conducted to date and their results is presented in Table 2.

Table 2. Summary of fermented cereal beverages as potential carriers form bioactive compounds, probiotics, prebiotics delivery to de gut.

Cereal Fermented Beverage	Probiotic Bacteria	Results	Reference
Oat	Human fecal cultures	Increase in SCFAs [1], increase of healthy intestinal bacteria, reduction of harmful bacteria	Kedia et al. [39]
Oat	Different *Lactobacillus* strains	High levels of antioxidant capacity, high polyphenols content, increase of β-glucan content during fermentation, decrease in the hydrolysis index of starch, high probiotic viability	Luana et al. [40], Bernat et al. [41], Gupta et al. [42], Gupta and Bajaj [43], Kedia et al. [44], Wang et al. [45]
Oat	*L. curvatus* P99	High probiotic viability after in vitro digestion, antimicrobial activity, blocking of the adhesion of pathogenic bacteria to epithelial cells, autoaggregation capacity	Funck et al. [46]
Oat	*L. plantarum* DSM9843	In vivo study: increase of lactic, acetic and propionic acid, high probiotic viability after digestion; decrease in flatulence; and softer stool consistency	Johansson et al. [47]
Rice	*L. fermentum* KKL1	Strong antioxidant capacity, glucoamylase and α-amylase production, phytase activity, high hydrosoluble vitamins, antibiotic susceptibility	Ghosh et al. [48]
Rice	*L. plantarum* L7	High antioxidant capacity; increase in lactic, succinic, and acetic acid during fermentation; high probiotic viability after in vitro digestion; antibiotic susceptibility; antimicrobial activities; increase in minerals and phytase activity	Giri et al. [49]
Maize	*L. paracasei* LBC-81 with *S. cerevisiae* CCMA 0731 and *L. paracasei* LBC-81 *S. cerevisiae* CCMA 0732	Probiotic viability above the minimum recommended, high production of lactic acid during fermentation, 70 volatile compounds identified	Menezes et al. [51]
Kwete	*L. rhamnosus* yoba 2012 and *S. thermophilus* C106	Decrease in aflatoxins content = detoxification of beverage	Wacoo et al. [52]
Cereals mixing	Mixed or single LAB	Malt was the best substrate for microbial growth used as single or mixed beverages	Rathore et al. [5]
Rice and maize	*L. acidophilus* LACA 4 and *L. pantarum* CCMA 0743 supplemented with FOS	High probiotic viability, increase in lactic and acetic acids during fermentation, good sensorial acceptance	Freire et al. [53]

[1] SCFAs: short chain fatty acids.

2.3. Fermented Pseudocereal Beverages

Several studies have focused on the development of non-dairy probiotic beverages using pseudocereals as vehicles for the delivery of bioactive compounds, probiotics, and prebiotics. Pseudocereals are viable potential substrates, as they contain nutrients easily metabolized by probiotic microorganisms. They are a good source of high-quality proteins comparable to those of cereals, minerals (Ca, Cu, Fe, Mg, Mn and Zn) in higher amounts than in conventional cereals, carbohydrates, and fiber [54]. Quinoa (*Chenopodium quinoa*, L.) is the pseudocereal most widely used as a food matrix. It is the only plant-based food that has all of the essential amino acids (lysine, methionine, and threonine), trace elements and vitamins, and its protein quality to matches that of milk [55]. It can also decrease the risk of type-2 diabetes and cardiovascular diseases [56]. Furthermore, it is gluten-free, so its consumption is suitable for celiacs and people with gluten-allergy problems.

One study reported the use of two varieties of quinoa (Rosada de Huancayo and Pasankalla) as suitable food matrices for the development of fermented beverages [57]. The fermentation was carried out by the probiotics *Lactobacillus plantarum* Q823, *Lactobacillus casei* Q11, and *Lactococcus lactis* ARH74 for 6 h at 30 °C. After 28 days of storage (5–7 °C), *L. plantarum* Q823 and *L. casei* Q11 were detected at levels higher than 9 Log CFU/mL, which is a concentration above the recommended minimum for probiotic effects, with initial concentrations of 8 Log CFU/mL. Vera-Pingitore et al. [58] have previously reported that *L. plantarum* Q823 can survive during the passage through the human gastrointestinal tract. In this study, seven healthy female volunteers consumed 20 mL of quinoa-based beverage containing 9.19 Log CFU/mL on a daily basis or 7 days, and microbial counts were analyzed in feces. Levels between 5 and 7 Log CFU/mL were detected for at least 7 days after the end of the intake. Therefore, quinoa-based fermented beverages contain high amounts of protein, fiber, vitamins and minerals, with probiotics which could exert health benefits on the human gastrointestinal microbiota. However, more long-term human clinical trial studies are needed to demonstrate that these beverages have probiotic properties.

There are few documented studies that have attempted to determine the in vivo effect of fermented pseudocereal beverages on the modulation of the gut microbiome in either animal or human investigations. However, one study has evaluated the impact of several beverages based on aqueous extracts of soy and quinoa with prebiotics (FOS) and/or with probiotics (*Lactobacillus casei* Lc-01) on the human intestinal microbiota, using the Simulator of the Human Intestinal Microbial Ecosystem (SHIME®) [59]. The SHIME is a five-stage sequential reactor system simulating the different parts of the gastrointestinal tract in vitro, representing the human gut microbiota [60]. The study of Bianchi et al. [59] reported that a synbiotic beverage fortified with both a probiotic and a prebiotic showed the best beneficial effect on the gut microbiota, as the oligosaccharides used were hydrocolloids, which protected the microorganism. The concentration used in the SHIME was a proportion equivalent to 8 Log CFU/mL in the beverage. *L. casei* Lc-01 of the synbiotic beverage survived the stomach and intestinal conditions and reached the colon, maintaining its functionality, and the concentration of SCFAs was stable during the in vitro gastrointestinal digestion. Furthermore, the growth of several species of *Lactobacillus* spp. and *Bifidobacterium* spp. in the colon were stimulated by the synbiotic beverage. At the same time, the growth of potential enteropathogenic bacteria such as *Clostridium* spp., enterobacteria and other pathogenic bacteria such as *Bacteroides* spp. and *Enterococcus* spp. was reduced. Another positive effect of the beverage on the gastrointestinal tract was the significant decrease in the ammonia ion production. Ammonia can stimulate the development of colon carcinogenesis, since it can affect intestinal cells, changing their morphology and intermediary metabolism by increasing DNA synthesis [61]. Therefore, this beverage based on quinoa and soybean with FOS and fermented by *L. casei* Lc-01 positively modulates the gut microbiota improving the diversity and richness of beneficial bacteria without affecting their functionality and reducing the growth of the pathogenic ones, and decreasing the production of toxic elements such as ammonia.

Some studies have investigated the use of other pseudocereals, such as chia (*Salvia hispanica*, L.), amaranth (*Amaranthus*, L.) or buckwheat (*Fagopyrum esculentum*, L.), as food carriers to develop pseudocereal probiotic beverages, obtaining interesting results. In a study on the elaboration of a beverage with the probiotic *Lactobacillus rhamnosus* GG (5–6 Log CFU/mL), using mashed buckwheat previously fermented with LAB, the results showed that the levels of the microorganism were higher than 6 Log CFU/mL after 14 days of cold storage at 6 °C [62]. Kocková and Valík [63] also produced beverages based on buckwheat or dark buckwheat fermented with *L. rhamnosus* GG ATCC 53,103 (6 Log CFU/mL) at 37 °C for 10 h. This probiotic was able to grow and metabolize buckwheat and dark buckwheat and to survive during 21 days of a refrigerated storage period at 5 °C, with the probiotic counts being above the minimum recommended (>7 Log CFU/mL). Kocková et al. [64] studied the use of different pseudocereals as substrates for the production of different beverages fermented with *L. rhamnosus* GG (5 Log CFU/mL) for 10 h at 37 °C, using amaranth flour, amaranth grain, buckwheat flour, or whole buckwheat flour. The results showed that the probiotic could grow and metabolize these pseudocereals and after 21 days of storage at 5 °C, the probiotic levels were higher than 6 Log CFU/mL, and thus over the limit required for probiotic food, except for the beverage with whole buckwheat flour. Another study reported that chia can be fermented by *L. plantarum* C8, and that after 24 h of fermentation, its overall characteristics were improved, such as the phenolic compound concentration and antioxidant activity [65]. Therefore, this pseudocereal could be a good matrix for the development of probiotic beverages. The main studies conducted to date on fermented pseudocereal beverages and their results are summarized in Table 3.

2.4. Fermented Fruit and Vegetable Beverages

Fruit and vegetable beverages are an excellent source of vitamins, antioxidants, minerals, and bioactives. At the same time they represent a good alternative to dairy matrices and a good choice for the entire human population, because they have hydration properties, are refreshing and have attractive flavors [21,66]. Therefore, different fruits and vegetable juices are used to develop fermented beverages in combination or alone as an alternative to fermented dairy products. The fermentation process can increase the shelf life of fruit and vegetable beverages, improving their nutritional and functional properties, with beneficial effects on health [16]. Recently, a wide variety of research has been focused on the production of fermented non-dairy synbiotic beverages, including different types of vegetables or fruits, such as blended carrot-orange juices and nectars with different inulin concentrations [67,68], pomegranate juices, and Cornelian cherry beverages using delignified wheat bran [69,70], clarified apple juice with oligofructose [71], orange juice with oligofructose [72], orange juices and hibiscus tea mixed beverage with oligofructose [73], and blended red fruit beverages (strawberry, blackberry and papaya) supplemented with three separate prebiotics: FOS, inulin and galactooligosaccharides [74]. Generally, the findings have indicated a good compatibility among prebiotic ingredients and vegetable beverage matrices. Furthermore, prebiotic supplementation can improve the viability of the different probiotic strains so that they are above the minimum concentration recommended during the beverages processing and storage and are also able to survive during gastrointestinal digestion in order to reach the colon, promoting the growth of beneficial bacteria. Furthermore, a recent randomized, controlled, triple-blinded, parallel trial study of polycystic ovarian syndrome (POCS) showed the effect of synbiotic pomegranate juice (containing inulin and three species of *Lactobacillus*) in terms of improving the testosterone level, body mass index, insulin, insulin resistance, weight, and waist circumference in POCS. However, neither group showed a significant change in the fasting blood sugar, luteinizing hormone, and follicle-stimulating hormone [75].

Table 3. Summary of fermented pseudocereal beverages as potential carriers for bioactive compound, probiotic, and prebiotic delivery to the gut.

Pseudocereal Fermented Beverage	Probiotic Bacteria	Results	Reference
Two quinoa varieties (Rosada de Huancayo, Pasankalla)	L. plantarum Q823, L. casei Q11, L. lactis ARH74	Probiotic viability above the minimum recommended after 28 days of storage	Ludena-Urquizo et al. [57]
Quinoa	L. plantarum Q823	High probiotic viability after the gastrointestinal digestion	Vera-Pingitore et al. [58]
Aqueous extracts of soybean and quinoa grains with FOS	L. casei Lc-01	Positive modulation of the gut microbiota, decrease in toxic elements (ammonia)	Bianchi et al. [59]
Mashed buckwheat previously fermented with LAB	L. rhamnosus GG	High probiotic viability after 14 days of cold storage, good sensorial acceptance	Matejčeková et al. [62]
Buckwheat, dark buckwheat	L. rhamnosus GG	Probiotic viability above the minimum recommended after 21 days of cold storage	Kocková and Valík [63]
Amaranth flour, amaranth grain, buckwheat flour, whole buckwheat flour	L. rhamnosus GG	High probiotic viability after 21 days of storage, except for the beverage with whole buckwheat flour	Kocková et al. [64]

Several LAB can biotransform polyphenols into phenolic compounds with an improved bioavailability and bioactivity during the fermentation time. Several studies have investigated phenolic compound biotransformation during fermentation and gastrointestinal digestion. The studies on fermented fruit or vegetable beverages have shown an improved antioxidant capacity and phenolic composition modification. Apple juice fermented with *L. plantarum* ATCC14917 at 37 °C improved the antioxidant capacity by increasing the quercetin, phloretin and 5-O-caffeoylquinic acid contents during 24 h of fermentation [76]. Yang et al. [77] reported an increase of the total flavonoids content as well as the antioxidant activity in fermented mixed beverages from apples, carrots, and pears during fermentation with two commercial *L. plantarum* 115 *L. plantarum* Vege Start 60. On the other hand, the biotransformation of phenolic compounds during fermentation and gastrointestinal digestion in fermented pomegranate juices ensured the survival of *L. plantarum* CECT220, *L. acidophilus* CECT903, *B. longum subsp. infantis* CECT4551, and *B. bifidum* CECT870, suggesting a prebiotic effect [78]. Furthermore, one study on a fermented tea infusion found an increase in the overall antioxidant capacity, a modification in the phenolic composition and an increase in their cellular uptake after in vitro digestion [79]. Oolong tea polyphenols have been reported to improve host health through the generation of SCFAs and modulation of the human gut microbiota, leading to potential applications for anti-obesity therapies [80]. Specifically, (-)-Epigallocatechin 3-O-(3-O-methyl) gallate showed a prebiotic effect with the modulation of gut microbiota and obesity prevention in high-fat diet-fed mice [81,82]. Phenolic compounds are recognized as antioxidants, but some of them also exhibit antimicrobial activity. Cueva et al. [83] showed that phenolic compounds generated from probiotic metabolism (phenylpropionic, benzoic and phenylacetic) can inhibit the growth of intestinal pathogens and prevent intestinal dysbiosis.

The ability of probiotic microorganisms to metabolize phenolic compounds is known to depend on the species or strains. However, differences in the total polyphenol content and antioxidant capacity have been shown between different vegetable beverages for the same probiotic strains. These differences may be related to the variability in the phytochemical composition of the different vegetable and fruit matrices [84,85]. In addition, the matrix also has an influence on the exopolysaccharides (EPS) production during fermentation, improving the consistency and antioxidant capacity of fermented juices [86]. At the same time, the EPS also have a significant role as prebiotics and can enhance probiotic colonization in the gut. They have also been used as immunomodulatory, immunostimulatory, antidiabetic, and hypocholesterolemic agents [87,88].

Bearing in mind the nutritional importance of fruit and vegetable beverages, some of them, such as fresh prickly pear juices, present hazardous volatile components in negligible quantities. Therefore, the reduction of risky compounds by modification or decomposition during the fermentation time is an interesting strategy. Panda et al. [89] demonstrated prickly pear quality enhancement by fermentation with *Lactobacillus fermentum* ATCC 9338 for 48 h at 28 °C. The study demonstrates the decomposition of several risky organic compounds present in the fresh juice, such as 2-propenenitrile, 2-(acetyloxy); furfuryl alcohol; acetaldehyde; 2,2-diethyl-3-methyloxazolidine; 4h-Pyran-4-one; 3,5-dihydroxy-2-methyl; and furan.

Beyond the nutritional and physicochemical advantages, recent studies have shown that different fermented fruit and vegetable beverages also have some physiological functions. For example, some studies have shown a stable α-glucosidase inhibitory activity with an anti-hyperglycemic in vitro effect in a pumpkin beverage fermented by *L. mali* K8 [90]. Gamboa-Gómez et al. [91] also showed an anti-hyperglycemic effect with an infusion of oak leaves and fermented beverages from *Quercus convallata* and *Q. arizonica* in vitro and in vivo studies with female mice. On the other hand, blended fermented blueberry pomace by *L. rhamnosus* GG, *L. plantarum*-1, and *L. plantarum*-2 showed in in vitro hypocholesterolaemic effect. In addition, this fermented beverage exhibited an outstanding performance in terms of anti-fatigue in a mouse weight swimming experiment [92]. According to Harima-Mizusawa et al. [93], citrus beverage fermented with *L. plantarum* YIT0132 had a good effect in relieving the perennial allergic rhinitis symptoms in a double-blind, placebo-controlled trial. Other fermented beverages, such as those of tomato, feijoa, blueberry-blackberry, cactus pear, and prickly pear fruits exhibit a great in vitro anti-inflammatory capacity and help maintain the integrity of intestinal barrier [85,86,94]. However, the results are influenced by the different vegetable beverage matrices. For example, Valero-Cases et al. [94] showed the best improvement of the intestinal barrier with fermented tomato juices with respect to fermented feijoa ones. The vasorelaxant capacity was proposed for fermented jabuticaba berry beverages through an in vivo study of vascular reactivity in male Wistar rats. Theses beverages could act as an interesting cardiovascular protector [95]. Cheng et al. [96] reported an increase of SCFAs production and an improvement of the fecal microbiota community structure in vitro with blueberry pomace fermented by *L. casei* CICC20280. Wang et al. [97] showed that the consumption of fermented beverages of Changbai Mountain vegetables and fruits can reduce the Firmicutes/Bacteroidetes ratio and increase the Bacteroidales S24–7 group, Bacteroidaceae, the genus *Bacteroides*, and Prevotellaceae in a mouse model study. However, these are results from in vitro and in vivo studies with animal models, so future research in humans is required to evaluate the physiological effects on health improvement. A summary of studies conducted to date on fruit and vegetable fermented beverages and their results is shown in Table 4.

Table 4. Summary of fruit and vegetable fermented beverages as potential carriers form bioactive compounds, probiotics, prebiotics delivery to de gut.

Fruits and Vegetables Fermented Beverage	Probiotic Bacteria	Results	Reference
Symbiotic beverages: Carrot+orange juices and nectars + inulin Orange + hibiscus tea + oligofructose Red fruit beverage + FOS, GOS, Inulin Pomegranate + Cornelian cherry + delignified wheat bran Clarified apple juice + oligofructose	Different LAB [1] strains	Prebiotic ingredients + vegetable beverage matrices = good compatibility Prebiotic supplementation = viability of probiotic strains above the minimum recommended. High viability of probiotic strains after gastrointestinal in vitro digestion	Valero-Cases and Frutos [67,68], Mantzourani et al. [69], Mantzourani et al. [70], Pimentel et al. [71], Miranda et al. [73], Bernal-Castro et al. [74]
Pomegranate + inulin	Three species of *Lactobacillus*	In vivo study: improve testosterone level, insulin, insulin resistance, body mass index, weight and waist circumference in polycystic ovarian syndrome	Esmaeilinezhad et al. [75]
Apple juice	*L. plantarum* ATCC14917	Improved antioxidant capacity, increasing quercetin phloretin and 5-O-caffeoylquinic acid contents	
Mixed beverages from apples, carrots and pears	*L. plantarum* 115 and Vege Start 60	Increase of total flavonoids content and the antioxidant activity	Yang et al. [77]
Pomegranate juices	*L. plantarum* CECT220, *L. acidophilus* CECT903, *B. longum* subsp. *infantis* CECT4551, *B. bifidum* CECT870	The biotransformation of phenolic compounds during fermentation and gastrointestinal digestion, suggesting a prebiotic effect	Li et al. [76]
Tea infusion	*L. plantarum* ASCC276, *L. plantarum* ASCC292, *L. acidophilus* CSCC2400, *L. plantarum* WCFS1, *L. rhamnosus* WQS, *L. brevis* NPS-QW145	Increase in the antioxidant capacity, modification of the phenolic composition, increase in cellular uptake after in vitro gastrointestinal digestion	Zhao and Shah [79]
Oolong tea	Fecal bacteria	Improved the host health generating SCFAs [2] and modulating the human gut microbiota, anti-obesity therapy	Zhang et al. [80]
Prickly pear	*Leuconostoc mesenteroides* strains	Production of EPS [3], improvement of consistency and antioxidant capacity	Di Cagno et al. [86]
Prickly pear	*L. fermentum* ATCC 9338	Decomposition of some risky organic compounds present in the fresh juice like: 2-propenenitrile, 2-(acetyloxy); furfuryl alcohol; acetaldehyde; 2,2-diethyl-3-methyloxazolidine, 4h-Pyran-4-one, 3,5-dihydroxy-2-methyl and furan	Panda et al. [89]
Pumpkin	*L. mali* K8	α-glucosidase inhibitory activity with anti-hyperglycemic effect	Koh et al. [90]
Infusion of oak leaves	Kombucha culture	Anti-hyperglycemic effect and antioxidant activity	Gamboa-Gómez et al. [91]
Blueberry pomace	*L. rhamnosus* GG, *L. plantarum-1* and *L. plantarum-2*	Hypocholesterolemic and anti-fatigue effect	Yan et al. [92]
Citrus	*L. plantarum* YIT0132	Good effect in relieving perennial allergic rhinitis symptoms	Harima-Mizusawa et al. [93]
Tomato, feijoa, blueberry-blackberry, cactus pear, and prickly pear fruits	Different LAB strains	Great in vitro anti-inflammatory capacity and help to maintain the integrity of intestinal barrier	Di Cagno et al. [86], Valero-Cases et al. [94], Filannino et al. [85]
Blueberry pomace	*L. casei* CICC20280	Increase of SCFA production and an improvement of fecal microbiota	Cheng et al. [96]
Changbai Mountain vegetables and fruits	Naturalized species of bacteria	Reduction of Firmicutes/Bacteroidetes ratio, increase of Bacteroidales S24-7 group, Bacteroidaceae, genus *Bacteroides* and Prevotellaceae in a mouse model study	Wang et al. [97]

[1] LAB: lactic acid bacteria; [2] SCFAs: short chain fatty acids; [3] EPS: exopolysaccharides.

3. Conclusions and Future Perspectives

The studies carried out to date have provided useful information and a deeper understanding of the metabolic mechanisms of growth, probiotic viability, and the microbial biotransformation or production of bioactive compounds in fermented non-dairy beverages. Non-dairy matrices (legumes, cereals, pseudocereals, fruits, and vegetables) represent potential carriers of probiotics, prebiotics, and bioactive compounds. They are a good alternative to dairy matrices because it has been proven that the fermentation of these vegetable matrices can improve the shelf life and their safety due to the organic acids generated during the fermentation period, their nutritional and functional composition, and their digestibility. Moreover, in all the matrices reviewed, the probiotic concentrations are above the minimum recommended (>7 Log CFU/mL). Therefore, they are a good alternative to the dairy products on the market that can also be consumed by people intolerant or allergic to milk proteins, those who are hypercholesterolemic, or those who are vegetarian, among others. However, to corroborate the health benefits of fermented non-dairy beverage consumption, further in vivo research, including human clinical studies addressing matrix combinations and doses in different populations, is needed.

Author Contributions: Conceptualization: E.V.-C.; methodology: E.V.-C and M.-J.F.; writing-original draft preparation: E.V.-C. and D.C.-B.; writing—review and editing: E.V.-C., D.C.-B., J.-J.P. and M.-J.F.; project administration: J.-J.P.; supervision: E.V.-C., D.C.-B. and M.-J.F. All authors have read and agreed to the published version of the manuscript.

Funding: E.V.-C.: Thanks to Generalitat Valenciana and the European Social Found for the Vali+d Postdoctoral fellowship. D.C.-B.: Thanks to the Spanish-Ministry of Education, Culture and Sport for the FPU-PhD fellowship.

Conflicts of Interest: The authors declare no conflicts of interest.

References

1. Ajmone Marsan, P.; Cocconcelli, P.S.; Masoero, F.; Miggiano, G.; Morelli, L.; Moro, D.; Rossi, F.; Sckokai, P.; Trevisi, E. Food for healthy living and active ageing. *Stud. Health Technol. Inform.* **2014**, *203*, 32–43.
2. Guerrero, C.; Wilson, L. Chapter 5—Enzymatic Production of Lactulose. In *Lactose-Derived Prebiotics*; Illanes, A., Conejeros, R., Eds.; Academic Press: London, UK, 2016; pp. 191–227.
3. Villaño, D.; Gironés-Vilapana, A.; García-Viguera, C.; Moreno, D.A. Chapter 10—Development of Functional Foods. In *Innovation Strategies in the Food Industry*; Galanakis, C.M., Ed.; Academic Press: Cambridge, MA, USA, 2016; pp. 191–210.
4. Gouw, V.P.; Jung, J.; Zhao, Y. Functional properties, bioactive compounds, and in vitro gastrointestinal digestion study of dried fruit pomace powders as functional food ingredients. *LWT Food Sci. Technol.* **2017**, *80*, 136–144. [CrossRef]
5. Rathore, S.; Salmeron, I.; Pandiella, S.S. Production of potentially probiotic beverages using single and mixed cereal substrates fermented with lactic acid bacteria cultures. *Food Microbiol.* **2012**, *30*, 239–244. [CrossRef] [PubMed]
6. Vieira da Silva, B.; Barreira, J.C.M.; Oliveira, M.B.P.P. Natural phytochemicals and probiotics as bioactive ingredients for functional foods: Extraction, biochemistry and protected-delivery technologies. *Trends Food Sci. Technol.* **2016**, *50*, 144–158. [CrossRef]
7. Yasmin, A.; Butt, M.S.; van Baak, M.; Shahid, M.Z. Supplementation of prebiotics to a whey-based beverage reduces the risk of hypercholesterolaemia in rats. *Int. Dairy J.* **2015**, *48*, 80–84. [CrossRef]
8. Marques, T.M.; Cryan, J.F.; Shanahan, F.; Fitzgerald, G.F.; Ross, R.P.; Dinan, T.G.; Stanton, C. Gut microbiota modulation and implications for host health: Dietary strategies to influence the gut–brain axis. *Innov. Food Sci. Emerg. Technol.* **2014**, *22*, 239–247. [CrossRef]
9. Marco, M.L.; Heeney, D.; Binda, S.; Cifelli, C.J.; Cotter, P.D.; Foligne, B.; Ganzle, M.; Kort, R.; Pasin, G.; Pihlanto, A.; et al. Health benefits of fermented foods: Microbiota and beyond. *Curr. Opin. Biotechnol.* **2017**, *44*, 94–102. [CrossRef]
10. Plé, C.; Breton, J.; Daniel, C.; Foligné, B. Maintaining gut ecosystems for health: Are transitory food bugs stowaways or part of the crew? *Int. J. Food Microbiol.* **2015**, *213*, 139–143. [CrossRef]

11. Food and Agriculture Organization of the United Nations and World Health Organization Expert Consultation Report (FAO/WHO). *Guidelines for the Evaluation of Probiotics in Food*; Joint FAO/WHO Working Group Meeting: London, ON, Canada, 2002.
12. Salminen, S.; von Wright, A.; Morelli, L.; Marteau, P.; Brassart, D.; de Vos, W.M.; Fonden, R.; Saxelin, M.; Collins, K.; Mogensen, G.; et al. Demonstration of safety of probiotics—A review. *Int. J. Food Microbiol.* **1998**, *44*, 93–106. [CrossRef]
13. Ricci, A.; Allende, A.; Bolton, D.; Chemaly, M.; Davies, R.; Girones, R.; Koutsoumanis, K.; Lindqvist, R.; Nørrung, B.; Robertson, L.; et al. Update of the list of QPS-recommended biological agents intentionally added to food or feed as notified to EFSA 6: Suitability of taxonomic units notified to EFSA until March 2017. *EFSA J.* **2017**, *15*, 4884.
14. Tripathi, M.K.; Giri, S.K. Probiotic functional foods: Survival of probiotics during processing and storage. *J. Funct. Foods* **2014**, *9*, 225–241. [CrossRef]
15. Ranadheera, C.S.; Evans, C.A.; Adams, M.C.; Baines, S.K. In vitro analysis of gastrointestinal tolerance and intestinal cell adhesion of probiotics in goat's milk ice cream and yogurt. *Food Res. Int.* **2012**, *49*, 619–625. [CrossRef]
16. Shori, A.B. Influence of food matrix on the viability of probiotic bacteria: A review based on dairy and non-dairy beverages. *Food Biosci.* **2016**, *13*, 1–8. [CrossRef]
17. Aljewicz, M.; Cichosz, G. The effect of probiotic *Lactobacillus rhamnosus* HN001 on the *in vitro* availability of minerals from cheeses and cheese-like products. *LWT Food Sci. Technol.* **2015**, *60*, 841–847. [CrossRef]
18. Mani-Lopez, E.; Palou, E.; Lopez-Malo, A. Probiotic viability and storage stability of yogurts and fermented milks prepared with several mixtures of lactic acid bacteria. *J. Dairy Sci.* **2014**, *97*, 2578–2590. [CrossRef]
19. O'Brien, K.V.; Aryana, K.J.; Prinyawiwatkul, W.; Ordonez, K.M.C.; Boeneke, C.A. Short communication: The effects of frozen storage on the survival of probiotic microorganisms found in traditionally and commercially manufactured kefir. *J. Dairy Sci.* **2016**, *99*, 7043–7048. [CrossRef]
20. Rutella, G.S.; Tagliazucchi, D.; Solieri, L. Survival and bioactivities of selected probiotic lactobacilli in yogurt fermentation and cold storage: New insights for developing a bi-functional dairy food. *Food Microbiol.* **2016**, *60*, 54–61. [CrossRef]
21. Granato, D.; Branco, G.F.; Nazzaro, F.; Cruz, A.G.; Faria, J.A.F. Functional foods and nondairy probiotic food development: Trends, concepts, and products. *Compr. Rev. Food Sci. Food Saf.* **2010**, *9*, 292–302. [CrossRef]
22. Vijaya Kumar, B.; Vijayendra, S.V.; Reddy, O.V. Trends in dairy and non-dairy probiotic products—A review. *J. Food Sci. Technol.* **2015**, *52*, 6112–6124. [CrossRef]
23. Marsh, A.J.; Hill, C.; Ross, R.P.; Cotter, P.D. Fermented beverages with health-promoting potential: Past and future perspectives. *Trends Food Sci. Technol.* **2014**, *38*, 113–124. [CrossRef]
24. Gibson, G.R.; Roberfroid, M.B. Dietary modulation of the human colonic microbiota: Introduccing the concept of prebiotics. *J. Nutr.* **1995**, *125*, 1401–1412. [CrossRef] [PubMed]
25. Sirisomboon, P.; Pornchaloempong, P.; Romphophak, T. Physical properties of green soybean: Criteria for sorting. *J. Food Eng.* **2007**, *79*, 18–22. [CrossRef]
26. Katz, Y.; Gutierrez-Castrellon, P.; Gonzalez, M.G.; Rivas, R.; Lee, B.W.; Alarcon, P. A comprehensive review of sensitization and allergy to soy-based products. *Clin. Rev. Allergy Immunol.* **2014**, *46*, 272–281. [CrossRef] [PubMed]
27. Osorio-Diaz, P.; Agama-Acevedo, E.; Mendoza-Vinalay, M.; Tovar, J.; Bello-Perez, L.A. Pasta added with chickpea flour: Chemical composition, in vitro starch digestibility and predicted glycemic index. *CyTA J. Food* **2008**, *6*, 6–12.
28. Rossi, E.A.; Vendramini, R.C.; Carlos, I.Z.; Pei, Y.C.; De Valdez, G.F. Development of a novel fermented soymilk product with potential probiotic properties. *Eur. Food Res. Technol.* **1999**, *209*, 305–507. [CrossRef]
29. Bedani, R.; Rossi, E.A.; Isay Saad, S.M. Impact of inulin and okara on *Lactobacillus acidophilus* La-5 and *Bifidobacterium animalis* Bb-12 viability in a fermented soy product and probiotic survival under in vitro simulated gastrointestinal conditions. *Food Microbiol.* **2013**, *34*, 382–389. [CrossRef]
30. Mridula, D.; Sharma, M. Development of non-dairy probiotic drink utilizing sprouted cereals, legume and soymilk. *LWT Food Sci. Technol.* **2015**, *62*, 482–487. [CrossRef]
31. Santos, C.C.A.A.; Libeck, B.S.; Schwan, R.F. Co-culture fermentation of peanut-soy milk for the development of a novel functional beverage. *Int. J. Food Microbiol.* **2014**, *186*, 32–41. [CrossRef]

32. Cabello-Olmo, M.; Oneca, M.; Torre, P.; Sainz, N.; Moreno-Aliaga, M.J.; Guruceaga, E.; Diaz, J.V.; Encio, I.J.; Barajas, M.; Arana, M. A fermented food product containing lactic acid bacteria protects ZDF rats from the development of type 2 diabetes. *Nutrients* **2019**, *11*, 2530. [CrossRef]
33. Topping, D.L.; Clifton, P.M. Short-chain fatty acids and human colonic function: Roles of resistant starch and nonstarch polysaccharides. *Physiol. Rev.* **2001**, *81*, 1031–1064. [CrossRef]
34. Nagino, T.; Kaga, C.; Kano, M.; Masuoka, N.; Anbe, M.; Moriyama, K.; Maruyama, K.; Nakamura, S.; Shida, K.; Miyazaki, K. Effects of fermented soymilk with *Lactobacillus casei* Shirota on skin condition and the gut microbiota: A randomised clinical pilot trial. *Benef. Microbes* **2018**, *9*, 209–218. [CrossRef] [PubMed]
35. Wang, S.; Chelikani, V.; Serventi, L. Evaluation of chickpea as alternative to soy in plant-based beverages, fresh and fermented. *LWT Food Sci. Technol.* **2018**, *97*, 570–572. [CrossRef]
36. Chavan, M.; Gat, Y.; Harmalkar, M.; Waghmare, R. Development of non-dairy fermented probiotic drink based on germinated and ungerminated cereals and legume. *LWT Food Sci. Technol.* **2018**, *91*, 339–344. [CrossRef]
37. Schwan, R.F.; Ramos, C.L. Chapter 10: Functional Beverages from Cereals. In *Functional and Medicinal Beverages*; Grumezescu, A., Holban, A.M., Eds.; Elsevier: Amsterdam, The Netherlands, 2019; pp. 351–379.
38. Angelov, A.; Yaneva-Marinova, T.; Gotcheva, V. Oats as a matrix of choice for developing fermented functional beverages. *J. Food Sci. Technol.* **2018**, *55*, 2351–2360. [CrossRef] [PubMed]
39. Kedia, G.; Vazquez, J.A.; Charalampopoulos, D.; Pandiella, S.S. In vitro fermentation of oat bran obtained by debranning with a mixed culture of human fecal bacteria. *Curr. Microbiol.* **2009**, *58*, 338–342. [CrossRef] [PubMed]
40. Luana, N.; Rossana, C.; Curiel, J.A.; Kaisa, P.; Marco, G.; Rizzello, C.G. Manufacture and characterization of a yogurt-like beverage made with oat flakes fermented by selected lactic acid bacteria. *Int. J. Food Microbiol.* **2014**, *185*, 17–26. [CrossRef]
41. Bernat, N.; Chafer, M.; Gonzalez-Martinez, C.; Rodriguez-Garcia, J.; Chiralt, A. Optimisation of oat milk formulation to obtain fermented derivatives by using probiotic *Lactobacillus reuteri* microorganisms. *Food Sci. Technol. Int.* **2015**, *21*, 145–157. [CrossRef] [PubMed]
42. Gupta, S.; Cox, S.; Abu-Ghannam, N. Process optimization for the development of a functional beverage based on lactic acid fermentation of oats. *Biochem. Eng. J.* **2010**, *52*, 199–204. [CrossRef]
43. Gupta, M.; Bajaj, B. Development of fermented oat flour beverage as a potential probiotic vehicle. *Food Biosci.* **2017**, *2017*, 104–107. [CrossRef]
44. Kedia, G.; Vazquez, J.A.; Pandiella, S.S. Fermentability of whole oat flour, PeriTec flour and bran by *Lactobacillus plantarum*. *J. Food Eng.* **2008**, *89*, 246–249. [CrossRef]
45. Wang, C.; Liang, S.; Wang, H.; Guo, M. Physiochemical properties and probiotic survivability of symbiotic oat-based beverage. *Food Sci. Biotechnol.* **2018**, *27*, 735–743. [CrossRef] [PubMed]
46. Funck, G.; Marques, J.; Cruxen, C.; Sehn, C.; Haubert, L.; Dannenberg, G.; Klajn, V.M.; Silva, W.; Fiorentini, A. Probiotic potential of *Lactobacillus curvatus* P99 and viability in fermented oat dairy beverage. *J. Food Process. Preserv.* **2019**, *43*, e14286. [CrossRef]
47. Johansson, M.L.; Nobaek, S.; Berggren, A.; Nyman, M.; Bjorck, I.; Ahrne, S.; Jeppsson, B.; Molin, G. Survival of *Lactobacillus plantarum* DSM 9843 (299v), and effect on the short-chain fatty acid content of faeces after ingestion of a rose-hip drink with fermented oats. *Int. J. Food Microbiol.* **1998**, *42*, 29–38. [CrossRef]
48. Ghosh, K.; Ray, M.; Adak, A.; Halder, S.K.; Das, A.; Jana, A.; Parua Mondal, S.; Vagvolgyi, C.; Das Mohapatra, P.K.; Pati, B.R.; et al. Role of probiotic *Lactobacillus fermentum* KKL1 in the preparation of a rice based fermented beverage. *Bioresour. Technol.* **2015**, *188*, 161–168. [CrossRef] [PubMed]
49. Giri, S.S.; Sen, S.S.; Saha, S.; Sukumaran, V.; Park, S.C. Use of a potential probiotic, *Lactobacillus plantarum* L7, for the preparation of a rice-based fermented beverage. *Front. Microbiol.* **2018**, *9*, 473. [CrossRef] [PubMed]
50. Ranum, P.; Pena-Rosas, J.P.; Garcia-Casal, M.N. Global maize production, utilization, and consumption. *Ann. N. Y. Acad. Sci.* **2014**, *1312*, 105–112. [CrossRef]
51. Menezes, A.G.T.; Ramos, C.L.; Dias, D.R.; Schwan, R.F. Combination of probiotic yeast and lactic acid bacteria as starter culture to produce maize-based beverages. *Food Res. Int.* **2018**, *111*, 187–197. [CrossRef]
52. Wacoo, A.P.; Mukisa, I.M.; Meeme, R.; Byakika, S.; Wendiro, D.; Sybesma, W.; Kort, R. Probiotic enrichment and reduction of aflatoxins in a traditional African maize-based fermented food. *Nutrients* **2019**, *11*, 265. [CrossRef]

53. Freire, A.L.; Ramos, C.L.; Schwan, R.F. Effect of symbiotic interaction between a fructooligosaccharide and probiotic on the kinetic fermentation and chemical profile of maize blended rice beverages. *Food Res. Int.* **2017**, *100*, 698–707. [CrossRef]
54. Reguera, M.; Haros, C.M. Structure and composition kernels. In *Pseudocereals Chemistry and Technology*; Haros, C.M., Schoenlechner, R., Eds.; Wiley-Blackwell: West Sussex, UK, 2017; pp. 28–48.
55. Bhargava, A.; Shukla, S.; Ohri, D. *Chenopodium quinoa*—An Indian perspective. *Ind. Crop. Prod.* **2006**, *23*, 73–87. [CrossRef]
56. Ranilla, L.G.; Apostolidis, E.; Genovese, M.I.; Lajolo, F.M.; Shetty, K. Evaluation of indigenous grains from the Peruvian Andean region for antidiabetes and antihypertension potential using in vitro methods. *J. Med. Food* **2009**, *12*, 704–713. [CrossRef]
57. Ludena-Urquizo, F.E.; García-Torres, S.M.; Tolonen, T.; Jaakkola, M.; Pena-Niebuhr, M.G.; von Wright, A.; Repo-Carrasco-Valencia, R.; Korhonen, H.; Plumed-Ferrer, C. Development of a fermented quinoa-based beverage. *Food Sci. Nutr.* **2017**, *5*, 602–608. [CrossRef] [PubMed]
58. Vera-Pingitore, E.; Jimenez, M.E.; Dallagnol, A.; Belfiore, C.; Fontana, C.; Fontana, P.; von Wright, A.; Vignolo, G.; Plumed-Ferrer, C. Screening and characterization of potential probiotic and starter bacteria for plant fermentations. *LWT Food Sci. Technol.* **2016**, *71*, 288–294. [CrossRef]
59. Bianchi, F.; Rossi, E.A.; Sakamoto, I.K.; Tallarico Adorno, M.A.; Van de Wiele, T.; Sivieri, K. Beneficial effects of fermented vegetal beverages on human gastrointestinal microbial ecosystem in a simulator. *Food Res. Int.* **2014**, *64*, 43–52. [CrossRef] [PubMed]
60. Molly, K.; Vandewoestyne, M.; Desmet, I.; Verstraete, W. Validation of the simulator of the human intestinal microbial ecosystem (SHIME) reactor using microorganism associated activities. *Microb. Ecol. Health Dis.* **1994**, *7*, 191–200.
61. Ichikawa, H.; Sakata, T. Stimulation of epithelial cell proliferation of isolated distal colon of rats by continuous colonic infusion of ammonia or short-chain fatty acids is nonadditive. *J. Nutr.* **1998**, *128*, 843–847. [CrossRef]
62. Matejčeková, Z.; Liptáková, D.; Valík, L. Functional probiotic products based on fermented buckwheat with *Lactobacillus rhamnosus*. *LWT Food Sci. Technol.* **2017**, *81*, 35–41. [CrossRef]
63. Kocková, M.; Valík, L. Development of new cereal-, pseudocereal-, and cereal-leguminous-based probiotic foods. *Czech J. Food Sci.* **2014**, *32*, 391–397. [CrossRef]
64. Kocková, M.; Dilongová, M.; Hybenová, E.; Valík, L. Evaluation of cereals and pseudocereals suitability for the development of new probiotic foods. *J. Chem.* **2013**, *2013*. [CrossRef]
65. Bustos, A.Y.; Gerez, C.L.; Mohtar Mohtar, L.G.; Paz Zanini, V.I.; Nazareno, M.A.; Taranto, M.P.; Iturriaga, L.B. Lactic acid fermentation improved textural behaviour, phenolic compounds and antioxidant activity of chia (*Salvia hispanica* L.) dough. *Food Technol. Biotechnol.* **2017**, *55*, 381–389. [CrossRef]
66. Kumar, H.; Salminen, S.; Verhagen, H.; Rowland, I.; Heimbach, J.; Banares, S.; Lalonde, M. Novel probiotics and prebiotics: Road to the market. *Curr. Opin. Biotechnol.* **2015**, *32*, 99–103. [CrossRef]
67. Valero-Cases, E.; Frutos, M.J. Effect of inulin on the viability of *L. plantarum* during storage and in vitro digestion and on composition parameters of vegetable fermented juices. *Plant Foods Hum. Nutr.* **2017**, *72*, 161–167. [CrossRef] [PubMed]
68. Valero-Cases, E.; Frutos, M.J. Development of prebiotic nectars and juices as potential substrates for *Lactobacillus acidophilus*: Special reference to physicochemical characterization and consumer acceptability during storage. *LWT Food Sci. Technol.* **2017**, *81*, 136–143. [CrossRef]
69. Mantzourani, I.; Terpou, A.; Bekatorou, A.; Mallouchos, A.; Alexopoulos, A.; Kimbaris, A.; Bezirtzoglou, E.; Koutinas, A.A.; Plessas, S. Functional pomegranate beverage production by fermentation with a novel synbiotic *L. paracasei* biocatalyst. *Food Chem.* **2020**, *308*, 125658. [CrossRef]
70. Mantzourani, I.; Terpou, A.; Alexopoulos, A.; Bezirtzoglou, E.; Bekatorou, A.; Plessas, S. Production of a potentially synbiotic fermented Cornelian cherry (*Cornus mas* L.) beverage using *Lactobacillus paracasei* K5 immobilized on wheat bran. *Biocatal. Agric. Biotechnol.* **2019**, *17*, 347–351. [CrossRef]
71. Pimentel, T.C.; Madrona, G.S.; Prudencio, S.H. Probiotic clarified apple juice with oligofructose or sucralose as sugar substitutes: Sensory profile and acceptability. *LWT Food Sci. Technol.* **2015**, *62*, 838–846. [CrossRef]
72. da Costa, G.; Silva, J.; Mingotti, J.; Barão, C.; Klososki, S.; Pimentel, T. Effect of ascorbic acid or oligofructose supplementation on *L. paracasei* viability, physicochemical characteristics and acceptance of probiotic orange juice. *LWT Food Sci. Technol.* **2016**, *75*, 195–201. [CrossRef]

73. Miranda, R.F.; da Silva, J.P.; Machado, A.R.F.; da Silva, E.C.; de Souza, R.C.; Marcolino, V.A.; Klososki, S.J.; Pimentel, T.C.; Barão, C.E. Impact of the addition of *Lactobacillus casei* and oligofructose on the quality parameters of orange juice and hibiscus tea mixed beverage. *Food Process. Preserv.* **2019**, *43*, e14249. [CrossRef]
74. Bernal-Castro, C.A.; Díaz-Moreno, C.; Gutiérrez-Cortés, C. Inclusion of prebiotics on the viability of a commercial *Lactobacillus casei* subsp. rhamnosus culture in a tropical fruit beverage. *J. Food Sci. Technol.* **2019**, *56*, 987–994. [CrossRef]
75. Esmaeilinezhad, Z.; Babajafari, S.; Sohrabi, Z.; Eskandari, M.H.; Amooee, S.; Barati-Boldaji, R. Effect of synbiotic pomegranate juice on glycemic, sex hormone profile and anthropometric indices in PCOS: A randomized, triple blind, controlled trial. *Nutr. Metab. Cardiovasc. Dis.* **2019**, *29*, 201–208. [CrossRef]
76. Li, Z.; Teng, J.; Lyu, Y.; Hu, X.; Zhao, Y.; Wang, M. Enhanced antioxidant activity for apple juice fermented with *Lactobacillus plantarum* ATCC14917. *Molecules* **2018**, *24*, 51. [CrossRef] [PubMed]
77. Yang, X.; Zhou, J.; Fan, L.; Qin, Z.; Chen, Q.; Zhao, L. Antioxidant properties of a vegetable-fruit beverage fermented with two *Lactobacillus plantarum* strains. *Food Sci. Biotechnol.* **2018**, *27*, 1719–1726. [CrossRef] [PubMed]
78. Valero-Cases, E.; Nuncio-Jauregui, N.; Frutos, M.J. Influence of fermentation with different lactic acid bacteria and in vitro digestion on the biotransformation of phenolic compounds in fermented pomegranate juices. *J. Agric. Food Chem.* **2017**, *65*, 6488–6496. [CrossRef]
79. Zhao, D.; Shah, N.P. Lactic acid bacterial fermentation modified phenolic composition in tea extracts and enhanced their antioxidant activity and cellular uptake of phenolic compounds following in vitro digestion. *J. Funct. Foods* **2016**, *20*, 182–194. [CrossRef]
80. Zhang, X.; Zhu, X.L.; Sun, Y.; Hu, B.; Sun, Y.; Jabbar, S.; Zeng, X.X. Fermentation in vitro of EGCG, GCG and EGCG300″Me isolated from Oolong tea by human intestinal microbiota. *Food Res. Int.* **2013**, *54*, 1589–1595. [CrossRef]
81. Cheng, M.; Zhang, X.; Miao, Y.; Cao, J.; Wu, Z.; Weng, P. The modulatory effect of (-)-epigallocatechin 3-O-(3-O-methyl) gallate (EGCG3″Me) on intestinal microbiota of high fat diet-induced obesity mice model. *Food Res. Int.* **2017**, *92*, 9–16. [CrossRef]
82. Yang, Y.; Qiao, L.; Zhang, X.; Wu, Z.; Weng, P. Effect of methylated tea catechins from Chinese oolong tea on the proliferation and differentiation of 3T3-L1 preadipocyte. *Fitoterapia* **2015**, *104*, 45–49. [CrossRef]
83. Cueva, C.; Moreno-Arribas, M.V.; Martin-Alvarez, P.J.; Bills, G.; Vicente, M.F.; Basilio, A.; Rivas, C.L.; Requena, T.; Rodriguez, J.M.; Bartolome, B. Antimicrobial activity of phenolic acids against commensal, probiotic and pathogenic bacteria. *Res. Microbiol.* **2010**, *161*, 372–382. [CrossRef] [PubMed]
84. Fessard, A.; Kapoor, A.; Patche, J.; Assemat, S.; Hoarau, M.; Bourdon, E.; Bahorun, T.; Remize, F. Lactic fermentation as an efficient tool to enhance the antioxidant activity of tropical fruit juices and teas. *Microorganisms* **2017**, *5*, 23. [CrossRef]
85. Filannino, P.; Cavoski, I.; Thlien, N.; Vincentini, O.; De Angelis, M.; Silano, M.; Gobbetti, M.; Di Cagno, R. Lactic acid fermentation of cactus cladodes (*Opuntia ficus*-indica L.) generates flavonoid derivatives with antioxidant and anti-Inflammatory properties. *PLoS ONE* **2016**, *11*.
86. Di Cagno, R.; Filannino, P.; Vincentini, O.; Lanera, A.; Cavoski, I.; Gobbetti, M. Exploitation of *Leuconostoc mesenteroides* strains to improve shelf life, rheological, sensory and functional features of prickly pear (*Opuntia ficus-indica* L.) fruit puree. *Food Microbiol.* **2016**, *59*, 176–189. [CrossRef] [PubMed]
87. Bhat, B.; Bajaj, B.K. Hypocholesterolemic potential and bioactivity spectrum of an exopolysaccharide from a probiotic isolate *Lactobacillus paracasei* M7. *Bioact. Carbohydr. Diet. Fibre* **2019**, *19*, 100191. [CrossRef]
88. Han, J.; Xu, X.; Gao, C.; Liu, Z.; Wu, Z. Levan-producing *Leuconostoc citreum* strain BD1707 and its growth in tomato juice supplemented with sucrose. *Appl. Environ. Microbiol.* **2016**, *82*, 1383–1390. [CrossRef]
89. Panda, S.K.; Behera, S.K.; Qaku, X.W.; Sekar, S.; Ndinteh, D.T.; Nanjundaswamy, H.M.; Ray, R.C.; Kayitesi, E. Quality enhancement of prickly pears (*Opuntia* sp.) juice through probiotic fermentation using *Lactobacillus fermentum*—ATCC 9338. *LWT Food Sci. Technol.* **2017**, *75*, 453–459. [CrossRef]
90. Koh, W.Y.; Uthumporn, U.; Rosma, A.; Irfan, A.R.; Park, Y.H. Optimization of a fermented pumpkin-based beverage to improve *Lactobacillus mali* survival and α-glucosidase inhibitory activity: A response surface methodology approach. *Food Sci. Hum. Wellness* **2018**, *7*, 57–70. [CrossRef]

91. Gamboa-Gómez, C.I.; Simental-Mendía, L.E.; González-Laredo, R.F.; Alcantar-Orozco, E.J.; Monserrat-Juarez, V.H.; Ramírez-Espana, J.C.; Gallegos-Infante, J.A.; Moreno-Jiménez, M.R.; Rocha-Guzmán, N.E. In vitro and in vivo assessment of anti-hyperglycemic and antioxidant effects of Oak leaves (*Quercus convallata* and *Quercus arizonica*) infusions and fermented beverages. *Food Res. Int.* **2017**, *102*, 690–699. [CrossRef]
92. Yan, Y.; Zhang, F.; Chai, Z.; Liu, M.; Battino, M.; Meng, X. Mixed fermentation of blueberry pomace with *L. rhamnosus* GG and *L. plantarum-1*: Enhance the active ingredient, antioxidant activity and health-promoting benefits. *Food Chem. Toxicol.* **2019**, *131*, 110541. [CrossRef]
93. Harima-Mizusawa, N.; Kano, M.; Nozaki, D.; Nonaka, C.; Miyazaki, K.; Enomoto, T. Citrus juice fermented with *Lactobacillus plantarum* YIT 0132 alleviates symptoms of perennial allergic rhinitis in a double-blind, placebo-controlled trial. *Benef. Microbes* **2016**, *7*, 649–658. [CrossRef]
94. Valero-Cases, E.; Roy, N.C.; Frutos, M.J.; Anderson, R.C. Influence of the fruit juice carriers on the ability of *Lactobacillus plantarum* DSM20205 to improve in vitro intestinal barrier integrity and its probiotic properties. *J. Agric. Food Chem.* **2017**, *65*, 5632–5638. [CrossRef]
95. Martins de Sá, L.; Castro, P.; Lino, F.; Bernardes, M.; Viegas, J.; Dinis, T.; Santana, M.; Romao, W.; Vaz, G.B.; Lião, L.; et al. Antioxidant potential and vasodilatory activity of fermented beverages of jabuticaba berry (*Myrciaria jaboticaba*). *J. Funct. Foods* **2014**, *8*, 169–179. [CrossRef]
96. Cheng, Y.; Wu, T.; Chu, X.; Tang, S.; Cao, W.; Liang, F.; Fang, Y.; Pan, S.; Xu, X. Fermented blueberry pomace with antioxidant properties improves fecal microbiota community structure and short chain fatty acids production in an in vitro mode. *LWT Food Sci. Technol.* **2020**, *125*, 109260. [CrossRef]
97. Wang, Y.; Yu, M.; Shi, Y.; Lu, T.; Xu, W.; Sun, Y.; Yang, L.; Gan, Z.; Xie, L. Effects of a fermented beverage of Changbai Mountain fruit and vegetables on the composition of gut microbiota in mice. *Plant Foods Hum. Nutr.* **2019**, *74*, 468–473. [CrossRef] [PubMed]

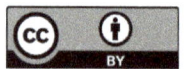

© 2020 by the authors. Licensee MDPI, Basel, Switzerland. This article is an open access article distributed under the terms and conditions of the Creative Commons Attribution (CC BY) license (http://creativecommons.org/licenses/by/4.0/).

MDPI
St. Alban-Anlage 66
4052 Basel
Switzerland
Tel. +41 61 683 77 34
Fax +41 61 302 89 18
www.mdpi.com

Nutrients Editorial Office
E-mail: nutrients@mdpi.com
www.mdpi.com/journal/nutrients

www.ingramcontent.com/pod-product-compliance
Lightning Source LLC
LaVergne TN
LVHW070156120526
838202LV00013BA/1303